Ulrich Bonk
Breast Cancer

Ulrich Bonk (Editor)

Breast Cancer

International Recommendations for an Objective Diagnosis

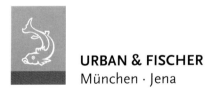

URBAN & FISCHER
München · Jena

All business correspondence should be made with:
Urban & Fischer Verlag, Lektorat Medizin, Karlstraße 45, 80333 München
Internet: http://www.urbanfischer.de

All rights including translation, are reserved. No part of this publication may be reproduced, stored in a retrieval system, or transmitted in any other form or by any means, electronic, mechanical, recording, or otherwise without the prior written permission of the publisher.
The Editors (or Author(s)) and the Publisher of this work have made every effort to ensure that the drug dosage schedules herein are accurate and in accord with the standards accepted at the time of publication. The reader is strongly advised, however, to check the product information sheet includes in the package of cach drug he or she plans to administer to be certain that changes have not been made in the recommended dose or in the contraindications for administration.
The Publishers have made an extensive effort to trace original copyright holders for permission to use borrowed material. If any has been overlooked, it will be corrected at the first reprint.

Die Deutsche Bibliothek – CIP-Einheitsaufnahme

Breast cancer : international recommendations for an objective
diagnosis ; with 80 figures / Ulrich Bonk (ed.). – München ; Jena :
Urban und Fischer, 1999
  ISBN 3-437-21726-7

© 2000 Urban & Fischer Verlag, München · Jena

Book production: Gudrun Kumbartzki, Sibylle Hartl
Typesetting department: Fotosatz Otto Gutfreund GmbH, Darmstadt
Printer and binder: Wilhelm Röck, Weinsberg

Printed in Germany

ISBN 3-437 21726-7

Dedication

Dedicated to Prof. Dr. Roland Bässler
German Register of Breast Diseases
Fulda

Dedication

"Quality of care is the degree to which health services for individuals and populations increase the likelihood of desired health outcomes and are consistent with current professional knowledge." (Lohr, 1990)

Preface

Mammography screening can reduce breast cancer mortality provided the diagnostic and therapeutic chain is performed in highest quality. This requires particular skills of all clinical partners, their intense collaboration and a continuous quality monitoring of the involved individuals and the program as a whole. Those countries which have reduced breast cancer mortality successfully have shown that these rather extreme requirements can be met under conditions of rather different health care systems. Nevertheless, it is a serious challenge to develop a screening approach which is compatible with the German health care system. As someone, who has given the fight against breast cancer highest priority in his own research, I very much appreciate the unique effort this book is undertaking to support the goals of furthering a German solution to meet the challenges of breast cancer screening from the point of view of pathology and genetics.

Prof. Dr. Heinz Otto Peitgen
Director Center for Medical Diagnostic Systems and Visualization
(MeVis at the University of Bremen)

Foreword

The increase in the percentage of elderly people in our society is the main reason for the rising numbers of women suffering from breast cancer. Whilst the incidence of the disease gives an indication of the frequency with which breast cancer occurs, the mortality is also influenced by such factors as treatment and early diagnosis. Unfortunately, the mortality rate for breast cancer has remained stable, especially in Germany; indeed, there is a slow but steady increase in the number of deaths from the disease. This is also true in the Free Hanseatic City of Bremen. As pathologists at an institute in that city we have been convinced for many years now that the only way of improving these figures is to develop a better early diagnostic programme. Our natural allies in this task have been the members of the local German Cancer Society, such as Prof. Dr. Schmidt, and scientists at the University of Bremen, such as Professor Bullerdiek and Professor Peitgen. For many years our Institute has recommended fine-needle biopsy of the female breast as a useful diagnostic step. Over the past years we have conducted training courses for this procedure.

On the recommendation of Professor Prechtel, the specialist in mammary pathology from Starnberg, and formerly of the University of Munich, the publishers sent me photographs and texts for a proposed atlas of fine-needle biopsy. The material was found amongst the papers left by the Hungarian surgeon and pathologist, Istvan Degrell, who had died more than ten years previously. My task was to attempt to adapt this material to present-day circumstances. I knew the works of Dr Degrell from medical literature, since he had published in 1976 a book on the clinical and pathological indications of breast cancer (Karger Verlag, Switzerland). In 1984 I published with the same company our manual describing methods of dealing with biopsies and operation preparations. Cytopathologists who were also friends of mine, such as Dr Bollmann and Dr Bosse, with whom I had conducted training courses in cytology here in Germany, suggested to me repeatedly that I should attempt an objective classification of breast-cancer diagnoses. As active supporters of applied DNA cytometry they place great value on this procedure, with the aim of establishing an objective genetic grading. Both colleagues recommend always on the visions of Virchow to have the tool of an objective genetical classification for all tumours one future day. Dr Bollmann is a member of the Papanicolaou Society USA. It is him whom we have to thank for the suggestions of this society for handling fine needle aspiration of the breast.

When we came to examine the genetic basis and current prognostic factors related to mammary carcinoma it became evident that, in some countries, recommendations, standards and guidelines laid down by various scientific bodies with a view to an early and objective classification of breast cancer do already exist, and indeed are already being put into practice.

The mammography screening programme as advocated by the German Cancer Society has already been successfully implemented for the benefit of women in, for example, the Netherlands, Sweden and especially in the United Kingdom. In connection with the mammography screening programme in the United Kingdom, an associated programme for the morphological diagnosis of breast cancer was begun ten years ago, with the attendant publicity and continuous improvements as recommended by British specialist bodies. It is encouraging to note that the European Parliament, on the advice of experts from the countries concerned, has adopted the British guidelines, including the recommendations for the morphological diagnosis of breast cancer. Nonetheless, these European recommendations are not universally known, since to date it has not been possible to adopt the mammography screening programme everywhere in Europe, including Germany. Our foreign colleagues, publishers and relevant scientific bodies proved most willing and helpful in making available their texts for our proposed purpose in propagating these recommendations. I should like to take this opportunity of thanking them all – especially Mrs Karin Jöns, member of the European Parliament, from the Social Democratic Party of Bremen, for supporting help and information. As a member of the American Society of Cytopathology I should like to make a larger circle of experts familiar with the Society's guidelines for fine-needle biopsy of the breast. It is a known fact that the mammography screening programme in the US is well developed and supported by many organisations. With regard to histological classification, we follow the recommendations of Dr Page from the US. I should like to express my profound thanks to Dr Page for permitting us to reproduce here his remarks on the important expression **atypical ductal hyperplasia**, as described in a slide seminar he held in Hong Kong in 1994. As explained elsewhere, like many American pathologists we follow the recommendations of Dr Page in the sphere of histological diagnosis.

Pathology has benefited from the classification, collation and evaluation of the various findings not only through the successful establishment of a mammography screening programme in England and the Netherlands. Using as a basis the results of the mammography screening programmes in these countries, the pathologists Dr Elston and Dr Ellis in Nottingham and Dr Holland in Nijmegen have been able to assume such a convincing role as pathologists and teachers for the rest of us.

Although at first sight it seems an obvious enough step to collate international recommendations for the diagnosis of breast cancer, at second sight it becomes evident that many contradictions are inherent in this procedure. Studies have produced differing results which, however, serve as food for discussion in the interests of an accurate evaluation of the matter. In some respects, the collation of results is a continuous struggle against the passage of time. We in Germany greatly regret that so much time continues to pass without the establishment of a mammography screening programme. The collation of these recommendations serves not only a protective function, but is also indicative of a certain apprehension. We regret not only that which we have failed to achieve in the past, but are also concerned about the uncertainties the future holds.

The philosopher Theodor W. Adorno commented that "Time reflects the desire to possess as a fear of loss, a fear of irretrievability. That which is, can be perceived in relation to the possibility of not being." Of course we must remain optimistic, even though we still keep encountering logical impasses with respect to the mammography screening programme in Europe. Of course we hope that new optical developments will permit an improved objective classification of breast cancer, as Harms's workgroup from Würzburg has indicated.

The diagnosis of breast cancer represents an attack on the female self-esteem and results in a radical change in a woman's life. The breast is part of a woman's identity and is the most prominent visual sign of her femininity. It is one of the fundamental subjects of myth, poetry and art. As a symbol of femininity it is both erotic and a source of nourishment. When disease occurs, the diagnosis applies to an individual woman; that is to say, she is affected as regards her own feminine identity on the one hand, whilst on the other she becomes caught up in a conflict regarding the perception of her femininity through the eyes of the outside world. My aim is to help women who are sick. In medicine, disease as such does not exist; sick people do.

I should like to offer my thanks to all my colleagues whose contributions and suggestions have helped me to bring this project to a successful conclusion. A particular word of thanks goes to Cornelia Blank and Kristine Glunde, the Project Manager, for keeping track of all aspects at all times, and to Jane Michael from Munich, for not losing sight of her English mother tongue despite the complexities of the text to be translated. I wish to thank the staff of Ullstein-Medical and in particular Dr J. Peter Prinz and Nathalie Blank.

Bremen, December 1997   ULRICH BONK

P. S.:
As readers of this book will realize, there has been a two years gap between my finishing the book and its publishing. This is due to a change of ownership of my publishers. This was resulted in a necessity to add my list of acknowledgements: There are the patient wives of our authors and Dr. Linda Deichert, pathologist; Susanne Krusche, medical student; Susanne Hischer, secretary; Gudrun Kumbartzki, Medical Tribune Wiesbaden; Gisela Heim, editorial office Munich and in particular Dr. Thomas Hopfe, chief editor Medicine, Urban & Fischer, Munich.

Tumour Centre of the Cancer Society
Bremen 1999   ULRICH BONK

Contributor List

- Abati, A., M.D., Chairman of the Committee of the Association of (Cyto)Pathologists, Radiologists, Obstetricians and Gynecologists, Surgeons and Cytotechnists in the scope of the National Cancer Institute-sponsored conference in Bethesda, Maryland, U.S.A., 1996, Cytopathology Section, National Cancer Institute/National Institutes of Health, Building 10, Room 2 A 19, 10 Center DR MSC 1500, Bethesda, Maryland 20892-1500, USA
- Albert, R., Dr. Ing., Institute of Virology, Laboratory for Image Processing, University of Würzburg, Versbacher Str. 7, 97078 Würzburg, Germany
- Bollmann, R., M.D., Institute of Pathology, Heilsbachstr. 15, 53123 Bonn, Germany
- Bonk, U., M.D., Director of the Institute of Pathology, Central Hospital Bremen-Nord, Hammersbecker Str. 228, 28755 Bremen, Germany
- Bosse, A., M.D., Professor, Institute of Pathology, Rheinisch-Westfälische TH Aachen, Aachen, Germany
- Bosse, U., M.D., Institute of Pathology, Carl-Stolcke-Str. 4, 49090 Osnabrück, Germany
- Brown, C.L., M.D., Chairman of the Cytology Sub-Group of the National Coordinating Committee for Breast Cancer Screening Pathology, The Royal London Hospital, Whitechapel, London, UK
- Bullerdiek, J., Dr. Biol., Professor, Center for Human Genetics and Genetic Couselling, University of Bremen, Leobenerstrasse, Bremen, Germany
- Connolly, J.L., M.D., Professor, Chairman of the Association of the ad hoc Committee of the Association of Directors of Anatomic and Surgical Pathology (ADASP), Department of Pathology, Harvard Medical School and Beth Israel Hospital, 330 Brookline Avenue, Boston MA 02215, USA
- Degrell, I., M.D. †, Surgeon and Pathologist, Hungary
- Gohla, G., M.D., Institute of Pathology, Central Hospital Bremen-Nord, Hammersbecker Str. 228, 28755 Bremen, Germany
- Hanisch, P., M.D., Institute of Pathology, Central Hospital Bremen-Nord, Hammersbecker Str. 228, 28755 Bremen, Germany
- Harms, H., Dr. Ing., Institute of Virology, Laboratory for Image Processing, University of Würzburg, Versbacher Str. 7, 97078 Würzburg, Germany
- Kristen, P., M.D., Department of Gynecology, University of Würzburg, Würzburg, Germany
- Kropp, S., M.D., Women Medical Center, St-Elisabeth-Hospital Ibbenbüren GmbH, P.O. 12 61, 49462 Ibbenbüren, Germany
- Michelaki, C., M.D., Institute of Pathology, Central Hospital Bremen-Nord, Hammersbecker Str. 228, 28755 Bremen, Germany
- Müller, J.G., M.D., Institute of Pathology, University of Würzburg, Würzburg, Germany

- Page, D. L., M. D., Professor, Director of Anatomic Pathology, Vanderbilt University Medical Center, Nashville, Tennessee, USA
- Rogalla, P., Dr. Biol., Center for Human Genetics and Genetic Couselling, University of Bremen, Leobenerstrasse, Bremen, Germany
- Rohen, C., Dr. Biol., Center for Human Genetics and Genetic Couselling, University of Bremen, Leobenerstrasse, Bremen, Germany
- Schenck, U., M. D., Professor, Laboratory for Clinical Cytology, Institute of Pathology, TU Munich, Prinzregentenplatz 14, 81675 Munich, Germany
- Schlotter, C. M., M. D., Women Medical Center, St-Elisabeth-Hospital Ibbenbüren GmbH, P. O. 12 61, 49462 Ibbenbüren, Germany
- Schwartz, G. F., M. D., M. B. A., Chairman of the International Consensus Conference on the Classification of Ductal Carcinoma In Situ, Jefferson Medical College, Philadelphia, PA, USA
- Sloane, J. P., M. D., Professor, Chairman of the National Coordinating Group for Breast Screening Pathology and the E.C. Working Group on Breast Screening Pathology, Department of Pathology, Duncan Building, Royal Liverpool University Hospital, Royal Liverpool University Hospital, Liverpool L69 3BX, UK
- Suen, K. C., M. D., Chairman of the Papanicolaou Society of Cytopathology Task Force on Standards of Practice, Department of Pathology, Vancouver Hospital, 855 West 12th Ave., Vancouver, British Columbia, V 5 Z 1 M 9, Canada
- Vogt, U., M. D., European Laboratory Association, Section Ibbenbüren, Ibbenbüren, Germany
- Wassmann, K., M. D., Women Medical Center, St-Elisabeth-Hospital Ibbenbüren GmbH, P. O. 12 61, 49462 Ibbenbüren, Germany

Acknowledgements

The Tumorzentrum Bremen acknowledges with deep gratitude the following foundations and companies for their generous contribution:

- Tönjes-Vagt-Stiftung, Bremen
- Wolfgang-Ritter-Stiftung, Bremen
- AMGEN
- Coulter-Immunotech Diagnostics, Hamburg
- DAKO, Diagnostika GmbH
- DIANOVA, Hamburg
- European Laboratory Association-ELA
- Essex Pharma GmbH
- Ethicon GmbH & Co KG
- Glaxo Wellcome GmbH & Co, Hamburg
- medac, Hamburg
- TAKEDA PHARMA GMBH
- Zeneca Oncology Germany, Osnabrück
- Pharmacia & Upjohn GmbH
- Zytomed, Berlin

Contents

1	**Introduction**	1
1.1	Anatomy and Physiology of the Breast, U. Bonk	1
1.2	Histopathology of Breast Tumours	7
1.2.1	Histopathology and Biology of the Invasive Mammary Carcinoma, U. Bonk	7
1.2.2	Ductal Pattern of Atypical Hyperplasia, D. L. Page	9
2	**Quality Assurance Recommendations for an Objective Diagnosis**	13
2.1	Mammography Screening Programmes and the Consequences for Pathologists	13
2.1.1	Guidelines for Breast Pathology Services, NCGBSP	13
2.1.2	Quality Assurance Guidelines for Pathology in Mammography Screening, E.C.	24
2.1.3	Recommendations for the Reporting of Breast Carcinoma, ADASP	47
2.1.4	Ductal Carcinoma In Situ (DCIS): A European Proposal for a New Classification, C. Michelaki	51
2.1.5	Consensus Conference on the Classification of Ductal Carcinoma In Situ	53
2.2	Fine Needle Aspiration Cytology	57
2.2.1	Fine Needle Aspiration Cytology of the Breast, U. Bonk, I. Degrell, G. Gohla, P. Hanisch	57
2.2.2	Fine Needle Aspiration and Mammary Secretion, Cytology and Core Biopsy, U. Schenck	67
2.2.3	Guidelines for Cytology Procedures and Reporting in Breast Cancer Screening, NHSBSP	70
2.2.4	The Uniform Approach to Breast Fine Needle Aspiration Biopsy, A. Abati	94
2.2.5	Guidelines of the Papanicolaou Society of Cytopathology for Fine-Needle Aspiration Procedure and Reporting, The Papanicolaou Society	101
2.3	Molecular Genetic and Molecular Biological Parameters	109
2.3.1	The Prognostic Significance of Genetic Parameters in Breast Cancer, C. Rohen, P. Rogalla, J. Bullerdiek	109
2.3.2	DNA Grading and DNA Typing of Mammary Carcinomas, R. Bollmann, U. Bosse	117
2.3.3	Quality Assurance in Mammary Cytology by Means of DNA Cytometry, R. Bollmann	122
2.3.4	Chromatin Arrangement as a Prognostic Marker in Node Negative Breast Cancer Patients, Measured in Different Thick Tissue Sections, R. Albert, J. G. Müller, P. Kristen, H. Harms	125

2.3.5 Cytometric Results of DNA Imaging and Established Prognostic Factors in Primary Breast Cancer,
C. M. Schlotter, S. Kropp, U. Bosse, U. Vogt, A. Bosse, K. Wassmann 132

2.3.6 The Influence of New Molecular Biological Parameters on Prognosis and Assessment in Primary Breast Cancers – Attempt at a Molecular Biological Classification,
U. Vogt, C. M. Schlotter, U. Bosse 147

Appendices 161
References 187
Index 213

Chapter 1

Introduction

1.1 Anatomy and Physiology of the Breast

Ulrich Bonk

The two mammary glands are situated above the pectoral muscles and consist of:
- A radial pattern of 15 to 20 tubulo-alveolar glands (= functional tissue + parenchyma)
- Connective tissue – a loose pallium and firm supportive tissue which gives the breast its shape.
- Adipose tissue surrounding the glands; this largely determines the size of the breast.

The skin of the breast is thin, translucent and elastic; it contains sebaceous and sweat glands.

The nipple (mamilla) is the conical projection at the tip of which the 15–20 mammary ducts come to the surface. It is covered with a multi-layer pigmented epithelium containing sebaceous and sweat glands and a large number of sensory nerve endings. Tufts of smooth muscle lead to the skin from the connective tissue between the mammary ducts, giving it the ability to become erect when stimulated. (This fact is important during lactation as it enables the infant to grasp and suck the nipple more easily.)

Additional features of the nipple: sweat glands, apocrine glands, hair follicles, bundles of smooth muscle tissue.

The Areola

In women who have not yet borne a child, the nipple and areola are light pink. In women who have borne a child, the areola darkens to a brownish colour. The skin of the areola contains sweat glands and fine hairs. Around the edge of the areola are the so-called Montgomery tubercles, some 15–20 small protuberances about the size of a pinhead. These are modified sebaceous glands which swell early in pregnancy and secrete a milk-like substance. They can become inflamed and form abscesses.

The Parenchyma

The mammary duct is a tubulo-alveolar gland consisting of a complex of similarly formed individual tubular glands with end-chambers which enlarge to form the alveoli before converging to form a common drainage duct.

A single mammary gland (lobe) consists of a segmental milk drainage duct (main mammary duct, ductus excretorius), a lactiferous sinus and a large number of lactiferous ducts, at the end of which lie the lobules containing the glandular alveoli (figure 1.1).

The narrow mammary ducts, which are enclosed by smooth muscle, expand behind the nipple and underneath the areola to form the lactiferous sinuses. During lactation these may become enlarged to a diameter of several millimetres. They serve as a reservoir for the milk so that the child can easily obtain nourishment by sucking (when breast-feeding, the child should be put to the breast in such a way that it grasps not only the nipple but also the areola). From the lactiferous sinus the ducts branch out into 20–40 smaller, subsegmental mammary ducts into which the alveoli within the lobules secrete milk at right angles.

The lobule forms a structural unit. It consists of a central duct and 10–100 acini. It is surrounded by intralobular tissue. Before a woman becomes pregnant for the first time, the smaller ducts are not properly channelled and the acini are either not present or are only present in rudimentary form.

The acini and the ducts are covered with a single-layer epithelium which is either cuboid

Figure 1.1: Mammary Duct. 1. Ductus excretorius; 2. Sinus lactiferus; 3. Ductus lactiferus; 4. Ductuli lactiferi; 5. Lobuli or acini; 4 and 5 = Terminal duct lobular unit

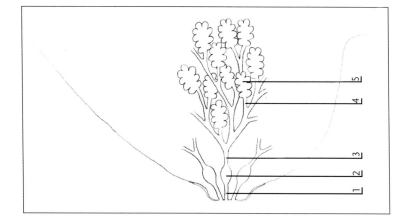

or cylindrical in shape. Its thickness depends on the functional state of the breast. In a virgin breast, the sections of gland often have no lumen; they are solid cones of epithelium. The epithelial cells surrounding the lumen proper are surrounded by an incomplete layer of myoepithelial cells (figure 1.2) along the surface. A basal membrane separates the parenchyma from the stroma.

The myoepithelial cells form a loose network which is arranged parallel to the longitudinal axis of the mammary ducts. They contain microfibrillae and hypertrophy during pregnancy and lactation. Contraction of the myoepithelia leads to a reduction in size of the lumen and squeezes the contents of the alveoli against the surrounding tissue (into the lactiferous sinus = milk reservoir) important for the emptying of the breast during lactation.

The deep mammary ducts are covered by a twin-layer epithelium which is cubo-cylindrical or prismatic in form. The lactiferous sinus is covered by a cylindrical epithelium. Towards the outside there are a decreasing number of myoepithelia. The excretory ducts expand somewhat towards the surface. They have a multi-layer, non-horny plate epithelium which gives way to the horny plate epithelium of the nipple.

Stroma

The interlobular connective tissue contains few cell types, consisting mainly of adipose cells and coarse collagen tissues. It encloses the individual lobes in such a way that each individual mammary duct constitutes a single lobe. The tela subcutanea, which lies immediately beneath the surface of the skin, consists of similar fat and connective tissue. They are separated by Cooper's ligaments, which are fibrous bands which attach the breast tissue to the skin. The interlobular connective tissue and the tela subcutanea give the breast firmness and largely determine its size. The mammary gland is attached to the pectoral muscle by loose connective tissue and can be moved from one side to the other.

The intralobular and periductular connective tissue immediately surrounding the mammary ducts is loose, rich in cells and composed of fine fibres (elastic fibres). It is characterised by its wealth of blood and lymph vessels and its ability to react to hormonal influences. It contains no fat cells. This connective tissue serves the metabolic supply. From here leucocytes, lymphocytes and histiocytes can enter the ductal system in order to fight infections or encourage resorption.

Lymphatic Flows of the Breast

As a result of the close contact of the lymphatic channels, which exist in large numbers, with the glandular parenchyma, in many cases it will be discovered when diagnosing breast cancer that the carcinoma has already metastasised into the local lymph nodes. It is well known that

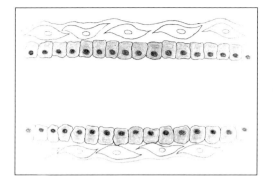

Figure 1.2: All ducts and ductules are lined by an inner layer of cuboidal or columnar epithelial cells and an outer layer of myoepithelial cells.

the principal route is via the armpit (plexus axillaris) and from there along the subclavian artery to the deep axillary and supraclavicular lymph nodes (truncus subclavius). Depending on the localisation of the primary tumour, however, the metastases can also travel via other routes directly into the thorax or the abdominal cavity.

Embryology

The mamillary gland develops from the so-called milk line, which runs ventrally on both sides from the buds, or beginnings, of the upper limbs to those of the lower limbs. From this milk line sprout a varying number of mammary glands in varying positions, depending on the species of animal in question. In the case of homo sapiens, in general only two mammary glands appear above the thorax. In the 5th month of gestation, up to 25 solid epithelial cones with sprouting ends appear in the region of the breast. In the 7th–8th month, the first lumina appear in these epithelial bands.

A greater or lesser degree of swelling and redness occurring at the commencement of lactation at any point on the milk line (most commonly in the armpit) can be a sign of an "additional" mammary gland (hypermasty). Sometimes a number of nipples, usually very small in size, can appear along the milk line (hyperthelia) (figure 1.3).

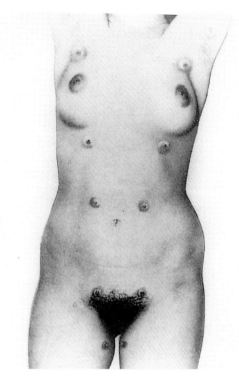

Figure 1.3: Milk line. Possible sites of supernumerary nipples along the milk line [1]

The Newborn Infant

During pregnancy, the placental estrogen, progesterone and prolactin levels are equally high in both the foetus and the mother, which also stimulates the development of the foetal mammary gland. At birth, the alveoli are filled with colostrum. As in the case of the mother, the breast is ready for lactation. It is approximately the size of a hazelnut and is often rough in texture.

The disappearance of the placental sex steroids in the days following birth and the production of a small amount of prolactin stimulates the mammary glands of the infant to secrete a milky substance. They swell to the size of walnuts, sometimes even larger. The swelling is accompanied by a greater or lesser degree of redness in the breasts and is the result of a local accumulation of blood, lymphatic fluid and oedema coupled with the fact that the alveoli are filled with milk. This phenomenon is not the result of an inflammation and corresponds to the commencement of lactation in the mother. No treatment is required (padding, alcohol compresses, camphor ointment, no antibiotics). This swelling of the breasts disappears spontaneously within three to four weeks and reverts during the next three to six months to the typical infant breast appearance.

Colostrum (= secretion + dead epithelial cells + phagocytes) is frequently excreted.

In the connective tissue in the area surrounding the nipple will be found 15–20 drainage ducts which enlarge to form the lactiferous sinuses. From here, a number of mammary ducts lead into the interior of the breast to the alveoli, which are filled with colostrum.

The Mammary Gland in Childhood

During the childhood years, when there is no ovarian activity, the breast remains flat and has a diameter of less than 1 cm. It consists of a small number of short, narrow, extended ducts covered with flattened epithelial cells and collagen connective tissue. The nipple is flat or slightly inverted.

Pre-Puberty

In girls, the ovarian follicles begin to grow during pre-puberty (approx. 8–10 years), secreting increasing quantities of estrogen. This stimulates the growth of the glandular cells and ducts in the breast and leads to a proliferation of the stroma connective tissue. The breast enlarges to form a "breast bud" (10–12 years); the nipples swell (12–14 years).

Puberty

As the ovaries mature (12–15 years), ovulation cycles begin to establish themselves, i. e. progesterone is also excreted. Together with the estrogen produced this leads to the development and extension of the glandular lobes and instigates the development of the structure of the mammary duct system. The breasts increase in size. The primary and secondary ducts lengthen and branch out. The connective and adipose tissue continues to increase. Epithelial proliferation also occurs at the end of the glandular ducts (formation of future lobules). The nipple and areola grow and become pink in colour.

Sexual Maturity

By the time a girl is approximately 16 years old the formation of the breast is largely complete, although it still contains only a small number of acini. It can continue to develop during each cycle until the age of 30 (Additional branching of the duct system and increase in the number of acini, growth of connective tissue and deposition of fat).

With the commencement of bi-phasic cycles, changes analogous to the menstrual rhythm can be observed:
- In the pre-menstrual phase: The breast increases in size as a result of increased blood circulation, increased water retention (oedema) and a dilatation of the acini. The woman experiences a pulling sensation and a tightness, sometimes even pain. The breast feels fuller and cysts may be palpable. Before and during menstruation, in some cases the secretion of a clear watery or milky substance can be observed (Weeping breast).
- In the postmenstrual phase, regressive changes take place in the parenchyma and the stroma. The lumina of the acini become narrower and the oedema in the tissues recedes. On the 4th–5th day of the cycle the breasts return to their "normal" size. They are soft and palpation is therefore easiest at this point in the cycle (self-examination following menstruation).

Changes to the Mammary Gland During Pregnancy

The corpus luteum in the ovary guarantees until the third month of pregnancy a high level of estrogen and progesterone, but then atrophies from this point. The placenta assumes progressively the function of the corpus luteum and also secretes lactogenic hormones. From the fifth month of pregnancy, the ovary is "dormant". Under the influence of the high estrogen levels during pregnancy, the mammary ducts and lobules proliferate and there is an increase of connective tissue.

The progesterone on the other hand leads to an oedematous loosening of the surrounding connective tissue, to an increase in blood volume and to an increased number of lymphocyte infiltrates in the stroma. The epithelial changes (increased mitosis, vacuolation of the cytoplasm by the epithelium of the acini etc.) are not uniform. The mammary ducts extend forwards into the intralobular connective and adipose tissue, branching out and forming new alveolar ends. Solid ends acquire a lumen, so that a large number of closely-packed alveoli are formed, which force the surface connective tissue proportionately into the background. The breast is prepared for milk production, but does not yet produce milk, because the estrogen and progesterone levels inhibit the reactivity of the alveoli to the lactogenic hormones. From the fourth month of pregnancy, the glands begin to produce a secretion (colostrum).

The epithelium of the alveoli and the lactiferous ducts is now in two layers and cuboid to cylindrical in form. The basal stem cells are large and transparent, the pre-secretory luminal cells on the surface somewhat darker. The basal cells of the glands are divided into either stem cells, which remain at the base of the epithelium, or pre-secretory luminal cells, which contain milk fat and protein. The latter separate from the mantle and appear in the alveolar lumen as colostrum particles together with the secretion and stray phagocytes (secretion of colostrum during the second half of pregnancy). The nuclei of the basal cells are relatively large and form oval-shaped vesicles. They have a clear, somewhat irregular chromatin structure and have nucleoli which are prominent in some cases. These changes in the cell structure are indicative of increased levels of secretion by the gland epithelia; they cannot be distinguished with certainty from the epithelia of certain proliferative mastopathies. The area surrounding the alveoli is rich in capillaries. Infiltrates of lymphocytes and mast cells are always to be found in the connective tissue of the mantle.

Clinical Indicators of Pregnancy

- Tension in the breasts in conjunction with swelling of the same following increased circulation coupled with growth of the glandular tissue and stroma.
- Loosening of the firm connective tissue.
- Increase in blood circulation. Veins which were previously not visible become clearly visible on the surface of the breast.
- Formation of striae (similar to stretch marks on the abdomen) following the stretching of skin and connective tissue.
- Nipple and areola increase in size and become brown in colour. This pigmentation continues after the pregnancy.
- Increased contractility of nipple and areola as a reaction to thermal and mechanical stimulation (sometimes even painful sensations).
- Growth of the Montgomery's follicles.
- Secretion of colostrum. Unlike milk, colostrum is not homogenous. It is sometimes watery, sometimes yellowish and cloudy and of a sticky consistency. Colostrum contains less fat than milk and contains so-called colostrum particles.

Milk Letdown. Lactation normally commences on the third or fourth day after parturition, under the influence of prolactin, which is produced by the anterior pituitary gland. During pregnancy the prolactin level rises continuously and reaches at the end levels which are 20–30 times higher than during a normal cycle. However, the prolactin can only act upon the acini once the estrogen and progesterone levels have sunk sufficiently (i. e. 3–4 days after delivery of the placenta). Once this stage is reached, it the prolactin can transform the "presecretory" alveoli into secretory cells, thus starting milk production. The prolactin level also sinks but is increased again at regular intervals by the stimulation of suckling as long as breast feeding continues.

During lactation, the enlarged alveoli and ducts are filled with secretion, as are the lactiferous sinuses. The alveoli are once more covered by a single layer cuboid to cylindrical epithelium, which is of varying depth depending on the functional state (highly prismatic and flattened cells). The glandular cells grow and release fine particles of fat into the interior of the cell. These migrate towards the pole on the lumen side and flow together to form droplets of fat, force the nucleus towards the base and finally separate off. In this way, the droplet of milk is released in a similar way to the apocrine secretions and is released into the lumen of the gland. This means that the cell is preserved and the cycle can begin once more. When empty of secretion, the cell mostly appears flat, and the nucleus is also flattened in shape. The particles of protein are secreted as in serous glands.

The milk letdown is frequently accompanied by a feeling of general physical discomfort and a slight rise in temperature and pulse. As a result of the changes in hormonal levels taking place, a temporary feeling of depression can occur.

The breasts swell and become hard and sensitive. The tension may be painful. The veins on the surface of the breasts are dilated and filled with blood. One to two days after lactation commences the hardening is reduced and the milk production gets under way.

Lactation Phase. The stimulation of the lacteal glands and the maintenance of their ability to produce milk is governed by the hormone prolactin, which is produced in the anterior pituitary. Stimulation of the sensory nerve ends in the nipple and areola by the suckling of the child lead via the hypothalamus to a synthesis and release of prolactin and oxytocin.

The oxytocin causes a contraction of the myoepithelia of the acini and the smaller lactiferous ducts and so transports the milk towards the surface (lactiferous sinuses). From here the child, if correctly positioned on the breast, can obtain the milk by sucking (creating a vacuum in the mouth cavity) and "biting" (compression of the lactiferous sinuses).

Oxytocin also leads to a contraction of the smooth muscle of the uterus and encourages it to return to its original size. However, it also influences the smooth muscle of the gastro-intestinal tract, the urethra and the blood vessels. Breast feeding is not only important for the newborn child, in that it provides it with optimal nourishment, but it also encourages the normalisation processes in the body of the mother.

Milk production is largely dependent on the demands made on the breast. Whether a woman can breast feed or not is dependent upon various factors:
- The woman's attitude towards breast feeding and to the child (Desire to breast feed).
- Her constitution and lifestyle (rest, sufficient sleep, nutrition, etc.).
- After approximately two weeks of breast feeding, the lacteal glands function independently. The prolactin and oxytocin levels rise each time the child is fed, and return afterwards to their normal resting levels.

Post-Lactation Phase. When breast feeding stops the breast begins to return to normal, although it will never return entirely to its original state. Normally the commencement of this process coincides with the start of the first menstrual period after delivery. During the early stages of stopping breast feeding there is a temporary expansion caused by an accumulation of milk, and the alveoli burst. Phagocytes remove the remaining milk. Remains of secretions and macrophages with particles of necrotic glandular epithelia may be present. The lobules atrophy in an irregular manner, and the lactiferous sinuses decrease in size. The connective tissue stroma increases. Over the next months the ducts become narrower, although ectasis may continue for some months.

Menopause

The mammary gland is subject to a physical involution which affects on the one hand the lobules (lobular involution) and the interlobular stroma on the other. In the case of the former, the acini become smaller and the interlobular connective tissue becomes more dense. Sometimes the acini join together to form microcysts. The involution of the stroma results from a gradual substitution of fat tissue for the interlobular connective tissue. Remains of the mammary parenchyma may be found in the fat tissue and may be erroneously diagnosed as tumours. In general, the breast of the menopausal woman can be easily palpated.

Juvenile Hyperplasia of the Mammary Gland

During puberty, an abnormal enlargement of the mammary gland on one or both sides may be observed (pubertal hyperplasia). The enlargement of the breast is the result of an increased proliferation of the glandular epithelia and an oedematous loosening of the surrounding connective tissue with an increase in collagen tissues and fat tissue.

Changes caused by hormones can be recognised both in the epithelia and in the connective tissue components. The glandular cells vary in size and shape depending upon whether the gland is dormant or active (menstrual cycle, pregnancy, post-parturition). The number of tubuli and acini vary between individuals and during the life of an individual, depending upon the hormonal stimulation. Milk production is not governed by the size of the breast but by the quantity and functionality of the glandular tissue. The sexual steroids and lactogenous hormones play an important role in the formation of benign and probably also of malignant changes. For this reason it seems important to describe in detail the changes which occur in the breast during a woman's life.

References: Page 187

1.2
Histopathology of Breast Tumours

1.2.1
Histopathology and Biology of the Invasive Mammary Carcinoma

ULRICH BONK

Almost a hundred putative prognostic factors for human breast-cancer patients have been reported. Faced with such a choice, the pathologist involved in assessing tissue samples in day-to-day practice will be wondering what status the histopathology method still has. Does it belong to brilliant quality management or shady risk management?

The American Joint Committee on Cancer has adopted criteria for the definition of a prognostic factor [1]. A prognostic factor must be statistically significant (i. e. its prognostic effect only rarely occurs by chance), independent (i. e. it retains its prognostic value when combined with other factors), and clinically relevant (i. e. it has a major impact on the accuracy of a prognosis).

With these criteria in mind, the College of American Pathologists (CAP) convened a multidisciplinary conference of invited participants, entitled the "CAP Conference XXVI: Clinical Relevance of Prognostic Markers in Solid Tumours", in Snowbird, Utah in June 1994 [2].

The participants identified two subsets of relevant prognostic factors for breast cancer that have been used clinically, as deemed appropriate by the managing physician.

Group I includes those prognostic factors that are well supported biologically and clinically in the scientific literature. These factors include the TNM variables, histologic type, grade (histologic/nuclear), and steroid receptors (oestrogen, progesterone).

Group II and III, with a large number of the latest prognostic factors – particularly using molecular biology – are still significant but not quite as meaningful as those in Group I.

The TNM staging system has been very useful, but although it is the best system available, it is not extremely accurate.

The recognized prognostic factors need to be integrated into the TNM staging system for greater accuracy in predicting the outcome. There is hardly any field of histopathological diagnosis which requires reliable cooperation between the physician in the clinic (or the practice) and the pathologist more than tumour diagnosis, which is increasing in quantity and becoming more and more differentiated in quality. The characteristics of individual tumours can now be recognized very much better and earlier with the aid of highly developed imaging methods, as a result of the knowledge gained from biochemical and immunohistochemical marker profiles and from a wide variety of test methods and also by including genetic data.

Even so, the status of histopathological diagnosis as a provable and retrospectively checkable prediction method has not been reduced. After all, the primary tumour, relapses and metastases have to be defined and classified histopathologically, so that comparisons between different manifestations of a tumour are possible, as well as deductions about the localization of occult primary tumours from the metastases. Our clinical partner expects a rapid and precise diagnosis: I should like to describe the most important criteria for breast cancer and those which can be worked out using conventional methods.

The European Union has produced quality-assurance guidelines for mammography screening [3]. Within this framework as it applies to pathology, guiding principles were developed under the chairmenship of Dr. J. P. Sloane of the University of Liverpool in England, based on a consensus of a large number of European pathologists. These current guidelines combine the preparatory recommendations. A standardized data record is used to poll the following types of invasive carcinoma:
- no special type (ductual) NST
- lobular, medullary, mucinous, tubular, mixed type
- miscellaneous primary carcinomas
- miscellaneous malignant tumours.

Further questions are:
- maximum diameter of the invasive tumour
- overall size of the tumour (including DCIS extending more than 1 mm beyond the invasive area)
- infiltration of the excision boundaries
- grading
- extent of the disease (localized or multiple)
- vascular invasion (blood vessels or lymph vessels).

It is also possible to add a comment or give addition information.

How should modern histopathological typing be applied to breast cancers?

The European Union's working party on pathology recommends the various internationally recognized publications as a basis. The International Academy for Pathology held two seminars at the 1994 World Pathology Congress in Hong Kong on the subject of the pathology of mammary carcinomas; these were chaired by David L. Page of the USA, and I. O. Ellis and C. W. Elston of the UK, respectively. These authors have kept track, over a very long period, of the fate of patients with widely differing mammary lesions. Their studies showed clear links between the histopathology and biology of invasive mammary carcinoma [4, 5, 6].

Categorizing a mammary lesion as "no special type (ductual)" is a negative diagnosis of exclusion. In histological assessment, the first step should always be to attempt to identify a specific type of invasive mammary carcinoma. The tubular, invasive cribriform, and mucinous types, in particular, are associated with a very good prognosis. The criteria for the various types of tumours have been dealt with in the literature [4, 6, 7, 8].

Analysis of subtypes of lobular carcinoma confirms differing prognoses. The classical, tubulo-lobular and lobular mixed types are associated with a better prognosis than carcinomas of no special type; this is not so for the solid variant.

As can be seen in table 1.1, the British working party has revealed the mixed types which in the meantime are familiar and established, with the various outcomes for the different histological types of mammary carcinoma.

For a tumour to be typed as ductal NST it must show that type in over 90% of its mass as judged by examination of representative sections of the tumour. If the ductal NST pattern comprises between 10% and 90% of the tumour (the rest being of a recognized special type) then it will fall into one of the mixed groups – tubular mixed, mixed lobular and ductal or mixed ductal and special type.

The result of these long-term studies is that the histological type provides highly significant

Table 1.1: Frequency and 10-Year-Survival of Each Histological Type [5]

Type of carcinoma	No. in study	Relative frequency [%]	10 year survival [%]
Ductal NST	760	47	47
Lobular	243	15	54
Tubular	38	2,3	90
Tubular mixed	220	13,6	69
Cribriform	13	0,8	91
Mucinous	14	0,9	80
Medullary	44	2,7	51
Atypical medullary	76	4,6	55
Mixed ductal/lobular	77	4,7	40
Mixed ductal/special	40	2,5	64
Miscellaneous	21	1,3	60
In situ (DCIS)	73	4,5	92
LCIS	2	0,1	NA
Total	1621	100	54

prognostic information. An evaluation of the prognosis of special types of carcinoma and tubulo-lobular carcinoma is shown in table 1.2.

Somewhere some of us got caught in a "no-win" debate of grading versus typing. This is over. We should do both, because it adds to the precision and understanding of the resultant diagnosis.

Grading is covered elsewhere in this congress, so I have confined myself to the significance of the histological type for mammary carcinomas.

Table 1.2: Evaluation of the Prognosis of Special Types of Carcinoma and Tubulo-Lobular Carcinoma [5]

Prognosis	Histological type
Excellent	Special (tubular, invasive cribriform, mucinous) Tubulo-lobular
Good	Tubular mixed Mixed ductal Special
Average	Classical lobular Medullary Atypical medullary
Poor	Solid lobular Ductal NST

The requirements for typing are relatively simple: good specimen fixation and preparation combined with strict application of the appropriate diagnostic criteria.

References: Page 187

1.2.2
Ductal Pattern of Atypical Hyperplasia (ADH)[1]

DAVID L. PAGE

The practical and philosophical aspects of ADH [1–3] may have been less than clear, and this presentation will clarify and focus on those aspects which we have found to be most effective in fostering understanding. Our approach to mammary proliferative lesions recognizes three categories of criteria [4]: Cytologic features, Histologic patterns, and semiquantitative extent of change. If there is some disagree-

---
[1] Talk held on the XX International Congress of the International Academy of Pathology, Hong Kong, 1994 Reprint by permission

ment among observers, the recognition that these three related but not completely overlapping categories need to be evaluated, brings a measure of precision to analyses and, thus, fosters agreement among observers. While there is considerable congruence between pattern and cytologic findings, low power pattern does not always predict cytology in these proliferative lesions. The minimal requirement involves a population of uniform, neoplastic-appearing cells.

Guidelines for Evaluation of Proliferative Ductal Pattern Lesions:
- Many of these lesions involve lobular units, but they are not of the "lobular" series of lesions recognized by ALH and LCIS (lobular carcinoma in situ) and are distinguished by cytologic and histologic patterns [5].
- Florid hyperplasia without atypia exhibits swirling (steaming) patterns of cells; Intercellular borders are usually ill-defined; there is irregularity of nuclear shape, chromasia and position; and there are irregular, often ragged, serpiginous slit-like secondary spaces, most marked central.
- Ductal carcinoma in-situ of non-comedo type (DCIS, NC) has a populated nuclear features, comprising without doubt, the entire population of cells throughout two membrane-bound spaces (a measure of the extent of lesion). Cytoplasm is usually pale and intercellular borders are usually distinct. Secondary spaces have smooth, rounded "punched-out" borders (cribriform architecture) and rigid, non-tapering bars can be found. The approach of Tavassoli and Norris [6] addresses this borderline between ADH and DCIS-NC with an overall size criterion which is a useful adjunct.
- Atypical ductal hyperplasia (ADH) exhibits partial involvement of basement membrane-bound space by a cell population of the type defined above for non-comedo ductal carcinoma in situ. Usually, the second (non-atypical) cell population consists of columnar, polarized cells, of the type usually seen in the ductal lamina positions immediately above the basement membrane.
- Upper limit of ADH. When in doubt (between atypical ductal hyperplasia and ductal carcinoma in-situ), the more benign diagnosis is appropriate (ADH).
- Lower limit of ADH (ADH vs. no AH).
- In order to qualify for atypical ductal hyperplasia (as opposed to florid hyperplasia without atypia), the bothersome cell population usually, but not always, has uniformly, hyperchromatic nuclei.
- In order to qualify for atypical ductal hyperplasia (as opposed to florid hyperplasia without atypia), the bothersome cells need to comprise an entire non-tapering bar crossing a space or at least comprise a cell population of similarly appearing "neoplastic" cells.

 Each upper and lower limit borderline has its own set of criteria, i.e., between PDWA (proliferative disease without atypia) v. ADH and ADH v. DCIS. One practical outcome of all of this is that a lesion recognized to be intermediate between PDWA and DCIS (i.e. ADH) is almost always a tiny lesion of less than 3 mm in largest size almost without exception.

Conclusions. In conclusion, one fact is without dispute: If diagnosticians agree not to agree on criteria, they will disagree. It is the criteria of ADH linked with the underlying biologic derivations and reproducible consequences which recognizes increased risk of cancer, not the words or the "experts" applying them.

Several confirming studies on the implications of specifically defined ADH have been done recently [6–8].

Special studies of molecular markers including DNA ploidy are in their infancy for ADH. Also, whereas the classic pattern discussed here has had verification in several studies noted above, there are other varieties of atypical ductal hyperplasia, or at least atypical hyperplasia of non-lobular pattern which are being considered currently. These consist of apocrine, unusual aspects of adenosis, hypersecretory and micropapillary as a special diagnostic consideration in some unusual cases. The slides submitted illustrate some of these features.

Figures 1.4 and 1.5 (see color plate) are from

the same case and illustrate involvement of a solitary lobular unit of 2,8 mm in greatest extent. Each basement membrane-bound space has a second population of luminal cells which are near the basement membrane. They are different in cytologic pattern from the characteristic "neoplastic-appearing" population centrally and thus deny a diagnosis of ductal carcinoma in situ.

Figure 1.6 (see color plate) demonstrates ADH in the wall of a cystically dilated space. Note cells present not forming the arches are a quite different second cells present not forming the Arches are a quite different second cell population that maintains normal polarity.

Figure 1.7 (see color plate) is a focus of atypical cells which may have been produced by some irregularity of processing but is not recognized as indicating an increased risk of later breast carcinoma beyond that of ordinary proliferative disease.

The last figure 1.8 (see color plate) illustrates the co-occurrence of apocrine [9] features, (at least suggested), and secretory activity [10]. The criteria for atypical hyperplasia with secretory features co-occurring is not well-developed.

References: Page 187

Chapter 2

Quality Assurance Recommendations for an Objective Diagnosis

2.1
Mammography Screening Programmes and the Consequences for Pathologists

2.1.1
Guidelines for Breast Pathology Services[1]

National Coordinating Group for Breast Screening Pathology, National Health Service Breast Screening Programme (NHSBSP), Chairman: J. P. SLOANE, UK

Introduction

Although the primary method of screening for breast cancer is a radiological rather than pathological technique, the quality of pathology services is of crucial importance as the definitive diagnosis of cancer is almost invariably made by pathologists. It is essential not only for them to distinguish cancer from benign conditions, but also to report histological features of prognostic significance in order to ensure that patients are treated appropriately and that screening programmes are properly monitored. Although the success of a breast screening programme is ultimately measured by a reduction in mortality in the invited population, statistically significant mortality data do not become available for many years. Other methods of monitoring programmes are thus required and these include the number of tumours detected and their prognostic features which should be more favourable than those of symptomatic cancers.

Figure 2.1 shows survival curves for symptomatic patients treated at the Nottingham Breast Unit, divided into good, moderate or poor prognostic groups based on a score (the Nottingham prognostic index) [1] calculated from the tumour size, grade and the presence of regional lymph node metastases. There is a marked difference in survival in patients assigned to these three groups. These pathological characteristics, however, can only have significant prognostic value if they are reported consistently by all pathologists participating in a screening programme.

Specimens from screened women provide pathologists with significantly greater prob-

---

[1] Publication: National Coordinating Group for Breast Screening Pathology (1997): Guidelines for Breast Pathology Services. NHSBSP Publication* No 2 (revised), 32 pages. (ISBN 1 871997 87 9) Copyright © 1997 by NHSBSP
This document replaces *Guidelines for Pathologists* which was published by the NHSBSP in 1989.
* NHSBSP Publications, National Breast Screening Programme, The Manor House, 260 Ecclesall Road South, Sheffield S11 9PS, UK.
Reprint by permission

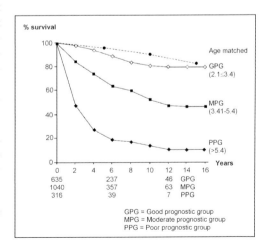

Figure 2.1: Survival according to the Nottingham Tenovus primary breast cancer study
Prognostic Index

lems than those from symptomatic women, both on macroscopic and histological examination. The main problem of macroscopic examination is localising impalpable lesions which require specimen radiography. This technique adds significantly to the length of time required to examine a biopsy specimen.

Problems encountered in histological examination are largely due to the disproportionate number of lesions that lie on the borderline between benign and malignant. Ductal carcinoma in situ (DCIS), for example, accounts for only about 5% of cancers in symptomatic women but for over 17% of all cancers so far detected in the UK screening programme [2]. It may be difficult to distinguish DCIS from ductal hyperplasia, particularly the atypical forms, and from minimally invasive carcinomas. These distinctions may require a great deal of expertise and experience as well as extensive tissue sampling. Furthermore, DCIS is a heterogeneous group of proliferations and there is now evidence that different morphological variants are associated with different recurrence rates. Reproducible classification is thus required. A relatively high proportion of invasive carcinomas detected by screening are small, well-differentiated low grade tumours which may be difficult to distinguish from benign pseudoinfiltrative lesions.

Finally, there is a need to avoid unnecessary surgery in breast cancer screening. In addition to needle core biopsies which may be very difficult to interpret, high quality cytology services are important as it has been shown that where these techniques are used at the assessment stage, they can help to reduce the number of unnecessary surgical operations by increasing confidence about benign diagnoses. There is also some evidence of a slight increase in the number of cancers detected.

In the light of the above considerations, a national coordinating group in breast pathology was set up in association with breast screening by the National Health Service Breast Screening Programme (NHSBSP) and the Royal College of Pathologists.

The terms of reference of this group are:
- to recommend minimum acceptable standards and provide guidelines and advice on pathological examination of breast tissues in order to maximise detection of malignant neoplasia and to achieve a high level of accuracy and consistency in reporting breast lesions
- to consider ways of achieving these objectives and to identify resource implications.

The group meets twice yearly to consider developments which impact on the practice of breast pathology.

In particular, it performs the following key functions:
- advising the NHSBSP on pathology related issues
- providing support and information for regional pathology coordinators
- identifying educational needs of pathologists and organising training including national courses
- monitoring the adequacy of data provided by pathologists
- continual review of the pathology information system
- monitoring consistency of reporting through the national breast External Quality Assessment (EQA) scheme
- monitoring the performance of pre-operative diagnostic services
- facilitating the exchange of information between pathologists and cancer registries, particularly to improve the detection of interval cancers
- facilitating the exchange of information and pathological material between pathologists and the wider research community
- fostering links with the private sector.

The membership of the group comprises:
- all the pathology regional coordinators of the NHSBSP
- the chairmen of the corresponding coordinating groups in radiology and surgery
- the national breast screening coordinator
- the chairman of the Royal College of Pathologists' Standing Advisory Committee in Histopathology
- a representative of the English Department of Health

- coopted pathologists with specialist expertise in breast histopathology and cytopathology (see Appendix 1, pg. 161).

Setting the Objectives

The quality of the pathological data generated by the screening programme will depend on the expertise of pathologists and the techniques and reporting methods they employ. They in turn will be influenced by managerial and administrative decisions which affect the ability of pathologists to achieve the necessary standards.

The objective for the pathology quality assurance programme associated with breast cancer screening are listed below. The methods of achieving these objectives, the required standard of performance and outcome measurements are set out in table 2.1.

Outcome Objectives

- To improve the identification and pathological characterisation of lesions producing mammographic abnormalities.
- To improve the consistency of diagnoses made by pathologists.
- To improve the quality of prognostic information in pathological reports.
- To minimise the number of unnecessary surgical operations.

Pathological Reporting of Breast Specimens

Macroscopic Examination. Macroscopic examination is a vital part of the screening process and should not be delegated to biomedical scientists (BMSS) or inexperienced pathologists.

Biopsies Containing Palpable Lesions Need not Involve Specimen Radiography.

Biopsies containing palpable lesions need not involve specimen radiography. Although there have been some reports that specimen radiography increases the detection of occult carcinomas in specimens containing benign palpable lesions, it is not regarded as essential. Some workers, however, have found it useful for assessing excision margins. In general, it is considered to add little to careful macroscopic examination and adequate sampling.

It is Mandatory to Undertake Specimen Radiography of Biopsies Containing Impalpable Lesions.

It is mandatory, however, for the surgeon to arrange for immediate specimen radiography of biopsies containing impalpable lesions in order to ensure that they contain the radiological abnormality. Further specimen radiography is highly desirable to select the correct blocks of tissue for histological examination. If convenient, specimen radiography may be carried out in the radiology department or operating theatre complex. However, it is usually necessary to use designated equipment in the pathology laboratory. It is essential that all histopathologists reporting specimens from screened women should have ready access to the necessary x-ray and developing equipment and receive proper training in its use. Where such equipment is located in the pathology laboratory, arrangements should be made to monitor its safety and performance through a radiation protection officer or a medical physics quality assurance scheme. The Medical Devices Directorate has produced a report on specimen radiography equipment to which potential purchasers are referred [5]. Appropriate high intensity viewing boxes are also necessary for examining mammographic films. Laboratories should have written protocols for examining breast specimens and for using and monitoring the associated equipment. Histological reporting of impalpable lesions should not be undertaken where specimen radiography cannot be performed.

Record Tissue Stored. A record should be kept of tissue taken from all types of specimens, particularly of frozen tissue which may be useful tot research purposes.

Refer to Pathology Reporting in Breast Cancer Screening. For detailed guidance on macroscopic examination of biopsy, local excision and mastectomy specimens, the reader is referred

Table 2.1: Quality Assurance Standards

Quality Assurance Objectives	Outcome Measurements	Targets	Methods of Achieving Objectives
1) To improve the identification and pathological characterisation of lesions producing mammographic abnormalities	Proportion of specimens containing the mammographic abnormality in which it is identified histopathologically	< 1 %	a) High quality specimen radiography for impalpable lesions b) Adequate macroscopic examination and sampling of biopsy specimens c) Multidisciplinary meetings or discussions to correlate radiological and pathological findings
2) To improve consistency of diagnoses made by pathologists	Diagnostic consistency measured in the UK breast EQA scheme: a) for invasive carcinoma b) for ductal carcinoma in situ (including microinvasive carcinoma) c) for benign lesions (including atypical ductal hyperplasia and radial scar)	a) Minimal $k = 0.8$, achievable $k = 0.9$ b) Minimal $k = 0.7$, achievable $k = 0.8$ c) Minimal $k = 0.8$, achievable $k = 0.9$	a) Use of the standardised terminology and diagnostic criteria High quality sections Participation in technical EQA schemes b) Continuing medical education in breast pathology c) Participation in the national breast EQA scheme d) Referral of difficult cases for second opinion e) Research and development work on borderline lesions
3) To improve the quality of prognostic information in pathological reports	a) Proportion of invasive carcinomas graded and sized b) Consistency of grading in national EQA scheme c) Consistency of tumour measurement in national EQA scheme	a) Minimal > 90 %, achievable > 99 % (except in inappropriate specimens)* b) Minimal $k = 0.5$, achievable $k = 0.7$ c) Minimal % of measurements ±3 mm of the median = 88 % achievable % of measurements ±3 mm of the median = 90 %	a) Following grading criteria** b) Following guidance on measuring tumour size**
4) To minimise the number of unnecessary surgical operations	For cytology*** a) Benign: malignant ratio at initial surgery b) Unsatisfactory smears from cancer-bearing breasts c) False positive rate**** d) False negative rate**** e) Needle core biopsies	a) Minimal 1:2, achievable 1:4 b) Minimal < 10 %, achievable < 5 % c) Minimal < 1 %, achievable < 0.5 % d) Minimal < 5 %, achievable < 4 % e) Insufficient data available	a) Training in breast fine needle aspiraton cytology b) Monitoring performance using the CQA system and correcting deficiencies c) Ensuring clinical staff are able to undertake satisfactory aspirations and check the quality of the preparations d) Development of EQA scheme using telepathology

* Inappropriate specimens include needle biopsies, carcinomas less than 10 high power fields in size and cases where section quality is too poor to assess the relevant histological characteristics.
** As given in *Pathology Reporting* in Breast *Cancer Screening* (2nd edition) [3].
*** Achieving the targets depends not only on the performance of the cytopathologist but upon the clinicians undertaking the aspirations.
**** For definitions see *Guidelines for Cytology Procedures and Reporting in Breast Cancer Screening* [4].

to the second edition of *Pathology Reporting in Breast Cancer Screening* [3] produced jointly by the NHSBSP and the Royal College of Pathologists.

Histological Examination

The Screening Programme Provides Pathologists With a Disproportionate Number of Borderline Lesions.

In attempting to detect carcinomas at an early stage, the NHSBSP provides histologists and cytologists with a higher proportion of borderline lesions with the consequent risks of over- and under-diagnosis of malignancy. Problems are encountered principally in distinguishing in situ carcinomas from atypical ductal hyperplasia and microinvasive carcinoma and in reporting consistently pathological features of prognostic significance [6].

It is Important to Identify Atypical Proliferative Lesions Accurately and Reproducibly.

In recent years evidence has been provided that some non-cancerous atypical proliferative lesions are associated with an increased risk of developing carcinoma. It is important to identify these lesions accurately and reproducibly so that appropriate patient management can be instituted and more can be learned about their biological potential.

Recording Features of Prognostic Significance is Important.

Recording histological features of infiltrating carcinomas that are of prognostic significance, i.e. tumour size, grade, vascular invasion and tumour type, may affect the patient's immediate management and will allow a comparison to be made between cancers detected by screening and those presenting symptomatically as interval cancers or in women who, for various reasons, have not been screened. The number of positive and negative lymph nodes should also be recorded. Careful clinical follow up is essential to enable clinicians and pathologists to correlate pathological features of tumours with clinical outcome.

A Major Objective of the QA Programme is to Standardise Terminology and Diagnostic Criteria.

A major objective of the quality assurance programme is to unify, as much as possible, the terminology and diagnostic criteria employed in reporting breast lesions from screened women. Appendix 2 (pg. 163) consists of the standard histopathology and cytopathology reporting forms for use in entering pathological data onto the national computer database. The reporting of features included in these forms ensures that a standard set of data is collected from each woman, using the same terminology. These reporting forms are not intended to replace existing reporting procedures in individual laboratories unless so desired. It is recommended that the forms be completed when the specimen is reported unless a second opinion is sought when completion should be delayed until the definitive diagnosis is reached. In order to minimise variation in diagnostic criteria, definitions of terminology and more detailed guidelines for using the forms are included in the NHSBSP/Royal College of Pathologists booklets *Pathology Reporting in Breast Cancer Screening* [3] and *Guidelines for Cytology Procedures and Reporting in Breast Cancer Screening* [4].

Frozen Section Examination Should not Generally be Undertaken on Impalpable Lesions.

Frozen section examination should generally be reserved for palpable abnormalities where a definitive diagnosis cannot be made preoperatively. This investigation is now used much less frequently as a consequence of the development of preoperative cytology and needle biopsy services.

Frozen sections should not usually be undertaken on impalpable lesions except under the strict conditions laid down in *Pathology Reporting in Breast Cancer Screening* [3] and only after prior consultation with the surgeon.

Guidance on the principles and practical aspects of fine needle aspiration cytology is given in the document *Guidelines for Cytology Procedures and Reporting in Breast Cancer Screening* [4]. Wide bore needle biopsies are increasingly being performed in some centres usually in association with fine needle aspiration cytology and may be highly effective where cytology is equivocal or where cytological expertise is not well developed. They have the advantage that when performed for the assessment of microcalcification, they can be subjected to specimen radiography to ensure that the calcification is present in the core. If benign calcification is identified in the core and this provides a satisfactory explanation for the calcification seen on the mammogram, diagnostic excision biopsy can be avoided, especially if a specific lesion such as sclerosing adenosis is identified. Another major advantage is that it is possible to make an unequivocal diagnosis of invasive carcinoma rather than simply of malignancy. It should be remembered, however, that wide bore needle procedures can distort the mammographic appearances for several months and that multiple cores may be required to localise small abnormalities. Fine needle aspiration cytology and wide bore needle biopsy are thus complementary techniques.

Preoperative Tissue Diagnosis Reduces Unnecessary Surgical Operations.

Current evidence indicates that the use of fine needle aspiration cytology and/or wide bore needle biopsy substantially reduces the number of unnecessary operations performed both for benign disease and for malignancy, with consequent financial savings and reduced discomfort and inconvenience to the patient. Definitive surgery for carcinoma can be decided preoperatively by the triple approach of mammography, clinical examination and cytology/needle biopsy, allowing treatment for many malignant lesions in a one-stage operation and avoiding the need for frozen sections. If cytology or needle biopsy is negative in the face of strong clinical and radiological evidence of malignancy then they should be repeated and, if still negative, an open biopsy performed.

Aspiration of Cyst Fluid. Aspiration of cysts is of diagnostic value in itself. Cyst fluid need be submitted for cytological examination only if:
- the fluid is bloodstained or cloudy
- the cyst is recurrent
- there is a projection from the wall of the cyst on ultrasound or
- there is a residual mass after aspiration.

Any residual mass should be subjected to further aspiration and cytological examination.

Cytology Specimens Should be Reported by Pathologists.

All fine needle aspiration cytology should be reported by a consultant or a trainee pathologist under consultant supervision. The practice of allowing BMSs to report negative smears is regarded as inappropriate as the recognition of tubular and cribriform carcinomas depends on a high degree of skill and a knowledge of the histological appearances which may be encountered. False negative cases associated with delay in diagnosis have been the subject of more litigation in the USA than false positive cases and, although it is recognised that these can never be totally avoided, all possible measures to reduce them to a minimum should be taken. Breast cytology is increasingly being reported by pathologists who also report the histology but, where this is not the case, close liaison between cytologist and histologist is essential.

The Skill of the Operator is Crucial.

The detection of carcinoma by cytology or needle biopsy depends not only on the ability of the pathologist to identify malignancy, but also on the skill with which the operator can localise the lesion with the needle, obtain an adequate sample and, in the case of cytology, make a satisfactory preparation. Guidance on the practical aspects of aspiration, including image-guided specimens, can be found in the *Guidelines for Cytology Procedures and Reporting in Breast Cancer Screening* [4]. The failure to detect carcinoma by needle techniques is often due to unsatisfactory specimens. In some centres aspiration is performed by pathologists or, for image-guided techniques, with the pathologist in attendance. This allows an immediate evaluation of the sample, meaning that the test can be repeated immediately not only if the specimen is inadequate but also if benign findings conflict with strong radiological evidence of malignancy. This immediate reporting reduces the length of time the patient has to wait for a diagnosis and can reduce anxiety. It also enables treatment to be planned at the first clinic visit, reducing the number of clinic attendances and hence lowering costs [7, 8].

Clinical Staff Performing Aspiration Should be Properly Trained to do so.

Pathologists without dedicated sessions will not be able to perform these duties and in this case aspiration could be performed by clinical staff. If this is the case, they should be properly trained to localise lesions, to assess the cellularity of specimens and to make satisfactory preparations. Insufficient training and experience of the aspirator have been clearly shown to lead to a high proportion of unsatisfactory and false negative specimens for which the pathologist cannot accept responsibility. A similar argument applies to needle biopsies.

Audit and Multidisciplinary Discussion are Important.

Adequate multidisciplinary discussion and unit audit of sensitivity and specificity can lead to the identification of problems of preoperative tissue diagnosis and allow appropriate corrective measures to be instituted. In units where smear preparation of cytological samples is a problem, the use of transport medium should be considered.

Image-Guided FNAC can be Effective.

Needle sampling of impalpable lesions guided by ultrasound or x-ray imaging has proved highly effective in many centres where it has become standard practice. Guidance on image-guided aspiration techniques aimed at maximising their effectiveness can be found in the *Guidelines for Cytology Procedures and Reporting in Breast Cancer Screening* [4].

Technical Quality of Sections and Smears

High Technical Quality is Necessary.

High technical quality is necessary in order to achieve accurate histological and cytological diagnosis. At present, conventional well-established methods for preparing slides are adequate for diagnosing breast diseases. Immunohistology is required in a small number of cases. There are minor differences in processing and staining methods from laboratory to laboratory but they do not significantly alter pathological interpretation. The great majority of laboratories prepare slides of adequate quality but all laboratories involved in breast cancer screening should participate in the national immunocytochemistry EQA scheme, particularly if they provide an oestrogen receptor service, and appropriate general histology technical schemes.

Managing Quality Assurance

Introduction

The Pathology Quality Assurance Programme is organised by the UK National Coordinating Group for Breast Screening Pathology on behalf of the NHSBSP and the Royal College of Pathologists and is part of a much larger exercise involving all professional groups within the NHSBSP. The National Coordinating Group has five small subgroups devoted to the following quality assurance activities:
- Education and training
- External Quality Assessment (EQA)
- Information
- Cytology
- Research and development.

These aspects are discussed individually below.

Laboratories involved in diagnosing symptomatic or screen-detected breast disease should be accredited by CPA UK Ltd, and should have a nominated lead pathologist with responsibility for breast pathology including that generated by screening. This pathologist should be a member of the multidisciplinary breast team and participate in regular case management meetings. They should have attended appropriate training courses, participate in the national breast EQA scheme and ensure that all data required by the screening programme are provided.

Pathologists should have easy access to specimen radiography facilities and adequate technical and secretarial support.

Laboratory procedures for handling breast specimens should be well documented.

A fine needle aspiration cytology service which meets the quality standards laid down in *Guidelines for Cytology Procedures and Reporting in Breast Cancer Screening* [4] should be provided where required. A wide bore needle biopsy service may also be needed. Clinicians and radiologists should be generally satisfied with the speed and quality of the pathology service. All histological and cytological specimens should be reported by a consultant or a trainee under consultant supervision.

Close liaison between pathology laboratories and cancer registries is mutually important. Data on interval cancers and cancers in unscreened women are essential for monitoring the screening programme.

Health authorities have a major role to play in ensuring the quality of pathology services by insisting on quality standards in agreements with hospitals. The formation of breast cancer units dealing with a minimum number of cases per annum will facilitate achieving the required standards in pathology as in other disciplines involved in the diagnosis and management of patients with breast cancer [9, 10].

Education and Training

National Training Centres. When the NHS-BSP began it was recommended that pathologists participating in the screening process should attend a course at one of the national training centres offering pathology training (Guildford, King's College Hospital, London, Edinburgh and Nottingham). In the great majority of cases this has now been achieved, although courses continue to be provided for trainees in the specialist registrar grade and consultants taking on breast screening responsibilities for the first time.

Continuing Medical. Education Pathologists who have already attended one of these basic courses are advised to keep up-to-date by participating in the update and refresher courses which are available at the national training centres. In addition a national breast pathology update course takes place every two years in the spring, alternating with a national breast fine needle aspiration cytology course. These are currently held in Nottingham on behalf of the national training centres. All courses form part of Continuing Medical Education (CME) recommended by the Royal College of Pathologists. Regular advertisements for breast screening pathology courses appear in the College's bulletin and in most pathology journals.

Multidisciplinary Approach. One of the main functions of the courses is to outline the multidisciplinary approach to breast screening. Methods for examining specimens from screened women are described and specific diagnostic problems are emphasised. In addition secondments to training centres for more individual tuition can be arranged through the coordinators at each training centre.

Participation in EQA. Following attendance at one of these courses, histological expertise should be developed further through participation in the National Breast EQA Scheme (see below "External Quality Assurance"). Seeking second opinions on difficult cases is also a useful educational exercise.

Cytology Training. At the outset of the NHS-BSP, expertise in fine needle aspiration cytology of the breast was limited to relatively few centres and there was an urgent need for the development of comprehensive training programmes. This has been achieved in a number of ways. Courses in fine needle aspiration cytology and its application to both screening and symptomatic breast disease are provided at the national training centres and at the Royal Marsden Hospital. Periods of attachment may be spent in laboratories where the level of expertise is high. Self-tuition can be undertaken by writing (but not issuing) reports on cytological preparations made from breast tissue of patients undergoing surgery and relating diagnoses to subsequent histological findings. This type of self-assessment enables pathologists to determine when their competence is of a sufficient level to issue reports on which clinical decisions will be made. As yet, few specialist registrar posts offering training in cytology have been established, but it is hoped that these will increase in the future. The Royal College of Pathologists now awards a Diploma in Cytopathology.

Role of Regional Coordinators. Regional coordinators should play an important role in facilitating education and training within regions by holding regular regional breast screening pathology meetings which should contain a slide seminar component (see Appendix 3, pg. 166). The discussion of slides circulated in the national EQA scheme together with the analyses of consistency produced by the Cancer Screening Evaluation Unit is regarded as an indispensable educational activity.

Training in Service Level Agreements. Participation in basic training courses has now been made mandatory in breast screening agreements in some regions. It is recommended that this should be made a requirement in all such agreements with the NHSBSP.

External Quality Assurance (EQA)

Pathology departments involved in the screening programme are visited periodically by regional quality assurance teams, who may inspect local facilities and ensure that performance meets the agreed targets. These visits should normally take place at least once during the agreement period (usually once every three years) and their outcomes are reported to the regional breast screening quality assurance committee, the host hospital, the commissioning health authorities and the national coordinating team [11]. Appropriate action is taken where performance is deemed inadequate.

National EQA Scheme. A national slide exchange scheme in histology was set up shortly after the onset of the national breast screening programme and is described in detail in Appendix 4, pg. 167. The scheme has been useful in identifying problems of reporting consistency which can be addressed through education and training, and research and development. There is evidence that participation in the scheme itself has improved consistency. The findings of the first six circulations have been published [6].

The approach to EQA in cytology is discussed below.

Information

The function of this subgroup is to address the problems in gathering reliable and internally consistent histological and cytological data from the NHSBSP.

Dealing with Different Software Systems. For historical reasons, different software systems are used to collect pathological information from women who have had cytological or histological examinations. The majority of English regions, Wales and Northern Ireland use software originally developed by the Oxford RHA – the National Breast Screening System. Other systems are also used (Scottish, Trent, HSS and South Thames [West] systems). The subgroup software developers, and recently has recruited representatives from the user groups utilising the various systems mentioned above.

Histology and Cytology Pro Formas. In order to gather relevant pathological information, pro formas have been approved by the National Co-ordinating Group for Breast Screening Pathology to cover both histological and cytological data (see Appendix 2, pg. 163). These have been continually modified during the course of the NHSBSP in an attempt to improve both the quality of the information and its ease of entry. The immediate result has been that it is now possible to obtain quality assurance information on the data from individual screening centres, regions and nationally. Such information is capable of many substratifications, but requires careful appraisal before statistically valid conclusions can be drawn.

General Functions of the Information Group.
Ancillary functions undertaken by the Information Group have been the preparation of a guide to the use and benefits of different specimen radiographic machines and ancillary apparatus [5], input to the cytology group in devising a cytology quality assurance system, and general advice to the main coordinating group. Software modifications recommended by the main group are also processed through the information group.

Interactions with Other Subgroups. There are obvious overlaps with other pathology subgroups, notably research and development and EQA. In addition, the information potentially affects activities in the training and education quarter. Cross-representation and membership of these other subgroups harmonises these different activities.

Cytology

Problems of Organising Cytology EQA. EQA in breast cancer screening cytology differs from histology EQA in that multiple copies of a patient smear cannot be made at present. There is also a large number of different preparation and staining methods which means that pathologists could justifiably say that they cannot assess a smear because it is stained or prepared differently.

Cytology Quality Assurance (CQA). Because of this, the cytology group of the National Coordinating Committee for Breast Cancer Screening Pathology has recommended that, at the present time, cytology EQA in breast screening is performed using the Cytology Quality Assurance routine (CQA) which is programmed into the national breast screening computer system. This routine is detailed in the NHSBSP publication *Guidelines for Cytology Procedures and Reporting in Breast Cancer Screening* [4]. The report produced by the computer gives measures of sensitivity and specificity for the test and detailed examination of the results as illustrated in the above publication and in a subsequent review article allows the performance of a unit to be assessed [12].

General Applicability of CQA. It is recommended that the CQA routine is programmed into computer systems dealing with symptomatic breast disease, as they are set up so that the same parameters described above can be assessed.

Telepathology may be a system which will, in the future, be able to overcome the numerous problems inherent in cytology EQA and allow this difficult area to be explored further.

Biopsy Quality Assurance (BQA). At the time of writing, there is increasing use in many centres of needle core biopsies in obtaining a preoperative tissue diagnosis, usually in association with fine needle aspiration cytology. A method of monitoring performance similar to CQA is being developed for wide bore needle biopsies (BQA).

Research and Development

Importance of Research. Research is a vital component of pathology in breast cancer screening which provides excellent opportunities to study the early stages of human breast cancer. Applied research aimed at refining diagnostic criteria is essential to improve reporting consistency. Improved methods for evaluating the prognostic significance of borderline lesions and features of established neoplasms are also essential to ensure that patients are managed appropriately. Fundamental research is required to improve understanding of the basic biology of lesions encountered in screened women and may eventually generate information which can be used by clinical pathologists to improve their evaluation of breast biopsies.

All Pathologists Can Contribute to the Research Effort.

All pathologists can make a contribution to research, not just those with specific research programmes. The provision of reliable and adequate pathological data is essential for local and national trials such as screening the under 50s and the management of screen-detected DCIS. The development of a national telepathology service will require the cooperation and enthusiasm of numerous pathologists. Established researchers clearly need ready access to pathological material from screened women and a high level of cooperation between research groups and those delivering the clinical service is essential. The level of this interaction will clearly be improved by the establishment of breast units within district general hospitals.

Role of Regional Coordinators. Regional coordinators should play a major role in facilitating research within their regions (see Appendix 3, pg. 166).

Resource Implications. Adequate resources are a prerequisite for high quality pathology services. Breast pathology will not reach the required standard without sufficient manpower, capital equipment and running costs.

Manpower

Histology Workload. All histology departments should have a minimum of two consultants. In a district general hospital department, workload should not exceed 4,000 surgical specimens and 300 autopsies per consultant per annum. A consultant histopathologist in a teaching hospital should be expected to deal with only half this workload given commitments to teaching, research and specialised practice [13].

Cytopathology Workload. A consultant cytologist should not be expected to examine personally more than 6000 cases per annum, taking into account the time required for laboratory and screening programme management, audit, teaching, continuing medical education and research. In teaching hospitals, consultants should be expected to deal with half this workload [13]. Fine needle aspiration cytology for breast screening is not a primary screening procedure and should be treated as a diagnostic test. Additional consultant sessions are needed for cytologists who report specimens in fine needle aspiration clinics, take their own fine needle aspirates or cover more than one hospital.

Lead Pathologists. Lead pathologists require additional sessions for audit and multidisciplinary team meetings. The standard of breast pathology in departments where these workload statistics are exceeded is likely to be significantly compromised.

Support for Regional Coordinators. Regional coordinators should be funded for an adequate number of sessions so that their activities can be specifically dedicated to local coordination of breast screening pathology services. They also need access to adequate teaching facilities including a closed circuit colour television system for discussing local and national EQA cases (see Appendix 4, pg. 167).

Technical and Secretarial Support. Adequate secretarial support is required not only to ensure high quality histology and cytology services but also to support regional coordinators in their coordinating activities. Three sessions per week are required for the latter (see Appendix 3, pg. 166). Adequate technical support is also required; breast screening pathology is particularly demanding of technical time, often requiring a large number of blocks, specimen radiography and film development. Regional coordinators require additional technical help to prepare material for QA purposes (one session per week).

Capital Equipment. All laboratories involved in breast screening need access to high quality specimen radiography equipment. Adequate funds need to be provided for maintaining such equipment and replacing it where necessary. Specimen radiography equipment should come within a physics quality control programme.

Formation of Breast Units. The formation of breast units, in addition to improving the standards of diagnosis and Management of patients with breast disease, should also improve cost efficiency. The publication of EL(96)66, *Improving Outcomes in Breast Cancer: Guidance for Purchasers* [14], stressed the importance of multidisciplinary working in breast units and of high quality pathology services as part of that process.

References: Page 188

2.1.2
Quality Assurance Guidelines for Pathology in Mammography Screening

E. C. Working Group on Breast Screening Pathology, Chairman: J. P. SLOANE, Luxembourg

Prologue

In the following, guidelines for pathology in mammography screening produced by the E. C. Working Group on Breast Screening Pathology[1] will be shown. Almost the same guidelines were also published by the Breast Screening Programme of the National Health Service, UK; (NHSBSP)[2]. The latter publication includes additionally detailed appendices about new developments in histological examination written as brief reviews with detailed reference lists. Thus, we completed the guidelines of the E. C. Working Group with additional remarks (written in italics) and with the appendices of the guidelines produced by the NHSBSP.

It should be noted that the publication of the NHSBSP also includes a number of histological photographs about different mammary tumours which are not shown in this book.

---

[1] Publication: E. C. Working Group on Breast Screening Pathology (Sloane J. as Editor) (1996): Quality Assurance Guidelines for Pathology in Mammography Screening. In: European Commission (de Wolf C. J. M., Perry N. M. as Editors): European Guidelines for Quality Assurance in Mammography Screening. Office for Official Publications of the European Communities*, Luxembourg, II-C-1–II-C-31. (ISBN 92-827-7430-9) Copyright © 1996 by ECSC-EC-EAEC, Brussels, Luxembourg
  * Office for Official Publications of the European Communities, 2985 Luxembourg, Luxembourg
[2] Publication: National Coordinating Group for Breast Screening Pathology (1997): Pathology Reporting in Breast Cancer Screening. NHSBSP Publication* No. 3, 2nd Edition, 65 pages. (ISBN 1 871997 22 4) Copyright © 1997 by NHSBSP
  * NHSBSP Publications, National Breast Screening Programme, The Manor House, 260 Ecclesall Road South, Sheffield S11 9PS, U. K.
  Reprint by permission

Introduction

The success of a breast screening programme depends heavily on the quality of the pathological service. Specimens from screened women provide pathologists with particular problems of macroscopic and histological examination; the former principally result from identifying impalpable radiological abnormalities and the latter from classifying borderline lesions which are encountered with disproportionate frequency. Accurate pathological diagnoses and the provision of prognostically significant information are important to ensure that patients are managed appropriately and that the programme is properly monitored and evaluated. A standard set of data from each patient, using the same terminology and diagnostic criteria is essential to achieve the latter objective. The opinions expressed represent the consensus view of the E. C. Working Group on Breast Screening Pathology and other pathologists who made written or verbal comments on this document and the United Kingdom document on which it is based. We hope that European pathologists involved in breast screening will find the guidance useful and the method of recording data convenient.

Macroscopic Examination of Biopsy and Resection Specimens

Biopsy Specimens

Optimal Handling. Biopsies of mammographically detected lesions may provide especial difficulty in histological interpretation and consequently require optimal fixation and careful handling. Sometimes a photographic record of the sliced specimen, with the guide wire in position may be necessary to maximize the value of case discussions with clinical and radiological colleagues. Provision for macroscopic photography must, therefore, be borne in mind, especially for difficult cases.

The surgeon should be discouraged from cutting the specimen before sending it to the pathologist and should ideally mark it with sutures in order to obtain proper orientation. Sutures are preferable to metal staples which often retract into the specimen, thus becoming impossible to recognize, and may obscure microcalcifications. A code of orientation for the sutures needs to be established and indicated on the request form.

Palpable Lesions. Palpable lesions detected in the screening programme may be dealt with by conventional methods and there is no especial virtue in specimen radiography, assuming that there is no doubt that the radiological and palpable lesions are one and the same.

Confirming Excision of Radiological Abnormality. After excision, the intact specimen – with guide wire in situ – must be x-rayed. Ideally this procedure is carried out by the staff of the radiological department, so that the radiologist or surgeon can determine whether the relevant lesion has been resected. It may be necessary on medicolegal grounds for centres to name consultants responsible for confirming that mammographic lesions have been removed. Ideally those consultants should be the radiologists who interpreted the clinical mammograms. A good working relationship between pathologists, surgeons and radiologists is essential. Two copies of the specimen radiograph at this time could be taken with benefit, one for the department of radiology and one for the pathologist.

If Mammographic Abnormality not Identified. Clearly there will be a few occasions when the mammographic abnormality cannot be identified in the specimen. This may result from the excision of a lesion producing only architectural change in the clinical mammogram or from unsuccessful surgical localisation. Detailed pathological examination should still be undertaken even in the latter case and the findings communicated to the surgeon. Clinical mammography can subsequently be repeated to determine if the lesion is still present in the breast.

Fresh Specimens. Specimens should be examined within 2–3 hours if received fresh. Samples for oestrogen receptor determination should be snap frozen in liquid nitrogen within 30 minutes of excision if a ligand binding assay is used. It should be remembered, however, that oestrogen receptor status can adequately be determined on standard formalin-fixed, paraffin-embedded sections [1, 2]. (For further guidance on steroid receptor determination, see Appendix 1, pg. 169)

Frozen Sections. Rapid frozen sectioning is generally inappropriate in the assessment of clinically impalpable lesions. Rarely, however, it may be justified to enable a firm diagnosis of invasive carcinoma to be made in order to allow definitive surgery to be carried out in one operation. Three essential criteria, however, must be fulfilled:
- The mammographic abnormality must be clearly and unequivocally identified on macroscopic examination.
- It must be large enough (generally at least 10 mm) to allow an adequate proportion of the lesion to be fixed and processed without prior freezing.
- It must have proved impossible to make a definitive diagnosis preoperatively.

Fixation. The intact specimen may be examined in the fresh state or after fixation. Good fixation is very important to preserve the degree of morphological detail needed to diagnose borderline lesions and report features of prognostic significance, particularly grade and vascular invasion. Small specimens may be fixed whole but larger ones should be examined and sliced within 2–3 hours of excision, if possible, to allow adequate penetration of fixative.

Excision Margins. In order to demonstrate adequacy of excision, the entire surface of the specimen should be painted with India ink, radiolucent pigments, dyed gelatin or other suitable material. An appropriate period of drying must be allowed if spread of the chosen reagent is to be avoided. For further guidance, see Appendix 2, pg. 170.

Naked Eye Examination. After determining its weight (and size if required), the specimen is then serially sliced at intervals of up to 4 mm. The cut surfaces are examined by careful visual inspection. Palpation may also be informative. The maximum diameter, contour, colour and consistency of any macroscopic lesion are recorded. The size of lesions measured macroscopically should be checked later on histological sections as the true extent of the abnormality is not always appreciated by macroscopic inspection alone. If different, the histological dimensions should be accepted as the true size. In the case of malignant lesions, adequacy of excision should be assessed by naked eye and later by microscopic examination.

Specimen Radiography. Unless a lesion obviously accounting for the radiological abnormality is identified, a second radiograph of the sliced specimen should be performed. It is desirable for the pathologist to give a brief description of the abnormality in the specimen radiograph during macroscopic examination. Blocks should then be taken from the areas corresponding to the mammographic abnormalities and any other macroscopically suspicious zones. This method allows precise correlations to be made between the radiological and histological appearances and may serve as a reference map for orientation and reconstruction purposes. It is thus the favoured method of specimen radiography. It has been found, however, to be too time-consuming for some laboratories to undertake. A number of shorter, one stage, methods have been reported. For reviews see Anderson (1989) and Armstrong & Davies (1991) [3, 4].

Histological Characterization of Mammographic Changes. Whichever method is adopted, pathologists must satisfy themselves that the pathological changes responsible for mammographic abnormalities have been identified in the histological sections; it may be necessary to consult with radiologists to be certain of this. If not, the residual unblocked tissue and/or blocks should be re-x-rayed. Any residual tissue should be stored until the mammographic changes have been characterized histologically. It is not recommended that tissue is simply taken from around a guide wire introduced preoperatively which may not necessarily be very close to the mammographic abnormality.

Choice of Specimen Mammography Equipment. Although it is possible to prepare adequate mammographs of specimens using a clinical mammography machine, this approach may present logistical difficulties. There are several dedicated specimen mammography cabinets on the market. Their characteristics, mode of operation and the use of accessories have been described in a recent publication by the English Department of Health (1991) [5].

Extent of Sampling. The precise number of blocks to be taken cannot be stated dogmatically and clearly depends on the size and number of lesions present. With small biopsies, all the tissue should be blocked and examined. For malignant tumours in excess of 20 mm, about 3 blocks of the tumour are desirable. Where possible, at least one block should include the edge of the tumour and the nearest excision margin to enable measurement of this distance, in mm, on the histological sections.

For larger biopsies which cannot be blocked in toto, some sampling of radiologically and macroscopically normal breast should be undertaken in order to increase the detection of small occult cancers (particularly **in situ** change) and atypical proliferative lesions. The frequency with which such lesions are detected incidentally in unscreened women depends on the number of blocks taken [6]. The extent of sampling of biopsies containing benign screen-detected mammographic abnormalities should be decided locally and will depend, amongst other things, on the extent of local resources. Additional sampling is more effective if restricted to fibrous parenchyma, ignoring the adipose tissue.

Large Blocks. Large blocks and sections are used in some laboratories where they are found to be of value in identifying screen-detected lesions as well as in determining their size, extent of spread and adequacy of excision. They facilitate orientation by obviating the need for mental reconstruction of the overall picture from several separate sections. They also reduce the number of blocks required [7]. Other workers, however, have encountered problems in achieving adequate fixation and good cytological detail in addition to the technical difficulties of cutting large sections and the problems in storing them. These drawbacks can be overcome, but large blocks, although of value, are not regarded as essential for examining specimens from screened women and their use should depend on local preference.

Mastectomy Specimens

Naked Eye Examination. Mastectomy specimens should be dealt with within 2 hours of removal and either examined in the fresh state or incised before fixation to allow adequate penetration of fixative. The favoured method of examination is by slicing the breast from the deep surface in the sagittal plane after measuring the dimensions or recording the weight. The slices should be about 10 mm thick and may be left joined by the skin or separated completely and arranged in order. The maximum diameter of the main lesion should be measured and the distance from the nearest margin of excision determined as for biopsies (see earlier).

Sampling. Blocks of tumour (the number depending on tumour size as above) should be taken to include the edges and should always be sufficient to represent the maximum extent of the lesion noted macroscopically. Blocks of the nearest excision margin should be taken. Painting with India ink or pigments may be helpful as in local excision specimens. If the tumour has been removed, then 3–4 blocks should be taken from the cavity wall. The breast slices should be examined by careful naked eye inspection and palpation. Blocks should be taken from any suspicious areas, noting the quadrant in which they are located. At least one block should be taken from each quadrant and ideally two from the nipple – one in the sagittal and one in the coronal plane through the junction with the areola.

Axillary Dissection Specimens

Axillary contents received with mastectomy or biopsy specimens should be examined carefully to maximize lymph node yield. This is usually achieved by cutting the specimen into thin slices which are then examined by careful inspection and palpation. The use of clearing agents or Bouin's solution may increase lymph node yield but are time-consuming and expensive of reagents and not regarded as essential. The axillary contents can be divided into three levels if the surgeon has marked the specimen appropriately.

Sampling. Pathological examination should be performed on all lymph nodes received and the report should state the total number and the number containing metastases. A representative complete section of any grossly involved lymph node is adequate. For nodes greater than 5 mm in maximum dimension, three slices should be taken and processed in a single block. Nodes less than 5 mm should be embedded in their entirety. They can be processed in groups and are ideally examined at two levels.

European Breast Screening: Histopathology-Form

Using the Histopathology Reporting Form

This section gives guidance on how to use the histopathology form and provides definitions of the terms used. The aim is not to replace standard texts on breast histopathology but to focus on diagnostic criteria for including lesions in the various categories and therefore help to achieve maximum uniformity of reporting.

The guidance in this section is drawn from standard textbooks of breast pathology and other published data. Reporting forms can be obtained from, or may be computer-generated in, screening offices. It is not necessary to use the form as it appears in this document. It may be found desirable to undertake modifications locally, particularly if the form is also to function as the definitive pathology report to be entered in patients' notes and laboratory records. It is, of course, **essential** to record all the information requested by the form for submission to screening offices using exactly the same terminology. Evaluation of breast screening programmes depends upon provision of accurate pathology data.

Recording Basic Information

Side: Indicate left or right. For specimens from both sides, use one form for each side.
Pathologist: The pathologist should enter their name.
Date: Enter the date the specimen was reported.
Histological calcification: Indicate if calcification observed radiologically is seen in histological sections and, if so, whether it is present in benign or malignant changes or both.
Specimen radiograph seen? Please indicate if you have seen a specimen radiograph.
Mammographic abnormality present in specimen? Are you satisfied that the mammographic abnormality is present in the specimen? This may necessitate consultation with the radiologist responsible for examining the specimen radiograph. It is worth remembering that breast calcification is occasionally due to oxalate salts (Weddelite) which can only be detected satisfactorily in histological sections using polarized light [8].
Specimen type. Please choose one of the following terms:
- Localization biopsy: biopsy of impalpable lesion identified by radiologically guided marking.
- Open biopsy: non-guided biopsy/excision, lumpectomy, tylectomy, dochectomy.
- Segmental excision: include: wedge excisions, partial mastectomies and re-excision specimens for clearance of margins.

Mastectomy. Where specimen includes all or nearly all of the breast parenchymal tissue. Include: subcutaneous mastectomy, total glandular mastectomy, simple mastectomy, extended simple mastectomy, modified radical mastectomy, radical mastectomy, Patey mastectomy, supra-radical mastectomy.
Wide bore needle core. Pre-operative diagnostic needle biopsy, e. g. trucut, screw, etc.

Specimen weight. Please record the weight and/or size of all biopsy and segmental excision specimens. Weight is a more reproducible method of estimating the size of a specimen than 3 dimensional measurements to determine volume, even taking into account the different densities of fat and fibrous tissue, which form varying proportions of breast specimens.
Benign/Malignant Lesions Present. Tick the appropriate "yes" box if any benign or malignant lesion is present and the "no" box if non is identified. Both may be ticked as "yes".

Recording Benign Lesions

Fibroadenoma. A benign malformation composed of connective tissue and epithelium exhibiting a pericanalicular and/or intracanalicular growth pattern. The connective tissue is generally composed of spindle cells but may rarely also contain other mesenchymal elements such as fat, smooth muscle, osteoid or bone. The epithelium is usually double-layered but some multilayering is not uncommon. Changes identical to those found in lobular epithelium elsewhere in the breast (e. g. apocrine metaplasia, sclerosing adenosis, blunt duct adenosis, hyperplasia of usual type, etc.) may occur in fibroadenomas but need not be recorded separately unless they amount to atypical hyperplasia or **in situ** carcinoma.

Sometimes individual lobules may exhibit increased stroma producing a fibroadenomatous appearance and occasionally such lobules may be loosely coalescent. These changes are often called fibroadenomatoid hyperplasia or sclerosing lobular hyperplasia but may be recorded as fibroadenoma on the reporting form if they produce a macroscopically visible or palpable mass. Consequently, fibroadenomas need not be perfectly circumscribed.

Old lesions may show hyalinization and calcification (and less frequently ossification) of stroma and atrophy of epithelium. Fibroadenomas are occasionally multiple.

For the purposes of the screening form, tubular adenomas can be grouped under fibroadenomas.

Fibroadenomas should be distinguished from phyllodes tumours. The high grade or "malignant" phyllodes tumours are easily identified by their sarcomatous stroma. The low grade variants are more difficult to distinguish but the main feature is the more cellular stroma. Phyllodes tumours may also exhibit an enhanced intracanalicular growth pattern with club-like projections into cystic spaces and there is often overgrowth of stroma at the expense of the epithelium. Adequate sampling is important as the characteristic stromal features may be seen only in parts of the lesion. Although phyllodes tumours are generally larger than fibroadenomas, size is not an acceptable criterion for diagnosis; fibroadenomas may be very large and phyllodes tumours small. For purposes of convenience, low grade phyllodes tumours should be specified under "other benign lesions" and high grade under "other malignant tumour" although it is recognized that histological appearance is often not a good predictor of behaviour.

Papilloma. A papilloma is defined as a tumour with an arborescent, fibrovascular stroma covered by epithelium generally arranged in an inner myoepithelial and outer epithelial layer. Epithelial hyperplasia without cytological atypia is often present and should not be recorded separately. Atypical hyperplasia is rarely seen and, when present, should be recorded separately under "Epithelial Proliferation". Epithelial nuclei are usually vesicular with delicate nuclear membranes and inconspicuous nucleoli. Apocrine metaplasia is frequently observed but should not be recorded separately on the reporting form. Squamous metaplasia is sometimes seen, particularly near areas of infarction. Sclerosis and haemorrhage are not uncommon

Table 2.2: Distinction of Papilloma from Encysted Papillary Carcinoma

Histological features	Papilloma	Encysted papillary carcinoma
1) Fibrovascular cores	Usually broad and extend thoughout the lesion	Very variable, usually fine and may be lacking in at least part of the lesion
2) Cells covering papillae		
a) basal	Myoepithelial layer always present	Myoepithelial cells usually absent but may form a discontinuous layer
b) luminal	Single layer of regular luminal epithelium OR features of regular usual type hyperplasia	Cells often taller and more monotonous with oval nuclei, the long axes of which lie perpendicular to stromal core of papillae. Nuclei may be hyperchromatic. Epithelial multi-layering frequent, often producing cribriform and micropapillary patterns of DCIS overlying the papillae or lining the cyst wall
3) Mitoses	Infrequent with no abnormal forms	More frequent; abnormal forms may be seen
4) Apocrine metaplasia	Common	Rare
5) Surrounding tissue	Benign changes may be present including regular epithelial hyperplasia	Surrounding ducts may show ductal carcinoma in situ
6) Necrosis and haemorrhage	May occur in either. Not a useful discriminating feature	
7) Periductal and intratumoural fibrosis	May occur in either. Not a useful discriminating feature	
NB: All the features of a lesion should be taken into account when making a diagnosis. No criterion is reliable alone.		

and where the former involves the periphery of the lesion, may give rise to epithelial entrapment with the false impression of invasion. The benign cytological features of such areas should enable the correct diagnosis to be made.

The term **"intracystic papilloma"** is sometimes used to describe a papilloma in a widely dilated duct. These tumours should simply be classified as papilloma on the form. (For distinction from encysted papillary carcinoma, table 2.2)

Papillomas may be **solitary** or **multiple**. The former usually occur centrally in sub-areolar ducts whereas the latter are more likely to be peripheral and involve terminal duct lobular units. The distinction is important as the multiple form is more frequently associated with atypical hyperplasia and ductal carcinoma **in situ,** the latter usually of low grade type which should be recorded separately. This malignant change may be restricted to small foci and extensive sampling may be required to detect it. Some sub-areolar papillomas causing nipple discharge may be very small and extensive sampling may be required to detect them.

Lesions termed **ductal adenoma** exhibit a variable appearance which overlaps with other benign breast lesions. They may resemble papillomas except that they exhibit an adenomatous rather than a papillary growth pattern. These cases should be grouped under papilloma on the form. Indeed, some tumours may exhibit papillary and adenomatous features. Some ductal adenomas may show pronounced central and/or peripheral fibrosis and overlap with complex sclerosing lesions (see p. 30).

The condition of **adenoma of the nipple** (sub-areolar duct papillomatosis) should not be classified as papilloma in the screening form but specified under "Benign Lesions, Other".

Diffuse microscopic papillary hyperplasia should be recorded under "Epithelial Proliferation" in the appropriate box depending on whether atypia is present or not.

Sclerosing Adenosis. Sclerosing adenosis is an organoid lobular enlargement in which increased numbers of acinar structures exhibit elongation and distortion. The normal two cell lining is retained but there is myoepithelial and stromal hyperplasia. The acinar structures may infiltrate adjacent connective tissue and occasionally nerves and blood vessels, which can lead to an erroneous diagnosis of malignancy. Early lesions of sclerosing adenosis are more cellular and later ones more sclerotic. Calcification may be present.

There may be coalescence of adjacent lobules of sclerosing adenosis to form a mass detectable by mammography or macroscopic examination. The term "adenosis tumour" has been used to describe such lesions [9]. It is recommended that sclerosing adenosis is not entered on the screening form if it is a minor change detectable only on histological examination. Although sclerosing adenosis often accompanies fibrocystic change (see below), this is not always the case and the two changes should be recorded separately.

Occasionally apocrine metaplasia is seen in areas of sclerosing adenosis (apocrine adenosis). It can produce a worrying appearance and should not be mistaken for malignancy [10].

Rarely, the epithelium in sclerosing adenosis may show atypical hyperplasia or **in situ** carcinoma. In such cases, please record these changes separately on the reporting form.

The differential diagnosis of sclerosing adenosis includes tubular carcinoma, microglandular adenosis and radial scar. In tubular carcinoma, the infiltrating tubules lack basement membrane, myoepithelium, a lobular organoid growth pattern and exhibit cytological atypia. Ductal carcinoma **in situ** is a frequent accompaniment. Microglandular adenosis differs from sclerosing adenosis in lacking the lobular organoid growth pattern and being composed of rounded tubules lined by a single layer of cells lacking cytological atypia. The glandular distortion of sclerosing adenosis is lacking. Radial scar is distinguished from sclerosing adenosis by its characteristic floret-type growth pattern with ducto-lobular structures radiating out from a central zone of dense fibro-elastotic tissue. Furthermore, the compression of tubular structures associated with myoepithelial and stromal hyperplasia is lacking.

Complex Sclerosing Lesion/Radial Scar. Under this heading are included sclerosing lesions with a pseudoinfiltrative growth pattern which have been called various names including infiltrating epitheliosis, rosette-like lesions, sclerosing papillary proliferation, complex compound heteromorphic lesions, benign sclerosing ductal proliferation, non-encapsulated sclerosing lesion, indurative mastopathy and proliferation centre of Aschoff.

The radial scar is generally 10 mm or less in diameter and consists of a central fibro-elastotic zone from which radiate out tubular structures which may be two-layered or exhibit intra-luminal proliferation. Tubules entrapped within the central zone of fibro-elastosis exhibit a more random, non-organoid arrangement. Lesions greater than 10 mm are generally termed complex sclerosing lesions. They have all the features of radial scars and, in addition to their greater size, exhibit more disturbance of structure, often with nodular masses around the periphery. Changes such as papilloma formation, apocrine metaplasia and sclerosing adenosis may be superimposed on the main lesion. Some complex sclerosing lesions give the impression of being formed by coalescence of several adjacent sclerosing lesions. There is a degree of morphological overlap with some forms of ductal adenoma.

If the intra-luminal proliferation exhibits atypia or amounts to **in situ** carcinoma, it should be recorded separately under the appropriate heading on the screening form.

The main differential diagnosis is carcinoma of tubular or low grade "ductal" type. The major distinguishing features are the presence of myoepithelium and basement membrane around the tubules of the sclerosing lesions. Cytological atypia is also lacking and any intra-tubular proliferation resembles hyperplasia of usual type unless atypical hyperplasia and/or **in situ** carcinoma are superimposed (see above). Tubular carcinomas generally lack the characteristic architecture of sclerosing lesions.

Fibrocystic Change. This term is used for cases with several to numerous macroscopically visible cysts, the majority of which are usually lined by apocrine epithelium. The term is not intended for use with minimal alterations such as fibrosis, microscopic dilatation of acini or ducts, lobular involution, adenosis and minor degrees of blunt duct adenosis. These changes should be indexed as normal.

It is not intended that cystic change or apocrine metaplasia occurring within other lesions such as fibroadenomata, papillomata or sclerosing lesions should be coded here.

Apocrine metaplasia occurring in lobules without cystic change may produce a worrisome appearance, occasionally mistaken for carcinoma. This change should be specified as "apocrine adenosis" under other benign lesions.

Papillary apocrine hyperplasia should be indexed separately under epithelial proliferation with or without atypia, depending on its appearance. It should be noted, however, that apocrine cells usually exhibit a greater degree of pleomorphism than is seen in normal breast cells. Hyperplasia should therefore be regarded as atypical only when the cytological changes are significantly more pronounced than usual.

Solitary Cyst. This term should be used when the abnormality appears to be a solitary cyst. The size is usually greater than 10 mm and the lining attenuated or apocrine in type. The latter may show papillary change which should be indexed separately under epithelial proliferation of appropriate type. If multiple cysts are present, it is better to use the term "fibrocystic change" as above. Intra-cystic papillomas and intra-cystic papillary carcinomas should not be entered here but under papilloma or carcinoma.

Periductal Mastitis/Duct Ectasia (Plasma Cell Mastitis). This process involves larger and intermediate size ducts, generally in subduct areolar location. The ducts are lined by normal or attenuated epithelium, filled with amorphous, eosinophilic material and/or foam cells and exhibit marked periductal chronic inflammation, often with large numbers of plasma cells. There may be pronounced periductal fibrosis. The inflammatory infiltrate may contain large numbers of histiocytes giving a granulomatous appearance. Calcification may be present. The process may ultimately lead to obliteration of ducts leaving dense fibrous masses. Persistence of small tubules of epithelium around the periphery of an obliterated duct result in a characteristic garland pattern. Duct ectasia is often associated with nipple discharge or retraction.

Cysts are distinguished from duct ectasia by their rounded rather than elongated shape, tendency to cluster, lack of stromal elastin, frequent presence of apocrine metaplasia and less frequent presence of eosinophilic material or foam cells in the lumina.

Mammary duct fistula (recurring sub-areolar abscess) should be coded under "Benign, Other".

Other (Specify). This category is intended for use with less common conditions which form acceptable entities but cannot be entered into the categories above, e.g. fat necrosis, lipoma, adenoma of nipple, low grade phyllodes tumours. The index at the end of the booklet should help as a reference for lesions difficult to place in any of the above categories.

Classifying Epithelial Proliferation

This section is for recording intra-luminal epithelial proliferation in terminal duct lobular units or inter-lobular ducts.

Not Present. This should be ticked if there is no epithelial multilayering (apart from that ascribed to cross-cutting) or if there is slight multilayering without atypia, not exceeding 4 cells in thickness.

Present Without Atypia. This term is used to describe all cases of intra-luminal proliferation showing no or only minor atypia where the epithelial cells are more than 4 thick. The change may involve terminal duct lobular units or inter-lobular ducts. The major features which distinguish hyperplasia from ductal carcinoma **in situ** of low nuclear grade are summarized in table 2.3, pg. 33.

Hyperplasia of usual type should be recorded if it occurs alone or in association with cystic change or other benign lesions, but not if it is confined to fibroadenomas, adenomas, papillomas or radial scars/complex sclerosing lesions. The term should be used for cases where there is no atypia or atypia of only minor degree, insufficient to raise the possibility of DCIS.

Present With Atypia (Ductal). If a diagnosis of atypical ductal hyperplasia (ADH) is contemplated, then extensive sampling should be undertaken to search for evidence of unequivocal DCIS with which it frequently co-exists.

ADH is a rare lesion often co-existing with fibrocystic change, a sclerosing lesion or a papilloma. Its current definition rests on identification of some but not all features of ductal carcinoma **in situ**. Most of the difficulties are encountered in distinguishing ADH from the low grade variants of DCIS. The main features of low grade DCIS are:
- a uniform population of cells
- even cellular placements
- smooth geometric spaces between "rigid" bars or micropapillary formations
- hyperchromatic nuclei.

ADH has some but not all of the features described above. A diagnosis of DCIS should be reserved for lesions having all these features present in at least two or more duct spaces.

Table 2.3 provides more details of features which serve to distinguish ADH from usual type hyperplasia and ductal carcinoma **in situ**.

Useful **rules of thumb** to distinguish atypical ductal hyperplasia from ductal carcinoma **in situ** are:
- restrict the diagnosis of ADH to cases where the diagnosis of DCIS is seriously considered but in which the features are not sufficiently developed for a confident diagnosis.
- DCIS usually extends to involve multiple duct spaces and is rarely under 2–3 mm in extent. In any lesion where the process with the above features extends widely, a diagnosis of atypical ductal hyperplasia should be questioned.

For further guidance, the reader is referred to Page & Rogers (1992) [11].

Present with atypia (lobular). This change is characterized by proliferation within terminal duct lobular units of characteristic small rounded cells similar to those seen in lobular

Table 2.3: Comparison of Histological Features of Ductal Hyperplasia and DCIS*

Histological features	Usual type ductal hyperplasia	Atypical ductal hyperplasia	Low nuclear grade DCIS
Size	Variable size but rarely extensive unless associated with other benign processes such as papilloma or radial scar	Usually small (less than 2–3 mm) unless associated with other benign processes such as papilloma or radial scar	Rarely less than 2–3 mm and may be very extensive
Cellular composition	Mixed. Epithelial cells and spindle-shaped cells** present. Lymphocytes and macrophages may also be present. Myoepithelial hyperplasia may occur around the periphery	May be uniform single population but merges with areas of usual type hyperplasia within the same duct space. Spindle-shaped cells may be intermingled with the proliferating cells	Single cell population. Spindle-shaped cells not seen. Myoepithelial cells usually in normal location around duct periphery but may be attenuated
Architecture	Variable	Micropapillary, cribriform or solid patterns but may be rudimentary	Well developed micropapillary cribriform or solid patterns
Lumina	Irregular, often ill-defined peripheral slit-like spaces are common and a useful distinguishing feature	May be distinct, well formed rounded spaces in cribriform type. Irregular, ill-defined lumina may also be present	Well delineated, regular punched out lumina in cribriform type
Cell orientation	Often streaming pattern with long axes of nuclei arranged parallel to direction of cellular bridges which often have a "tapering" appearance	Cell nuclei may be at right angles to bridges in cribriform types, forming "rigid" structures	Micropapillary structures with indiscernible fibrovascular cores or smooth, well-delineated geometric spaces. Cell bridges "rigid" in cribriform type with nuclei orientated towards the luminal space
Nuclear spacing	Uneven	May be even or uneven	Even
Epithelial/tumour cell character	Small ovoid but showing variation in shape	Small uniform or medium sized monotonous cell populations present at least focally	Small uniform monotonous cell population
Nucleoli	Indistinct	Single small	Single small
Mitoses	Infrequent with no abnormal forms	Infrequent, abnormal forms, rare	Infrequent, abnormal forms, rare
Necrosis	Rare	Rare	If present, confined to small particulate debris in cribriform and/or luminal spaces

Major diagnostic features are shown in bold type.
* See Page & Rogers [11]
** These cells are usually called myoepithelial cells but immunohistological studies have shown that they have characteristics of basal keratin type epithelial cells [12]

Table 2.4: Distinction of Atypical Lobular Hyperplaisa from Lobular Carcinoma in Situ [12]

Histological features	Atypical lobular hyperplasia	Lobular carcinoma in situ
Cellular composition	Polymorphic. Cells similar to those seen in LCIS accompanied by spindle-shaped cells, leucocytes and other epithelial cells	Monomorphic proliferation of characteristic small rounded cells with granular or hyperchromatic nuclei, inconspicuous nucleoli and high nucleo-cytoplasmic ratio
Cell cohesioin	Usually good	Often poor
Cell spacing	Irregular	Regular
Luminal occlusion	Partial	Complete
Lobular distension	Slight	Moderate to marked
Pagetoid spread into interlobular ducts	Very common	Common

NB: All the features of a lesion should be taken into account when making a diagnosis. No criterion is reliable alone.

carcinoma in situ. The major points of distinction from the latter are summarized in table 2.4. Like the ductal variety, atypical lobular hyperplasia occurs in about 2% of non-cancer containing biopsies from unscreened women.

Classifying Malignant Non-Invasive Lesions

Ductal carcinoma *in situ*. Ductal carcinoma in situ (DCIS) is defined as a proliferation of epithelial cells with cytological features of malignancy within parenchymal structures of the breast and is distinguished from invasive carcinoma by the absence of stromal invasion across the basement membrane.

DCIS varies in cell type, growth pattern and extent of disease and may thus represent a group or spectrum of related **in situ** neoplastic processes. Classification has traditionally been according to growth pattern but has been carried out with little enthusiasm given a perceived lack of clinical relevance. More recently, evidence has emerged that lesions composed of cells of high nuclear grade are more aggressive [13, 14]. There is currently no generally accepted method of classifying DCIS but distinction between common histological subtypes is of value for correlating pathological and radiological appearances, improving diagnostic consistency, assessing the likelihood of invasion and determining the probability of recurrence after local excision. Despite the name, most DCIS is generally considered to arise from the terminal duct lobular units. The main points of distinction from lobular carcinoma **in situ** are summarized in table 2.5. For measurement of size see p. 50.

The nuclear grading system adopted below is derived from that employed by Holland et al. (1994) [15].

High Nuclear Grade DCIS. This is composed of cells with pleomorphic, irregularly-spaced and usually large nuclei exhibiting marked variation in size, irregular nuclear contours, coarse chromatin and prominent nucleoli. Mitoses are frequently present and abnormal forms may be seen.

High nuclear grade DCIS may exhibit several different growth patterns. It is often **solid** with central, **comedo**-type necrosis which frequently contains deposits of amorphous calcification. This is the easiest pattern to recognize. Sometimes a **solid** proliferation of malignant cells fills the duct without necrosis but this is relatively rare and is usually confined to nipple ducts in cases presenting with Paget's disease. High nuclear grade DCIS may also exhibit **micropapillary** and **cribriform** patterns frequently

Histological features	Ductal carcinoma in situ	Lobular carcinoma in situ
Cells	Variable, depending on nuclear grade (see p. 34)	Small, rounded with granular or hyperchromatic nuclei, inconspicuous nucleoli and high nucleo-cytoplasmic ratio
Intracytoplasmic lumina	Rare	Common
Growth pattern	Very variable, e.g. solid, comedo, papillary, cribriform	Diffuse monotonous with complete luminal obliteration
Cell cohesion	Usually good	Usually poor
Degree of distension of involved structures	Moderate to great	Slight to moderate
Pagetoid spread into interlobular ducts	Absent	Often present
Necrosis	Common with high nuclear grade, uncommon with low nuclear grade	Absent
Mitoses	Common with high nuclear grade, uncommon with low nuclear grade	Infrequent
Abnormal mitoses	Common with high nuclear grade, rare with low nuclear grade	Rare
Calcification	Common	Rare

Table 2.5: Distinction of Ductal from Lobular Carcinoma in Situ [12]

NB: All the features of a lesion should be taken into account when making a diagnosis. No criterion is reliable alone.

associated with central, comedo-like necrosis. Unlike low nuclear grade DCIS, there is rarely any polarization of cells covering the micropapillae or lining the intercellular spaces.

Low Nuclear Grade DCIS. This is composed of monomorphic, evenly-spaced cells with roughly spherical, centrally-placed nuclei and inconspicuous nucleoli. The nuclei are usually, but not invariable small. Mitoses are few and there is rarely individual cell necrosis.

The cells are generally arranged in **micropapillary** and **cribriform** patterns which are frequently present within the same lesion, although the latter is more common and tends to predominate. There is usually polarization of cells covering the micropapillae or lining the intercellular lumina. Less frequently, low nuclear grade DCIS has a **solid** growth pattern. When terminal duct lobular units are involved, the process can be very difficult to distinguish from lobular carcinoma **in situ**. Features in favour of DCIS are greater cellular cohesion and lack of intracytoplasmic lumina. Occasionally, however, there may be a combination of both processes.

Intermediate Nuclear Grade DCIS. Some cases of DCIS cannot be assigned easily to the high or low nuclear grade categories. The nuclei show mild to moderate pleomorphism which is less than that seen in high grade DCIS but they lack the monotony of the small cell type. The nucleus:cytoplasm ratio is often high and one or two nucleoli may be identified.

The growth pattern may be **solid, cribriform** or **micropapillary** and the cells usually exhibit some degree of polarization covering papillary processes or lining intercellular lumina although this is not as marked as in low nuclear grade DCIS.

Mixed Types. A proportion of cases of DCIS exhibit features of more than one histological subtype. One of the advantages of classifying DCIS according to nuclear grade is that, although variations of growth pattern are frequent, there is usually a dominant cell type and the lesion is fairly easily classified into one of the above main groups.

Rarely, cells of different nuclear grade may be seen within a single lesion. This should be recorded but **the case should be classified according to the highest nuclear grade observed.**

Other Histological Types. The main features of **encysted papillary carcinoma** are listed in table 2.2, pg. 29. Ductal carcinoma **in situ** of **signet ring cell**, pure **apocrine cell, cystic hypersecretory** and **neuroendocrine** types have been described and may be classified separately. For further details of these rare variants, the reader is referred to recent standard textbooks of breast pathology.

Lobular Carcinoma *In Situ*. The histological features of lobular carcinoma **in situ** are compared with those of atypical lobular hyperplasia in table 2.4, pg. 34, and with ductal carcinoma **in situ** in table 2.5, pg. 35. To maximize consistency of diagnosis, it is recommended that the term lobular carcinoma **in situ** be used when the characteristic uniform cells comprise the entire population of the lobular units, that there are no residual lumina and that there is expansion and/or distortion of at least one half the acini in the lobule. Otherwise the lesion should be classified as atypical lobular hyperplasia.

Paget's Disease. In this condition, there are adenocarcinoma cells within the epidermis of the nipple. Cases where there is direct epidermal invasion by tumour infiltrating the skin should be excluded. Paget's disease should be recorded regardless of whether or not an underlying **in situ** or invasive carcinoma is identified. The underlying carcinoma should be recorded separately.

Diagnosing Microinvasion

A microinvasive carcinoma is defined for the purposes of the reporting form as a tumour in which the dominant lesion is DCIS but in which there are one or more clearly separate foci of infiltration of non-specialized interlobular or interductal fibrous or adipose tissue, none measuring more than 1 mm (about 2 hpf see below) in maximal diameter. This definition is very restrictive and tumours fulfilling the criteria are consequently very rare. If there is sufficient doubt about the presence of invasion, the case should be classified as DCIS. Where the evidence is equivocal, tick the "Microinvasion – Possible" box on the reporting form. Possible microinvasion includes separate islands of appropriately abnormal epithelium which are embedded in periductal fibrosis or inflammation, where the true boundary of the specialized periductal or lobular stroma is not clear. The term "possible" microinvasion completely excludes merely ultrastructural evidence of basement membrane breach, histochemical or immunohistochemically identified basement membrane discontinuities and lesions in which there is demonstrable continuity in a 5 µm section with the parent DCIS. Microinvasion is largely restricted to high nuclear grade types of DCIS, mainly of comedo type. Cases of apparently pure comedo DCIS should thus be extensively sampled to exclude invasion. Microinvasive carcinomas should likewise be extensively sampled in order to exclude the possibility of larger invasive foci. Where such foci are found, the lesion should be classified as an invasive carcinoma and the approximate number and size range of the invasive foci stated under "Comments/Additional Information". Small invasive carcinomas without an **in situ** component are classified as invasive.

Classifying Invasive Carcinoma

Typing invasive carcinomas has established prognostic value [16, 17]. Some caution should be exercised in typing carcinomas in inadequately fixed specimens or if they have been removed from patients who have been treated primarily by chemotherapy or radiotherapy. The more common types are described below.

"Ductal" – No Specific Type (Ductal-NST). This group contains infiltrating carcinomas which cannot be entered into any **type** other category on the form, or classified as any of the less common variants of infiltrating breast carcinoma. Consequently, invasive ductal carcinomas exhibit great variation in appearance and are the most common carcinomas, accounting for up to 75% in most series.

Infiltrating Lobular Carcinoma. Infiltrating lobular carcinoma is composed of small regular cells identical to those seen in the **in situ** form. In its classical form, the cells are dissociated from each other or form single files or targetoid patterns around uninvolved ducts. Several variants have been identified in addition to this classical form but in each case the cell type is the same:
- the **alveolar** variant exhibits small Aggregates of 20 or more cells [18]
- the **solid** variant consists of sheets of cells with little stroma [19]
- the **tubulo-lobular** type exhibits microtubular formation as part of the classical pattern [20].

Tumours that show mixtures of typical tubular and classical lobular carcinoma should be classified as mixed (see below):
- the **pleomorphic** variant is uncommon and exhibits the growth pattern of classical lobular carcinoma throughout but the cytological appearances are more pleomorphic.
- Mixtures of above.

At least 90% of the tumour should exhibit one or more of the above patterns to be classified as infiltrating lobular.

Tubular Carcinoma (Including Cribriform Carcinoma). Tubular carcinomas are composed of round, ovoid, or angulated single layered tubules in a cellular fibrous or fibro-elastotic stroma. The neoplastic cells are small, uniform and may show cytoplasmic apical snouting. At least 90% of the tumour should exhibit the classical growth pattern to be classified as tubular. If the co-existent carcinoma is solely of the invasive cribriform type, however, then the tumour should be typed as tubular if the tubular pattern forms over 50% of the lesion. **Invasive cribriform carcinoma** is composed of masses of small regular cells similar to those seen in tubular carcinoma. The invasive islands, however, exhibit a cribriform rather than a tubular appearance. Apical snouting is often present. More than 90% of the lesion should exhibit the cribriform appearance except in cases where the only co-existent pattern is tubular carcinoma when over 50% must be of the cribriform appearance in order to be so classified. If a diagnosis of cribriform carcinoma is preferred, then tick the **"tubular"** box and make the appropriate comment under **"Comments/Additional Information"**.

Medullary Carcinoma. These rare tumours are composed of syncytial interconnecting masses of large pleomorphic cells with vesicular nuclei and prominent nucleoli; they are of histological grade 3. The stroma may be sparse but always contains large numbers of lymphoid cells. The border of the tumour is well-defined. The whole tumour must exhibit these features to be typed as medullary. Surrounding **in situ** elements are very uncommon.

The term **atypical medullary carcinoma** may be specified under "other primary carcinoma" for lesions which do not fulfil all the criteria for medullary carcinoma. The atypical medullary group has been defined by both Fisher et al. (1975) [21] and Ridolfi et al. (1977) [22]. These tumours show less lymphoid infiltration, less circumscription or areas of dense fibrosis while still having the other features of a medullary carcinoma. A well circumscribed tumour is also classified as atypical medullary if up to 25% is composed of "ductal" type and the rest comprises classical medullary carcinoma. If in doubt, classify as "Ductal-NST".

Mucinous Carcinoma. This type is also known as mucoid, gelatinous or colloid carcinoma. There are islands of uniform small cells in lakes of extracellular mucin. An **in situ** component is uncommon. At least 90% of the tumour must exhibit the mucinous appearance to be so classified.

Mixed Tumours. Tubular or cribriform mixed carcinomas have a usually central tubular or cribriform zone, which amounts to 75–90% of the area, with a ductal-NST or infiltrating lobular component usually at the periphery accounting for the remainder [23]. Such tumours have a good prognosis but less so than the pure types. The **mixed NST** and **mucinous carcinomas** include any mixtures of mucinous with ductal NST where the former accounts for 10–90%. In **mixed NST and lobular carcinomas** distinct and separate ductal NST and lobular elements must be present; the former occupies between 10% and 90% of the tumour area. These tumours are regarded as biphasic and are distinct from mixed and pleomorphic lobular carcinomas (see above). Mixtures of NST and specific types not listed on the form should be classified as "**other primary carcinoma**".

Other Primary Carcinoma. Other primary breast carcinomas should be entered under this heading and will include variants such as **atypical medullary, spindle cell, infiltrating papillary, argyrophil, secretory, apocrine**, etc.

Other Malignant Tumour. Please include non-epithelial tumours and secondary carcinomas in this category. For purposes of convenience, all high grade **phyllodes** tumours should be recorded here.

Not Assessable. This category should be ticked only if an invasive carcinoma cannot be assigned to any of the previous groups for technical reasons, e.g. the specimen is too small or poorly preserved.

Recording Prognostic Data

Maximum Diameter. All lesions should be measured in the fresh or fixed state and on the histological preparation. If the two measurements are discrepant then that obtained from histological examination should be recorded where tumours are small enough to be visualized in cross-section. This may give a small underestimation of size due to shrinkage of the tissue in processing. It is considered, however, that the slight but consistent underestimation in the size of all tumours is preferable to the larger and less predictable errors that may result from measuring poorly delineated tumours macroscopically. Clearly, sufficient blocks should be taken from the periphery of larger tumours to allow accurate estimates of their size to be made from combined histological and macroscopic examination. The largest dimension should be recorded to the nearest millimetre.

For non-invasive carcinomas, the maximum diameter should be entered in the "Non-Invasive" section only where the tumour is of ductal type; lobular carcinoma **in situ** is not measured. For invasive carcinomas, the invasive component only needs to be recorded unless accompanying ductal carcinoma **in situ** extends more than 1 mm beyond the periphery of the infiltrative component, when the size of the infiltrative component and the overall size should be stated in the appropriate spaces of this section. This is to allow the identification of invasive carcinomas, where the **in situ** component forms a significant proportion of the lesion and may be important in determining the risk of recurrence after local excision (see Appendix 3, pg. 170). The largest dimension, to the nearest millimetre, is recorded in each case. The diagrams below illustrate whole and invasive tumour measurements in a variety of circumstances. Foci of lymphatic and blood vascular invasion are not included in the whole tumour measurement (figure 2.2).

If a carcinoma (either infiltrative or ductal **in situ**) is insufficiently delineated to measure reliably, make an appropriate comment in the "Comments/Additional Information" section and give an approximate estimate of the maximum dimension of the area over which the changes extend. It may be necessary to use combined histological, macroscopic and radiological information to make a reliable estimate.

Lymph Nodes. All lymph nodes should be examined histologically. The use of immunohistology is most appropriate in cases where there

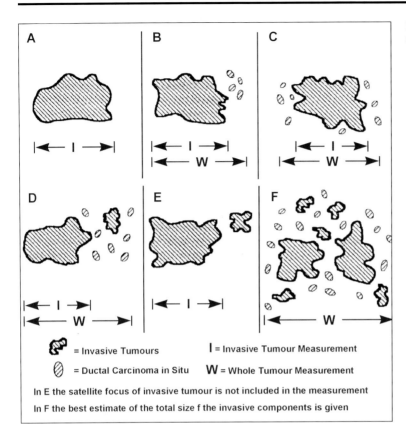

Figure 2.2, explanation see page 38

In E the satellite focus of invasive tumour is not included in the measurement
In F the best estimate of the total size f the invasive components is given

is doubt about the presence of small metastases. The clinical relevance of metastases detected solely by this means remains controversial. Please record data from **axillary** nodes separately from nodes from other sites. The presence of extracapsular spread can be noted under "Comments/Additional Information". (For further information on examining lymph nodes, see Appendix 4, pg. 171)

Excision. For infiltrative tumours, the distance from the nearest resection margin should be recorded and checked from the histological sections. Other margins can be reported if required. This normally refers to the infiltrative component but, if associated ductal carcinoma **in situ** extends nearer to the margin than the infiltrative component, then enter its distance from the margin and state in the "Comments" section that this measurement refers to the **in situ** component. The information should be related to orientation markers if used.

For pure ductal carcinoma **in situ**, the distance from the nearest excision margin should be recorded if the lesion is sufficiently delineated. If not, make a comment under "Comments/Additional Information". The presence of non-neoplastic breast parenchyma between the DCIS and the margin is usually associated with adequate excision. The specimen radiograph is also a useful adjunct in assessing surgical clearance. In cases where the adequacy of excision is uncertain, please tick the relevant box and state the reason for uncertainty under "Comments/Additional Information". See earlier for guidance on macroscopic examination.

Grade. Grading can provide powerful prognostic information. It requires some commitment and strict adherence to a recommended protocol. The following protocol is based on that described by Elston & Ellis (1991) [24]. The method involves the assessment of three components of tumour morphology: tubule formation, nuclear pleomorphism and frequency of mitoses. Each is scored from 1–3. Adding the scores gives the overall histological grade as shown below.

Tubule Formation:
1 majority of tumour (greater than 75%)
2 moderate amount (10–75%)
3 little or none (less than 10%).

Nuclear Pleomorphism:
- nuclei small, with little increase in size in comparison with normal breast epithelial cells, regular outlines, uniform nuclear chromatin, little variation in size.
- cells larger than normal with open vesicular nuclei, visible nucleoli and moderate variability in both size and shape.
- vesicular nuclei, often with prominent nucleoli, exhibiting marked variation in size and shape, occasionally with very large and bizarre forms.

Mitoses. The score depends on the number of mitoses per 10 high power fields assessed at the tumour periphery. The size of high power fields is very variable and hence it is necessary to standardize the mitotic count using the graph below. In order to determine the mitotic count for an individual microscope, the following procedure should be adopted (fig. 2.3):
- measure the field diameter of the microscope with a graticule
- plot this value on the vertical axis of the graph
- draw a vertical line at this value
- read off the value **a** on the horizontal axis where the line intersects the lower bold line
- read of the value **b** on the horizontal axis where the line intersects the upper bold line
- the count is then
  o Score Count
  o >**b**
  o between **a**+1 and **b**
  o 0 to **a**

For example, for a field diameter of 0,48, **a** = 6, **b** = 12 from graph – therefore:
- Score 3 = >12 mitoses/10hpf
- Score 2 = 7–12 mitoses/10hpf
- Score 1 = 0–6 mitoses/10hpf

This needs to be done only once for each microscope.

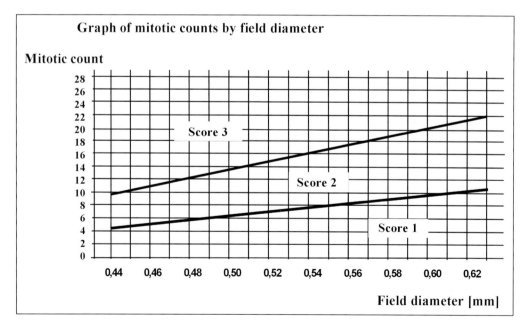

Figure 2.3: Graph of mitotic counts by field diameter

Overall Grade. The scores for tubule formation, nuclear pleomorphism and mitoses are then added together and assigned to grades as below:
- Grade 1 = score 3–5
- Grade 2 = score 6–7
- Grade 3 = score 8–9

It is recommended that grading is not restricted to invasive carcinoma NST but is undertaken on all histological subtypes. There are two major reasons for this recommendation:
- there are occasionally problems in deciding whether to classify a tumour as NST or some other type
- there may be significant variation within certain subtypes, e. g. invasive lobular carcinoma.

Tick "Not assessable" if for any reason the grade cannot be determined, e. g. specimen poorly preserved or too small. It must be clearly stated if a grading system other than that described above is used.

Disease Extent. The term **"localized"** is used to describe a single focus of tumour with defined borderlines of **any size.** It should also be used where the exent of the tumour cannot accurately be defined although all of it appears to be part of a single lesion.

The term **"multiple"** is used to describe multiple foci of **in situ** or infiltrating carcinoma which are widely separated (at least 40 mm) and present in quadrants or segments other than that of the main tumour. **"Multiple"** is preferred to **"multifocal"** or **"multicentric"** as there is currently a lack of agreement on how these terms should be used.

Tick "Not assessable" if the extent of the disease cannot be determined or if it is not clear whether the tumour is localized or multiple.

Vascular Invasion. The presence of unequivocal tumour in vascular spaces should be recorded. If there is doubt about diagnosing vascular invasion, please tick the "not seen" box. The difficulty in identifying small blood vessels as blood or lymphatic precludes accurate recording of their type and specification of lymphatic or venous invasion is not required. Ideally, a clear rim of endothelium should be identified around the tumour before vascular invasion is recorded. The use of immunostaining for endothelial markers may be helpful in confirming vascular invasion in difficult cases but is not recommended on a routine basis (see Appendix 5, pg. 171). Morphological features which may be helpful when diagnosing vascular invasion are:
- clumps of tumour in spaces outside the main tumour mass are more likely to indicate vascular invasion.
- nests of tumour separaten from the stroma by shrinkage artefact usually conform better to the shape of the space in which they lie.
- the proximity of larger veins and arteries in the diagnosis of lymphatic invasion.
- the presence within the space of erythrocytes and/or thrombus.

Comments/Additional Information. Any relevant additional information may be entered here as free text. Please also state if any further special investigations have been undertaken, e. g. steroid hormone receptor determination, oncogene analysis, etc.

Histological Diagnosis. If normal, tick the normal box and do not complete the rest of the form. "Normal" includes minimal alterations such as fibrosis and microscopic dilatation of acini or ducts, lobular involution and enlargement and blunt duct adenosis.

If malignant and benign changes are found, tick only the malignant box. Tick the benign box when the breast is neither normal nor exhibits malignancy.

References: Page 188

Membership: Page 161

Index for Screening Office Pathology System

Term	Place to classify on form
A	
Abscess	Other benign pathology (specify)
Adenocarcinoma (no special type)	Invasive ductal n. s. t.
Adenoid cystic carcinoma	Other primary carcinoma (specify)
Adenoma, apocrine	Other benign pathology (specify)
Adenoma intraduct	Enter as papilloma
Adenoma of nipple	Other benign pathology (specify)
Adenoma, pleomorphic	Other benign pathology (specify)
Adenoma, tubular	Fibroadenoma
"Adenomyoepithelioma"	Other primary carcinoma (specify) or Other benign pathology (specify)
Adenosis, NOS	Histology normal
Adenosis, apocrine	Other benign pathology (specify)
Adenosis, apocrine (atypical)	Other benign pathology (specify) Epithelial proliferation-atypia (ductal)
Adenosis, blunt duct	Histology normal
Adenosis, microglandular	Other benign pathology (specify)
Adenosis, sclerosing	Sclerosing adenosis
with atypia	Epithelial proliferation atypia ductal or lobular
Adnexal tumours	Other benign pathology (specify)
Alveolar variant of lobular carcinoma	Invasive lobular
Aneurysm	Other benign pathology (specify)
Angiosarcoma	Other malignant tumour (specify)
Apocrine adenoma	Other benign pathology (specify)
Apocrine adenosis	Other benign pathology (specify)
Apocrine carcinoma (in-situ)	Non-invasive malignant, ductal (specify)
Apocrine carcinoma (invasive)	Other primary carcinoma (if pure) or ductal n. s. t.
Apocrine metaplasia	Fibrocystic change
(multilayered/papillary)	Epithelial proliferation present
Argyrophil carcinoma	Other primary carcinoma (specify)
Arteriitis	Other benign pathology (specify)
Atypical blunt duct adenosis	Fibrocystic change Epithelial proliferation-atypia (ductal)
Atypical ductal hyperplasia	Epithelial proliferation-atypia (ductal)
Atypical epitheliosis (ductal)	Epithelial proliferation-atypia
Atypical lobular hyperplasia	Epithelial proliferation-atypia (lobular)
B	
B-cell lymphoma	Other malignant tumour (specify)
Benign phyllodes tumour	Other benign pathology (specify)
Blunt duct adenosis	Histology normal
Blunt duct adenosis (atypical)	Epithelial proliferation-atypia (ductal)
Breast abscess	Other benign pathology (specify)

Term	Place to classify on form
C	
Calcification (benign)	Calcification present, benign
Calcification (malignant)	Calcification present, malignant
Carcinoma, apocrine (in-situ)	Non-invasive malignant, ductal (specify type)
Carcinoma, apocrine (invasive)	Other primary carcinoma (if pure) or ductal n. s. t.
Carcinoma, clear cell	Other primary carcinoma (specify)
Carcinoma, colloid	Invasive mucinous carcinoma
Carcinoma, comedo-in-situ	Non-invasive malignant, ductal (specify type)
Carcinoma, cribriform (in-situ)	Non-invasive malignant, ductal (specify type)
Carcinoma, cribriform (invasive)	Invasive tubular or cribriform
Carcinoma, ductal in-situ	Non-invasive malignant, ductal (specify sub-type)
Carcinoma, lobular in-situ	Non-invasive malignant, lobular
Carcinoma, lobular (invasive)	Invasive lobular
Carcinoma, lobular variant	Invasive lobular
Carcinoma, medullary	Invasive medullary
Carcinoma, metastatic	Other malignant tumour (specify)
Carcinoma, mixed	Other primary carcinoma (specified types)
Carcinoma, mucinous	Invasive mucinous carcinoma
Carcinoma, papillary	Other primary carcinoma (specify)
Carcinoma, signet ring	Other primary carcinoma (specify)
Carcinoma, spindle cell	Other primary carcinoma (specify)
Carcinoma, squamous	Other primary carcinoma (specify)
Carcinosarcoma	Other primary carcinoma (specify)
Cellular fibroadenoma	Fibroadenoma
Clear cell carcinoma	Other primary carcinoma (specify)
Clear cell hidradenoma	Other benign pathology (specify)
Clear cell metaplasia	Other benign pathology (specify)
Collagenous spherulosis	Other benign pathology (specify)
Comedocarcinoma	Non-invasive malignant, ductal
Comedocarcinoma invasive	Invasive ductal n. s. t.
Complex sclerosing lesion	Complex sclerosing lesion/radial scar
Cribriform carcinoma (in-situ)	Non-invasive malignant, ductal (specify type)
Cribriform carcinoma (invasive)	Invasive tubular or cribriform
Cyclical menstrual changes	Histology normal
Cyst, epidermoid	Other benign pathology (specify)
Cyst, single	Solitary cyst
Cyst, multiple	Fibrocystic change
Cystic disease	Enter components
Cystic mastopathia	Enter components
Cystic hypersecretory hyperplasia	Other benign pathology (specify)
Cystic hypersecretory carcinoma	Non-invasive malignant, ductal
D	
Ductal carcinoma in-situ	Non-invasive malignant, ductal
Ductal carcinoma invasive	Invasive ductal n. s. t.
Ductal hyperplasia (regular)	Epithelial proliferation present without atypia
Ductal hyperplasia (atypical)	Epithelial proliferation, atypical (ductal)
Duct ectasia	Periductal mastitis/duct ectasia

Term	Place to classify on form
Duct papilloma	Papilloma, single
Dysplasia, mammary	Enter components

E
Eccrine tumours	Other benign pathology (specify)
Epidermoid cyst	Other benign pathology (specify)
Epitheliosis (regular)	Epithelial proliferation present without atypia
Epitheliosis (atypical)	Epithelial proliferation, atypical (ductal)
Epitheliosis (infiltrating)	Complex sclerosing lesion/radial scar

F
Fat necrosis	Other benign pathology (specify)
Fibroadenoma	Fibroadenoma
Fibroadenoma, giant	Fibroadenoma
Fibroadenoma, juvenile	Fibroadenoma
Fibrocystic disease	Enter components
Fibromatosis	Other benign pathology (specify)
Fistula, mammillary	Other benign pathology (specify)
Focal lactational change	Histology normal
Foreign body reaction	Other benign pathology (specify)

G
Galactocoele	Other benign pathology (specify)
Giant fibroadenoma	Fibroadenoma
Glycogen-rich carcinoma	Other primary carcinoma (specify)
Grading of carcinomas	See page 38
Granulomatous mastitis	Other benign pathology (specify)

H
Haematoma	Other benign pathology (specify)
Haemangioma	Other benign pathology (specify)
Hamartoma	Other benign pathology (specify)
Hyaline epithelial inclusions	O ther benign pathology (specify)
Hyperplasia, ductal (regular)	Epithelial proliferation present without atypia
Hyperplasia, ductal (atypical)	Epithelial proliferation-atypia (ductal)
Hyperplasia, lobular (= adenosis)	Histology normal
Hyperplasia, lobular (atypical)	Epithelial proliferation-atypia (lobular)

I
Infarct	Other benign pathology (specify)
"Inflammatory carcinoma"	Specify by type (usually ductal n. s. t.)
Invasive carcinoma	Specify by type
Invasive comedocarcinoma	Invasive ductal n. s. t.
Invasive cribriform carcinoma	Invasive tubular or cribriform
Involution	Histology normal

Term	Place to classify on form
J	
Juvenile fibroadenoma	Fibroadenoma
Juvenile papillomatosis	Other benign pathology (specify)
L	
Lactation	Histology normal
Lactational change, focal	Histology normal
Lipoma	Other benign pathology (specify)
Lipid-rich carcinoma	Other primary carcinoma (specify)
Lobular carcinoma in-situ	Non-invasive malignant, lobular
Lobular carcinoma invasive	Invasive lobular
Lobular hyperplasia (= adenosis)	Histology normal
Lobular hyperplasia (atypical)	Epithelial proliferation-atypia (lobular)
Lymphoma	Other malignant tumour (specify)
M	
Malignant phyllodes tumour	Other malignant tumour (specify)
Mammary duct ectasia	Periductal mastitis/duct ectasia
Mammillary fistula	Other benign pathology (specify)
Mastitis, acute	Other benign pathology (specify)
Mastitis, granulomatous	Other benign pathology (specify)
Mastitis, plasma cell	Periductal mastitis/duct ectasia
Mastopathia, cystic	Enter components
Medullary carcinoma	Invasive medullary
Menopausal changes	Histology normal
Metaplasia, apocrine (single layer)	Fibrocystic change
Metaplasia, apocrine (multilayered/papillary)	Fibrocystic change Epithelial proliferation present
Metaplasia, clear cell	Other benign pathology (specify)
Metaplasia, mucoid	Other benign pathology (specify)
Metaplasia, squamous	Other benign pathology (specify)
Metastatic lesion	Other malignant tumour (specify)
Microcysts	Histology normal
Microglandular adenosis	Other benign pathology (specify)
Microinvasive carcinoma	Code by in-situ component and specify microinvasion present
Micropapillary change	Epithelial proliferation present
Mixed carcinoma	Other primary carcinoma (specify types)
Mondar's disease	Other benign pathology (specify)
Mucinous carcinoma	Invasive mucinous carcinoma
Mucoele-like lesion	Other benign pathology (specify)
Mucoid metaplasia	Other benign pathology (specify)
Multiple papilloma syndrome	Papilloma, multiple
Multiple papilloma syndrome with atypia	Papilloma, multiple Epithelial proliferation-atypia (ductal)
Myoepithelial hyperplasia	Other benign pathology (specify)

Term	Place to classify on form
N	
Necrosis, fat	Other benign pathology (specify)
Nipple adenoma	Other benign pathology (specify)
Nipple – Paget's disease	Non-invasive malignant Paget's disease
Normal breast	Histology normal
P	
Paget's disease of nipple	Non-invasive malignant, Paget's disease
Non-invasive malignant, Paget's disease	Other benign pathology (specify)
Panniculitis	Non-invasive malignant, ductal (specify type)
Papillary carcinoma (in-situ)	Other primary carcinoma (specify)
Papillary carcinoma (invasive)	Papilloma
Papilloma, duct	Epithelial proliferation (with or without atypia)
Papillomatosis	Other benign pathology (specify)
Papillomatosis, juvenile	Specify under other benign pathology as adenoma of nipple
Papillomatosis, sclerosing	
Phyllodes tumour (low grade)	Other benign pathology (specify)
Phyllodes tumour (high grade)	Other malignant tumour (specify)
Pregnancy changes	Histology normal
R	
Radial scar	Complex sclerosing lesion/radial scar
Regular hyperplasia	Epithelial proliferation present without atypia
S	
Sarcoidosis	Other benign pathology (specify)
Sarcoma	Other malignant tumour (specify)
Sclerosing adenosis	Sclerosing adenosis
Sclerosing adenosis with atypia	Sclerosing adenosis Epithelial proliferation-atypia
Sclerosing subareolar proliferation	Specify under other benign pathology as adenoma of nipple
Squamous carcinoma	
Squamous metaplasia	Invasive malignant, other (specify)
Spindle cell carcinoma	Other benign pathology (specify)
Scar, radial	Invasive malignant, other (specify) Complex sclerosing lesion/radial scar
T	
Trauma	Other benign pathology (specify)
Tuberculosis	Other benign pathology (specify)
Tubular adenoma	Fibrodenoma
Tubular carcinoma	Invasive malignant, tubular or cribriform
W	
Wegener's granulomatosis	Other benign pathology (specify)

2.1.3
Recommendations for the Reporting of Breast Carcinoma[1]

Association of Directors of Anatomic and Surgical Pathology (ADASP), Chairman: J. L. CONNOLLY, USA

The Association of Directors of Anatomic and Surgical Pathology (ADASP) has named several committees to develop recommendations regarding the content of the surgical pathology report for common malignant tumours. A committee of individuals with special interest and expertise write the recommendations, and they are reviewed and approved by the council of ADASP and subsequently by the entire membership.

The recommendations have been divided into four major areas:
- items that provide an informative gross description
- additional diagnostic features that are recommended to be included in every report if possible
- optional features that may be included in the final report
- a checklist (see Appendix 2.1.3, pg. 175).

The purpose of these recommendations is to provide an informative report for the clinician. The recommendations are intended as suggestions and adherence to them is completely voluntary. In special clinical circumstances, the recommendations may not be applicable. The recommendations are intended as an educational resource rather than a mandate.

Invasive Carcinoma

Features the Association recommends should be included in the final report because they are generally accepted as having prognostic importance, are required for staging or therapy and/or are traditionally expected.

Gross Description

- How the specimen was received: fresh, in formalin, intact, cut, margins inked not, etc.
- How the specimen was identified and procedure used: labeled with (name, number), designated as breast, right or left, and procedure (core biopsy, incisional biopsy, excisional biopsy [lumpectomy], re-excision, quadrantectomy, simple mastectomy, modified mastectomy, other).
- Size: the overall size of the excised specimen should be measured in three dimensions.

Tumour Description

- Presence of mass(es) or absence of mass(es)
- Margins of mass(es) (circumscribed, infiltrative)
- Distance of mass(es) from nearest surgical margins (measured and recorded)
- Location of mass(es); e. g., quadrant if the specimen is a mastectomy
- Size of mass(es); at least greatest diameter should be recorded, three dimensions are preferable
- Texture of mass(es); e. g., soft, fleshy hard, gritty, etc.
- Description of prior biopsy site if present
- Description of the remainder of the breast tissue, nipple, and skin if present
- Number and appearance of lymph nodes if received
- It is recommended that tissue submitted for special investigation (e. g., estrogen receptor/progesterone receptor [ER/PR], flow cytometry, etc.) be specified if this information is known.
- Whether a diagnostic frozen section was performed and the diagnosis made.

Diagnostic Information

- Laterality of the breast and procedure
- Histologic type
- Ductal (usual, no special type, not otherwise specified)

---

[1] Publication: Association of Directors of Anatomic and Surgical Pathology (1995): Recommendations for the Reporting of Breast Carcinoma. American Journal of Clinical Pathology 104 (6): 614–619. Copyright © 1995 by the American Society of Clinical Pathologists. Reprint by permission

- Lobular (specify subtype)
- Classic
- Variant (alveolar, solid, pleomorphic, tubulo-lobular)
- Tubular
- Medullary
- Mucinous
- Secretory
- Infiltrating papillary
- Adenoid cystic
- Metaplastic
- Infiltration cribriform
- Other (specify)

Histologic grade. All ductal (NOS) carcinomas should be graded; some also advocate grading lobular carcinomas. The histologic type for the others (e. g., tubular, medullary replaces the grade). The Scarff-Bloom-Richardson grading scheme that evaluates the following three parameters is recommended: degree of tubule formation, nuclear grade, and mitotic rate. Points are assigned to each parameter as follows.

Tubules:
- 1 = 75% or more of tumour is composed of tubules
- 2 = 10% to 75% of tumour is composed of tubules
- 3 = < 10% of tumour is composed of tubules

Nuclei:
- 1 = small and uniform
- 2 = moderate variability in size and shape
- 3 = marked increase in size and marked irregularity

Mitotic rate. The mitotic rate is dependent on the area of the field selected. For a 40 X objective with a diameter of 0,44 mm (area of 0,152 mm^2), scoring of the number of mitoses per 10 fields (at the tumour edge) is as follows:
- 1 = 0 to 5
- 2 = 6 to 10
- 3 = > 11

The field of the microscope used should be measured and the counts adjusted proportionately [1].

The histologic grade is determined by summing the points:
- grade I = 3 to 5 points
- grade II = 6 to 7 points
- grade III = 8 to 9 points

Margins of resection. The Association recognizes that at the present time, the clinical relevance of a positive margin is not clear, and further recognizes there is no standard definition of what constitutes a positive or negative margin. However, margin involvement is used by many clinicians in forming therapeutic recommendations.

In reporting the margins of resection, state (1) whether sections of the margins have been taken parallel (shaved) or perpendicular to the surgical margin; and (2) whether tumour is at margin (grossly or microscopically). If tumour is not present at a shaved margin or at an inked margin, the distance from the margin should be specified.

Lymph nodes status. Lymph nodes status, given as numbers of nodes involved and the total number of nodes. If metastases are ≤ 2 mm, this fact and the size should be recorded. Any node larger than 2 cm should be recorded. The presence or absence of perinodal extension of tumour into axillary fat should be recorded. Nodes that are fixed to one another or other structures should be recorded. The Association does not recommend immunoperoxidase techniques to detect micrometastases.

Peritumoural angiolymphatic invasion (whether tumour cells involve peritumoural vascular spaces or not) should be recorded.

If vascular spaces in the skin are involved, this should be recorded. Although some prefer to separate lymphatic from blood vessel invasion, it is prognostically not necessary to distinguish between lymphatic vessels and blood vessels. The Association does not recommend the routine use of immunohistochemical stains to detect intravascular invasion.

Size of the carcinoma. Although this is recorded in the gross description, the Association recommends it be reported again in the diagnosis line because of the prognostic importance of this parameter.

In situ component. The presence or absence of an in situ component should be recorded. If the in situ component is ductal and is prominent within the main tumour mass and is present outside the mass or the tumour is primarily intraductal with only focal invasion, the in situ ductal carcinoma is considered to be "extensive" [2]. The Association recommends recording this finding if the patient is to be treated by less than total mastectomy. When ductal carcinoma in situ is present, the distance of the in situ process from the nearest margin should be recorded as at the margin, or the specific distance from the margin, even if the specimen also contains invasive carcinoma. Because lobular carcinoma in situ is often multifocal, the Association recommends that no specific comments on margin involvement be made.

Microcalcifications. If present on the mammogram, their presence in the sections should be sought (to be sure a calcified lesion was not missed), and a statement made about their presence and location or their absence.

Other significant disease. Atypical hyperplasia, papillomas, Paget's disease of the nipple, biopsy site changes, etc.

If information required for prognosis or therapy is not available or cannot be adequately assessed (eg, no nodes submitted with a mastectomy specimen, margins not assessable because specimen was cut before inking, etc.), should be stated specifically in the report.

Features considered optional in the final report.

These features are considered optional because they represent specific institutional preferences or they are considered inconclusive vis-à-vis prognostic significance.
- Stage. The data provided above should provide sufficient information for clinicians to determine stage. The Association does not consider inclusion of a specific tumour stage in the pathology report to be required.
- Results of ancillary investigations (eg, flow cytometry, ER/PR, oncogenes, p 53)
- Specific level or location of axillary lymph node unless marked and specific identification is requested by the surgeon.
- Identification of specific margins unless the surgeon precisely identifies them.
- Perineural infiltration
- Microvessel quantification.

In situ carcinoma

Features the Association recommends be included in the final report because they are generally accepted as having prognostic importance, are required for therapy, and/or are traditionally expected.

Gross Description

- How the specimen was received: fresh, in formalin, intact, cut, margins inked or not, etc.
- How the specimen was identified and procedure: Labeled with (name, number), designated as breast, right or left, and procedure (needle localization for calcifications, core biopsy, incisional biopsy, excisional biopsy [lumpectomy], re-excision, quadrantectomy, simple mastectomy, modified mastectomy, other).
- Size. The overall size of the excised specimen should be measured in three dimensions.

Tumour description

- Presence of mass(es) or absence of mass(es)
- Margins of mass(es) (circumscribed, infiltrative)
- Distance of mass(es) from nearest surgical margins (measured and recorded)
- Location of mass(es) (e.g., quadrant if the specimen is a mastectomy)
- Size of mass(es) (at least greatest diameter should be recorded, three dimensions are preferable)
- Texture of mass(es) (e.g., soft, fleshy hard, gritty, etc.)

- Description of prior biopsy site if present
- Description of the remainder of the tissue (breast)
- Number and appearance of lymph nodes if received
- It is recommended that fresh tissue should not be submitted for special investigation because the most important information is the presence or absence of invasion [3–6]. Blocks may be sectioned for special investigation if that information is desirable in an individual case.
- Whether a diagnostic frozen section was performed and the diagnosis made.

Diagnostic Information

Laterality of the breast and procedure

Histologic type. The Association recognizes that different terms are sometimes used for microscopically identical lesions [e.g., the term "lobular neoplasia" includes cases of atypical lobular hyperplasia). Moreover, ADASP recognizes that although the majority of cases of in situ carcinoma are readily categorized, there are borderline lesions. The criteria for diagnosing the small borderline lesions as to either lobular carcinoma in situ (LCIS) or ductal carcinoma in situ (DCIS) vary. Different authors use different qualitative and quantitative criteria in arriving at the diagnosis of LCIS or DCIS in these circumstances.

The Association realizes that the classification system for ductal carcinoma in situ (DCIS) (intraductal carcinoma) is in a state of flux; because of this, it is recommended that the lesion be graded using the traditional system based primarily on architectural pattern as well as assigning a specific nuclear grade [7, 8].

Architectural type. Ductal carcinoma in situ (intraductal carcinoma) (specify subtype):
- Cribriform
- Micropapillary
- Solid (microacinar)
- Papillary (includes most cases of intracystic)
- Comedo (requires high grade nuclei; necrosis usually present)
- Lobular carcinoma in situ

Nuclear grade. Because the architectural pattern may vary from area to area in the individual case and because nuclear grade may be important in regard to the potential for recurrence, the Association recommends that the ductal carcinoma in situ be divided into high, low, or intermediate nuclear grade in addition to providing type. Lobular carcinoma in situ is not routinely graded.

For ductal carcinoma in situ lesions only: Margins of resection.

The Association recognizes that at the present time, the clinical relevance of a positive margin is not clear, and further recognizes there is no standard definition of what constitutes a positive or negative margin. However, margin involvement is used by many clinicians in forming therapeutic recommendations.

Reporting the margins of resection. State (1) whether sections of the margins have been taken parallel (shaved) or perpendicular to the surgical margin; and (2) whether tumour is at margin (grossly or microscopically). If tumour is not present at a shaved margin or at an inked margin, the distance from the margin should be specified. Assessment of margins for lobular carcinoma is not recommended.

For ductal carcinoma in situ lesions only: Size.

If a mass is present, obtain this from gross observations; if not, several methods can be used to measure the size of an in situ process:
- sectioning the biopsy from one end of the specimen to the other at 3–4 mm intervals and submitting the sections in sequence thus allowing for an estimate of the size of the lesion based on the sections in which the lesion is present
- in small lesions, a measurement of size of the lesion may be obtained directly from the slide.

Microcalcifications. If the specimen was removed because of mammographic identification of microcalcifications, these should be identified in the tissue sections and reported. A correlation with the location of the microcalcifications in the mammogram also should be reported. It should be stated in which lesion the calcifications were identified (DCIS, adenosis, etc.). If they are not found or if the microcalcifications in the sections are not in the location indicated by the mammogram, this should be reported.

Other significant disease. Atypical hyperplasia, papillomas, Paget's disease of the nipple, biopsy site changes, etc. are other significant diseases. If information required for prognosis or therapy is not available or cannot be adequately assessed (margins not assessable because specimen was cut before inking, etc.), this should be stated specifically in the report.

References: Page 189

2.1.4
Ductal Carcinoma In Situ (DCIS): A European Proposal for a New Classification[1]

C. MICHELAKI

Increased use of mammography has led to an increased percentage of detected DCIS due to the frequent presence of calcification. Three-dimensional studies of breast tissue, expression of biological markers, studies upon cytogenetical features, incidence of recurrence and upon appearance of DCIS associated with infiltrating mamma carcinoma point to heterogeneous nature and biological behaviour of DCIS related to various histological types. The classification presently used is meant to be inadequate because it is just based on architectural pattern and the presence or absence of necrosis. The result is marked interobserver variation in the classification of DCIS.

Therefore Holland et al. have suggested a new classification with three categories based upon, primarily, cytonuclear differentiation (nuclei, chromatin, nucleoli, mitoses) and, secondarily, on architectural differentiation (cellular polarization): poorly differentiated DCIS, intermediately differentiated DCIS and well-differentiated DCIS. This classification also shows relation to cytogenetical features, mammography, precursor stages and receptor status, as described at the following.

Poorly differentiated DCIS. The first category, poorly differentiated DCIS, shows poor cytonuclear differentiation: Nuclei with marked pleomorphism, variation in size and shape and usually a large size. The chromatin is coarse, clumped and prominent. The nucleoli are prominent and sometimes multiple. Mitoses are frequent. Polarization of cells as a sign of architectural differentiation is absent or minimal. The architectural or growth pattern is solid, clinging, pseudomicropapillary or pseudocribriform. Central necroses is usually present and often prominent. Individual cell necroses and autophagocytosis are usually present. Calcification that is usually present in necrosis is amorphous.

Microcalcifications appearing in mammography show branching or coarse granular pattern. Three-dimensional studies of breast tissue demonstrate a usually continuous and segmental growth pattern of DCIS within the mammary tree. Expression of oestrogene and progesterone receptors seem to be less frequent than in DCIS of intermediate or well differentiation. As cytogenetical features neu (c-erbB-2) oncoprotein and p53 protein are usually positive and level of proliferation is high. When poorly differentiated DCIS appears as a component of an infiltrating tumour, it is nearly always associated with grade II or III infiltrating ductal carcinoma. In contrast to intermediately and well-differentiated DCIS there is no recognizable precursor stage but an amplification of the neu (c-erbB-2) oncogene seems to appear in an early step of these lesions.

Intermediately differentiated DCIS. The second category, intermediately differentiated DCIS, shows less pleomorphic nuclei than the poorly differentiated DCIS with some variation in size

---

[1] Based on the publication: Holland R., Peterse J. L., Millis R. R., Eusebi V., Faverly D., van de Vijver M. J., Zafrani B. (1994): Ductal carcinoma in situ : a proposal for a new classification. Semin. Diagn. Pathol. 11: 167–180.

and shape. The chromatin is fine to coarse, nucleoli are evident and mitoses are occasionally present. Polarization of cells as an evidence of architectural differentiation is present but less marked than in well-differentiated. An a sign of architectural differentiation cells show an orientation towards intercellular spaces, or around the luminal surface or micropapillae. The architectural pattern may be clinging, cribriform, micropapillary and solid. In solid pattern rosette-like appearance of cells surrounding small intercellular spaces can be found. Central necrosis may be present but is variable. Individual cell necrosis and autophagocytosis may be focally present. Calcification is either amorphous, when caused by necroses, or laminated/psammonalike, when caused by secretion.

Microcalcifications in mammography, that are less common than in the poorly-differentiated DCIS, show coarse-granular of fine-granular patterns. Three-dimensional studies of breast tissue show a segmental and usually continuous growth pattern within the mammary tree. Expression of oestrogene and progesterone receptors is more often then in poorly differentiated DCIS, bur less often than in well-differentiated DCIS. As cytogenetical features neu (c-erbB-2) oncoprotein and p53 protein may be positive. As a component of an infiltrating ductal carcinoma, intermediately differentiated DCIS is usually associated with grade II infiltrating ductal carcinoma. Intermediately differentiated DCIS may be the result of loss of differentiation in a well-differentiated lesion.

Well-differentiated DCIS. The third category, well-differentiated DCIS, shows pronounced cytonuclear differentiation: monomorphic round or oval nuclei, that are usually, but not always small, equally sized and with a smooth nuclear membrane. The chromatin is fine and uniform. Nucleoli are absent or inconspicuous. Mitoses are rare. Architectural differentiation is also marked: The cells show a well-defined apex and polarization with marked orientation of the apical side towards intercellular spaces, showing round intercellular spaces in the cribriform growth pattern or orientation towards duct lumen in the clinging or micropapillary growth pattern. In rare cases solid growth pattern with pronounced cytonuclear differentiation can be found and has to be distinguished from lobular carcinoma in situ. Central necroses is absent or minimal. Calcification may be rarely amorphous in cases of central necrosis, but in most cases calcification is laminated or psammonalike within secretion. Individual cell necrosis and autophagocytosis is absent.

In mammography well-differentiated DCIS of non-solid growth-pattern is associated with multiple clusters of fine-granular, sand-like microcalcifications. Three-dimensional studies of breast tissue show segmental and often discontinuous growth pattern within the mammary tree. Expression of oestrogene and progesterone receptors is frequently positive, whereas expression of neu (c-erbB-2) oncoprotein, p53 protein is rare. There is also a low level of staining with antibodies to cell cycle associated antigens. Well-differentiated infiltrating ductal carcinoma, often of tubular, tubulolobular or cribriform type, is frequently associated with well-differentiated DCIS. Well-differentiated DCIS can develop from recognizable stages of atypical hyperplasia.

This classification does not include rare DCIS types as endocrine, apocrine, mucinous, signet ring and cystic hypersecretory type.

In most cases the lesions consist of cells with homogeneous cytonuclear differentiation and architectural pattern and division into the classification is clear. Occasional cases, that show feature components of different categories in the same lesion, should accurately be noted. Whether biological behaviour of DCIS of mixed type depends upon the category type, representing the majority of the lesion. or upon the category type, representing the worst differentiated type of the lesion, even if it forms just a small part, has to be investigated.

2.1.5
Consensus Conference on the Classification of Ductal Carcinoma In Situ[1]

Conference Chairman Dr. GORDON SCHWARTZ, Jefferson Medical College, Philadelphia

Ductal carcinoma in situ (DCIS) constitutes a spectrum of noninvasive proliferative epithelial lesions with a predilection for the terminal duct-lobular units of the breast. Influenced by the ubiquitous use of screening mammography and emerging from relative obscurity only a generation ago, DCIS now represents up to one-fourth of breast cancer diagnoses in some institutions. Because it is noninvasive, it lacks the ability to metastasize, but it has been considered an initial step in a process that has the potential to progress to invasive cancer if not treated. For this reason, mastectomy, until recently, was the standard treatment for this disease.

Because it has been documented that only a minority of patients develop invasive cancer after excision of DCIS, some physicians have been treating selected patients with DCIS by local excision only, or local excision and radiation therapy, rather than by mastectomy. Differences in treatment recommendations abound because physicians have been unable to determine precisely which patients with DCIS fit best into each of these treatment categories, and if any women are well served by a recommendation for treatment that does not include the whole breast. Furthermore, pathologists do not universally agree on the features that define DCIS or those that might predict the subsequent risk of local recurrence or invasive cancer. Therefore, it is not surprising that optimal treatment is equally controversial.

To address these various issues, an international consensus conference was convened in Philadelphia, sponsored by The Breast Health Institute and The Fashion Group International, Philadelphia, and held at Thomas Jefferson University on April 25–28, 1997. Co-sponsor was the Department of Pathology of Jefferson Medical College/Thomas Jefferson University Hospital. The panelists named earlier, representing the disciplines of surgical pathology, surgery, breast imaging (radiology), radiation oncology, and biostatistics constituted the panel.

The panelists attempted to reach consensus on the following issues:
- The pathological classification of DCIS
- The identification of specific features that may convey prognostic significance
- Methods for determining size or extent of DCIS
- Margin assessment and the confirmation of complete local excision
- The appropriate manner in which surgical specimens from patients with suspected DCIS (mammographic abnormalities) should be processed from the time they are removed from the patient until the final microscopic slides are reviewed by the pathologist and a report rendered.

The conference participants recognized that there are situations in which the distinction between DCIS and atypical ductal hyperplasia, on one end of this spectrum, and between DCIS and DCIS with "microinvasion", on the other end, is difficult. Nevertheless, for the purposes of this conference, the panel limited its focus to DCIS. Atypical duct hyperplasia was excluded from consideration, as was microinvasive carcinoma. Any lesion that has any evidence of microinvasion, however limited, is classified as invasive carcinoma (pT1mic).

Classification

In the past several years, a number of new classification systems for DCIS have been proposed. In contrast to the traditional system of classification, primarily based on architecture, newer classification systems stratify DCIS primarily on the basis of nuclear grade, and secondarily, on the presence and amount of necrosis and cell polarization. Any classification system for DCIS should reflect the biological

---
[1] Published: Cancer Vol. 80, No. 9, 1997, pp 1798–1802. Reprint by permission of Wiley-Liss, Inc., a subsidiary of John Wiley & Sons, Inc.

potential of these lesions for local recurrence and/or progression to invasive carcinoma. Although the panel did not endorse any one system of classification, the consensus reached by the panel did recommend that the following features be documented in a pathology report that confirms the presence of DCIS:
- Nuclear grade
- Necrosis
- Polarization
- Architectural pattern(s).

The panel also recommended that the following information associated with the DCIS also be documented in the report:
- Margins (distance from any margin to the **nearest** focus of DCIS; focal or diffuse involvement of margins)
- Size (extent and distribution of DCIS)
- Microcalcifications associated with DCIS and calcifications outside the area of DCIS
- Correlation of the tissue specimen with specimen radiographic and mammographic findings
- Consideration of a synoptic report for DCIS was suggested.

The classification of DCIS should reflect its biology by establishing a grading system with definable clinical outcomes. Endpoints to consider in the assessment of the biology of DCIS include, but are not limited to, the following:
- Probability of local recurrence (LR)
- Risk of subsequent mastectomy
- Probability of subsequent invasive carcinoma
- Breast carcinoma specific mortality.

Such a classification would be a standard for studying (1) the natural history of the disease, including average time intervals to the various outcomes, and (2) treatment options, including the need for mastectomy after failed breast conservation.

Definitions

Nuclear Grade

The panel recommended that DCIS should be stratified primarily by nuclear grade.

Low Grade Nuclei (NG 1)
- **Appearance:** monotonous (monomorphic)
- **Size:** 1.5–2.0 normal RBC or duct epithelial cell nucleus dimensions
- **Features:** Usually exhibit diffuse, finely dispersed chromatin, only occasional nucleoli and mitotic figures. Usually associated with polarization of constituent cells.

Caveat. The presence of nuclei that are of similar size but are pleomorphic precludes a low grade classification.

High Grade Nuclei (NG 3)
- **Appearance:** markedly pleomorphic
- **Size:** Nuclei usually > 2.5 RBC or duct epithelial cell nuclear dimensions
- **Features:** Usually vesicular and exhibit irregular chromatin distribution and prominent, often multiple nucleoli. Mitoses may be conspicuous

Intermediate Grade Nuclei (NG 2). Nuclei that are neither NG 1 nor NG 3.

Necrosis

Necrosis has been shown in a number of studies to modify the risk associated with nuclear grade. The participants recommend that it be included in the features cited in the pathology report.

Definitions of Necrosis. Presence of ghost cells and karyorrhectic debris. The panel agreed that these are important features distinguishing necrotic debris from secretory material.

Necrosis Quantification. Comedonecrosis: Any central zone necrosis within a duct, usually exhibiting a linear pattern within ducts if sectioned longitudinally.

Punctate. Nonzonal-type necrosis (foci of necrosis that do not exhibit a linear pattern if longitudinally sectioned)

Cell Polarization

Polarization reflects the radial orientation of the apical portion of tumour cells towards intercellular (lumen-like) spaces, wither larger lumina or minute "microacinar" spaces which produce a rosette-like appearance. Such polarization is characteristic of lower grade DCIS with cribriform and solid architecture, but can also be recognized in epithelial protuberances, bridges, arcades and micropapillae of DCIS of lower grades with micropapillary architecture.

The group recognized that these features, A through C, would apply to the majority of recognized DCIS, but that a small proportion of cases, such as apocrine and signet ring cell types are not so easily classified. For these subtypes stratification is not yet established.

Architectural Pattern

The consensus panel recognized that architectural pattern alone does not stratify DCIS satisfactorily with regard to outcome. Moreover, there is not a consistent association with nuclear grade, so that any pattern may contain any nuclear grade. However, there is some evidence that micropapillary architecture, when present in its pure form, is more commonly associated with more extensive, multifocal and multicentric disease. Therefore, the panel agreed that architectural patterns present within a DCIS lesion should be cited in the report. In cases of a multiplicity of patterns within the same lesion, they should be listed in order of decreasing amounts, and the notation made that there are several patterns.

The following architectural patterns were accepted by the committee:
- Comedo
- Cribriform
- Papillary
- Micropapillary
- Solid

Necrosis may occur in any of these patterns. The term **comedo** refers specifically to solid intraepithelial growth within the basement membrane with central (zonal) necrosis. Such lesions are often but not invariably of high nuclear grade. This is a major departure from prior systems of classification that use the term comedo to indicate both central necrosis and high grade nuclear features. This current system permits the separation of nuclear grade from architecture, when appropriate.

Heterogeneity of Nuclear Grade

The nomenclature used should reflect the highest nuclear grade, but the panel recognized that some DCIS exhibits heterogeneity of nuclear grade. It is presently unknown if the relative proportion of each nuclear grade affects outcome. The panel agreed that a report could cite additional nuclear grades present in the lesion and include the apparent proportion of the highest grade component in such circumstances.

Size (Extent, Distribution) and Margins. The panel unanimously concurred that the size or extent of DCIS and the status of margins should be addressed in the pathology report regardless of the methods of assessment. Both, but particularly margin status, have been shown to be related significantly to outcome.

However, the panel also recognized that several methods to assess size and margins exist. These depend on surgical orientation and various processing techniques in individual surgical pathology laboratories.

Optimal Tissue Processing. The traditional surgical procedure has been a needle-guided (wire directed) localization and excision of an area of calcifications or mass with calcifications, with a specimen radiograph confirming the successful excision of the suspicious area. The following steps are considered requisite for the processing of the specimen.

1. Whenever feasible, the specimen should be oriented by the surgeon for the pathologist. Addressing the segmental anatomy of the ductal system of the breast, some panelists recommended identifying the radial axis with a suture sewn into the nipple edge of the specimen.
2. Whenever feasible, correlation of the specimen radiograph with the preoperative mammograms should be performed, usually by the radiologist, and this information

should be communicated to the pathologist. The specimen radiograph must be available to the pathologist for radiographic-pathological correlation. It is often helpful to place a metallic clip on the specimen near the site of the calcifications if they are faint or only within a very small area of the entire specimen. The additional specimen radiograph with the clip in place is then sent to the pathologist to aid the orientation of the specimen.

3. If the surgical margins are not submitted as separate specimens (vide infra), the surfaces of the specimen should be inked to permit orientation of the histological sections. Some pathologists find that different colored inks are preferable to a single color to facilitate orientation when the tissue is examined microscopically. However used, the principle is the careful identification of the margins of the specimen to be able to measure distance from the surgical margins to any focus of DCIS.

4. There are several ways in which the surgical specimen may be processed. When feasible and practical, the entire specimen should be processed in sequence in separate cassettes. This is the best way to assess the size of the area of DCIS encountered. Using this technique, the entire specimen is sectioned transversely (bread-loafed) by the pathologist into uniform sections, preferably 2 to 3 mm. Such an exhaustive examination may not be possible in all cases. Alternatively, the specimen should be sectioned, the slices radiographed, and only the slices showing the mammographic abnormality and the immediately adjacent slices are submitted for the initial histological examination. The remaining tissue may then be processed only in cases in which ductal carcinoma in situ is identified in these initial sections. This will then determine the size and extent of the lesion, evaluate the microscopic margins, and rule out invasion.

5. Determination of size or extent of DCIS is usually an estimate. This may be approximated by the number of segments, each approximately 2 to 3 mm thick, that contain DCIS microscopically. If DCIS is present only on a single slide, the greatest dimension of the lesion should be measured and reported. However, if DCIS is present on more than one slide, determination of size and/or extent of DCIS depends on the manner in which the specimen has been processed.

If DCIS is associated with characteristic linear, branching, casting-type microcalcifications, and margins are involved, the preoperative mammograms may provide a minimum estimate of DCIS size or extent. When the mammograms are used to estimate the size of DCIS, the largest area of calcifications may be measured. A single measurement of the maximum extent of calcifications should be recorded. The method of determining tumour size should be noted in the report, i.e., clinical palpation, mammogram, tissue specimen macroscopic or microscopic.

6. When the margins are not separately submitted by the surgeon (see number 7, below), the margins of the single specimen are determined by measurements of the distance between the DCIS and an inked resection margin. This narrowest (closest) margin will determine the margin status for a particular resection.

7. Some breast surgeons among the panelists believe that the current technique of inking the margins of a single specimen was not the optimal method to examine margins. An alternative technique of margin assessment was presented.

When the surgical specimen is excised in the operating room and removed from the operative field, a cavity remains. Rather than ink the excised tissue to see what has been removed, arcs of additional tissue following the contour of the cavity are excised by shaving the edges of the cavity as if one were peeling an onion from the inside out. These are separately excised, labeled, and submitted, usually from medial, lateral, superior, inferior, and deep margins (base of wound). These are processed by the pathologist separately. Any involvement within the tissue submitted as a "marginal biopsy" is considered a positive margin. Because many separate specimens may be submitted as desired, although most of the group accepted the five additional specimens as sufficient. Moreover, if a single margin is positive, it can be addressed at a subsequent procedure if breast conservation is to be used, because the exact location of the positive margin is unequivocal.

Invasion

This consensus statement applies to DCIS only and assumes the absence of any invasion, including that which is called "microinvasion". Criteria, definitions, and significance of microinvasion were not considered. As noted earlier, the presence of any invasion, however, "micro", confers a different degree of risk that has not been addressed by these proceedings. If present, it should be identified and quantified in the diagnosis.

Biological Markers

Biological markers currently have no uniquely definitive role in the management (i.e., the evaluation of therapeutic options or prognosis) of a patient with DCIS. However, the group recognized that this statement may change as data accumulate concerning correlations between the value of these different markers and patient outcome. Several participants in the consensus shared their experience to date, using estrogen and progesterone receptors, nuclear antigen Ki-67, gene products p53 and C-erB2 as examples.

Now that virtually all markers can be determined using slides made from the paraffin blocks of formalin-fixed tissue, irrespective of time between biopsy and these determinations, discarding the paraffin blocks after any length of time was strongly discouraged.

Future Directions

Further studies are essential to determine how best to combine the features of DCIS, as described earlier, into a universally acceptable, reproducible, and clinically useful system of classification.

The identification of biological and molecular markers that predict recurrence, progression to invasion, and response to therapy is an important goal and merits continued study.

Although the lesions discussed here traditionally have been considered "ductal carcinoma in situ", a few of the participants questioned the categorization of these lesions as "carcinoma in situ", recognizing the uncertain biological potential of these lesions, the difficulty in distinguishing low-grade DCIS from atypical hyperplasia in some cases, and the trend away from the use of this term in other organ systems. One suggestion was to use the term, "mammary intraepithelial neoplasia" to encompass the entire spectrum of proliferative breast lesions, including those lesions currently designated as DCIS.

Acknowledgement and Conference Participants: see Appendices 2.1.5, pg. 178

2.2
Fine Needle Aspiration Cytology

2.2.1
Fine Needle Aspiration Cytology of the Breast

U. BONK, I. DEGRELL†, G. GOHLA, P. HANISCH

Introduction

Fine Needle Aspiration (FNA) cytology is now increasingly performed and should be a fast, inexpensive and reliable method for accurate diagnosis of malignancy. This can only be achieved if several prerequisites are met.

The aspiration

The aspiration should:
- be non-traumatic
- offer optimal representativity
- yield as much material as possible.

If thin needles are used (0.6 mm, 22 Gauge) trauma is minimal. These needles are thinner than those used for venepuncture. The procedure should be adequately explained to the patient. There is no need for anaesthesia; the needle would hurt as much as the needle used for the aspiration.

Optimal representativity depends on the localisation of the lesion, its size, and the ability to fixate and "stereotactic" skill of the aspirator. An inexperienced aspirator often judges the localisation of lesions too superficially. With increasing skill cyst walls, fibrotic lesions and tumour margins can be easily recognised.

A high cell yield can be obtained by moving the needle during aspiration in several directions within the target. Some prefer to perform several aspirations in different directions.

The centre of lesions may be sclerotic or necrotic; in both cases the aspirate will be poorly cellular. The margins of lesions often offer the best target for cellular and representative aspirates.

The smear

The optimal smear should:
- be thin
- contain no blood clots
- show no mechanical artefacts.

Optimal smears are essential for reliable cytodiagnostics. If the clinicians perform the aspirates and prepare the smears, they should be regularly shown the quality (cellularity, representativity, lysis, etc.). Clinicians often do not realize the problems they create by providing cytologists with thick smears that have overstained clusters in blood clots, or with mechanically induced dissociation and smear artefacts. Aspiration and smear techniques can only be optimal if there is a direct feedback between aspirator and microscopist.

For the diagnosis "tumour positive" the smear should be highly cellular, and the cells should be well preserved and optimally evaluable.

The cytologic diagnosis "no tumour cells" should be no reason for the clinician to reassure the patient, unless the aspirate shows characteristics of a benign lesion appropriate to the clinical context.

In the case of clinical suspicion and negative cytology the FNA should be repeated or the lesion should be biopsied for histology.

Although FNA of the breast is often mainly used to confirm the clinical diagnosis malignancy, it can be a very valuable diagnostic tool of clinically benign palpable lesions, for instance to:
- distinguish a cyst from a solid tumour
- drain cysts therapeutically
- evaluate new lesions after therapy (scar, fat necrosis, suture granuloma)
- obtain material for bacteriology
- obtain material for receptor analysis
- confirm diagnosis benignancy (fibroadenoma, gynecomastia, fibrocystic changes), allowing a wait-and-see policy.

Clinical information

Reliable diagnostic results can only be obtained if complete, relevant clinical information is available. Although it is useful to study smears "blindly", unbiased by clinical information, the ultimate diagnosis should fit the clinical context.

The best results are obtained if the cytologist performs the aspiration: the clinical impression while palpating and aspirating the lesion will play a role in making the diagnosis. The cytologist might make a diagnosis "tumour positive" in case of a poorly cellular smear with few atypical cells, if his clinical impression was that of a malignant tumour and the characteristic grittiness was encountered at the aspiration.

Relevant clinical information consists of:
- sex
- age
- localisation ("breast" may vary from skin to thoracic wall)
- palpatory findings
- clinical diagnosis
- previous therapy (surgery, radiotherapy)
- pregnancy, lactation.

Mammographical findings may influence the cytodiagnosis; radiological suspicion of ductal carcinoma in situ may be cytologically confirmed (see: DCIS).

Staining

We prefer both Giemsa-staining and Papanicolaou-staining for all FNA smears. Giemsa smears are air dried (which is easy for clinicians) and fixation artefacts are avoided. The staining procedure is simple and fast, and can be easily adapted in case of under- or overstaining.

During air-drying the cells attach and spread on the glass; therefore, differences in cell- and nuclear sizes are magnified. On one hand this is an advantage, as well differentiated breast carcinomas show only slight anisonucleosis and polymorphism. On the other hand, the nuclear enlargement of benign proliferative lesions is conspicuous in Giemsa-stained smears and may be overinterpreted.

"Quick-stains" should be used mainly to evaluate cellularity and representativity. Optimal stains are essential for reliable diagnosis.

Cytodiagnosis

If clinicians want to use FNA as a diagnostic method, a lot of skill and background knowledge (clinical, cytological and histopathological) is required from the cytologist. Moreover the cytologist is responsible for all above mentioned quality aspects. Reliable cytodiagnosis should be based on simple, clear, reproducible criteria. However, criteria are never absolute; problem areas should be known to the cytologist.

The diagnostic interpretation should be reported with a clear conclusion. There should be clear agreements between cytologist and clinicians about the consequences of the conclusions. We use five basic categories; if possible, these may be supplemented by a more definite specification of the lesion:
- no diagnosis (inadequate material, too few cells or unevaluable material; consequence: repeat FNA)
- no tumour cells (adequate material, cytologically benign cells; policy depends on clinicalmammographical findings)

Table 2.6, explanation see below

Palpation	+	+	−	−	+	+	−
Mammography	+	−	+	−	+	−	+
FNA	+	+	+	+	−	−	−
Frozen section	−	?	?	+	+	+	+

- atypia; biopsy for histologic study indicated (cytological distinction between malignancy and benignancy not possible)
- suspicious of malignancy; biopsy for histologic study (with frozen section) indicated (too few tumour cells for definite diagnosis, or: unusual tumour type, or: unexpected finding)
- tumour positive, breast carcinoma. If the cytological diagnosis "tumour positive" confirms the clinical and mammographical findings ("triple diagnosis"), at our hospital definite surgery is performed without frozen section studies. In case of discrepancy frozen section studies are required (table 2.6).

Diagnostic criteria for malignancy and benignancy in FNA of the breast

Malignancy. General criteria for the diagnosis malignancy in FNA's of the breast are (table 2.7, pg. 60):
- dissociated intact cells with enlarged, polymorphic nuclei
- high cellularity
- three dimensional clusters, varying in number of cells. Microacinar and papillary formations.
- dirty background; debris, calcifications, "red stipling", lymphocytes, plasma cells, macrophages
- irregular nuclei, irregular chromatin, variation in size, number and form of nucleoli, high N/C ratio
- absence of naked bipolar nuclei
- mixture of fat and epithelial clusters.

Benignancy. General criteria for the diagnosis benignancy are (table 2.7):
- many naked bipolar nuclei
- poor or moderate cellularity

Table 2.7: Diagnostic and Cytological Prognostic Features for Benignancy and Malignancy of Breast Tumors

Features	Benignant	Malignant
Cellularity	• Usually low, can be high	• Usually high, can be low
Mitoses	• Usually absent or few in proliferative lesions possible	• Many (anormal) mitoses (per 10 hpf): Grade I 0–1 Grade II 2–4 Grade III >5
Cells:		
Type	• Variable cell types (myoepithelial, epithelial, apocrine metaplasia, macrophages, leucocytes, papillary, tubular, colloid, medullary, adenoid cystic, secretory, cribriform)	• Uniform or obvious atypia (lobular carcinoma) • Single cell population • No myoepithelial cells • No benign pairs (myoepithelia occur often as pairs) • Metaplastic, Inflammatory, sarcomas, lipid laden, signet-ring-like
Size	• Usually small	• Usually large with increased nucleus/plasma ratio: Grade I small Grade II medium Grade III large
Shape	• Usually circular, variable within limits • Conspicious cell lines	• Deformated • Often large intranuclear vacuoles
Groupings	• Cohesive, large clusters • Few single cells	• Loose clusters vs marked molding Gland formation: Grade I >75 % Grade II 10–75 % Grade III <10 % Clusters: Grade I predominate Grade II increasec single cells Grade III many single cells
Arrangement	• Relatively orderly, honeycomb-like • Branching monolayers with evenly distributed nuclei • Partly aspiration of complete three dimensional lobular structures • Rare acinar tissues which are more common in carcinoma	• Disorderly • Three dimensional clusters, varying in number of cells • Microacinar and papillary formation
Pleomorphism	• Usually little • Monomorphic	• Usually more Grade I monomorphic Grade II moderate variation Grade III pleomorphic

- branching monolayers with evenly distributed nuclei
- clean background
- monomorphic nuclei, smooth nuclear membrane, no or isomorphic inconspicuous nucleoli
- apocrine metaplasia, macrophages, leucocytes.

If all prerequisites for quality are met, at least 75% of all breast carcinomas can be reliably and definitely diagnosed, using above mentioned criteria.

In large literature series this number varies from 66 to 92%. It depends on diagnostic experience and the general set up of FNA in a hospital.

Table 2.7: Diagnostic and Prognostic Cytological Features for Benignancy and Malignancy of Breast Tumours (continued)

Features	Benignant	Malignant
Nucleus:		
Size (RBC diameter)	• Usually small (<2 x)	• Usually larger Grade I small (<2 x) Grade II medium (2–3 x) Grade III large (>3 x)
Shape	• Usually circular or oval	• Deformed
Pleomorphism	• Usually little • Usually more monomorphic	• Usually pleomorphic: Grade I slight Grade II moderate Grade III marked/bizzare
Membrane	• Smooth	• Usually irregular: Grade I smooth Grade II slightly irregular Grade III irregular
Nucleoli	• Usually absent or small, circular isomorphic inconspicious	• Often prominent: Grade I inconspicuous Grade II conspicuous Grade III prominent occupying more than one third of the nucleus, multiple
Chromatin	• Vesicular or fine reticular Even	• Often dark, coarse, irregular Grade I fine Grade II granular Grade II coarse, irregular with **lightened nuclei**
Naked bipolar nuclei	• Present	• Usually absent
Background	• Usually clean	• Usually necrotic, dirty; debris, calcifications, "red stipling", lymphocytes, plasma cells, macrophages
More features	• Granular detritus in cysts and ductal ectasia • Lipid accumulation in lactating mamma (more visible in air-dried smears)	• Accumulation of mucus in mucinous carcinoma
Summary	• Dual population • Cohesive	• Homogeneous population • Dispered

Usually approximately 10% of all breast carcinomas are underdiagnosed, either because no tumour cells are aspirated (small or fibrotic target), or because tumour cells are not recognised by the cytologist (mixtures of benign and malignant cells, or well differentiated carcinomas).

Retrospective studies show that in half of the underdiagnosed cases tumour cells can be recognised. These cases should be considered as true false negative.

In the same series 3 to 24% of the breast carcinomas are not definitely diagnosed; the conclusion is "atypia" or "suspicious of malignancy".

In these cases the smears may be quantitatively or qualitatively insufficient However, in a certain percentage suspicion of malignancy can

Table 2.8: Cytomorphologic Features: Presence (%) in FNA Smears from 49 Benign and 55 Malignant Breast Lesions

	Benign	Malignant	P
Epithelial arrangement			
Monolayer	76	23	< 0.001
Cluster	18	83	< 0.001
> 15 cells/group	88	30	< 0.001
Dissociation	12	67	< 0.001
Nucleus			
Size < 2 x erythrocyte	80	40	< 0.001
Anisonucleosis	25	40	NS
Smooth contour	84	15	< 0.001
Nucleolus	15	79	< 0.001
Regressive changes	50	50	NS
Cytoplasm			
Vacuoles	24	50	NS
Inclusion	4	10	NS
Apocrine metaplasia	14	10	NS
Columnar metaplasia	18	4	NS
Background			
Debris	2	30	< 0.001
Calcification	2	4	NS
Blood	12	30	NS
Mucin	2	3	NS
Stroma	20	17	NS
Miscellaneous			
Solitary naked bipolar nuclei	47	27	NS
Bipolar nuclei in epithelium	77	20	< 0.001
Macrophages	32	20	NS
Lymphocytes	2	4	NS
Fibroblasts	2	3	NS

Abbreviation: NS, not specific

be aroused although the diagnostic criteria are not met. These cases form the "grey area" in which the general criteria fail to distinguish benignancy and malignancy.

It is very important to recognise this "grey area of uncertainty". Although overtreatment due to false positive cytology will almost never occur if the "triple diagnosis" is followed, the categories "atypia" and "suspicious of malignancy" contain many benign lesions.

The aspirates in this grey area are mainly from benign proliferative lesions (adenosis, fibroadenoma) and from well differentiated carcinomas with small monomorphic nuclei (tubular carcinoma, invasive lobular carcinoma, DCIS cribriform). In these cases different morphologic features have different diagnostic values (table 2.8).

However, none of these criteria can be used to distinguish malignancy and benignancy definitely. An area of uncertainty will always remain; its extent depends on the experience of the cytologist. In these cases a biopsy for histologic study is indicated.

FNA patterns of Malignant Breast Lesions

FNA of the breast is, in the first instance a diagnostic procedure distinguishing benign from malignant lesions. A cytologic classification of breast tumours, comparable with the WHO-classification, does not exist. Although some proposals for cytologic-prognostic grading exist these never have been generally accepted.

No Special Histologic Subtypes

No Special Histologic Subtypes are shown in figures 2.4, 2.5 and 2.6 (see color plate).

Special Histologic Subtypes

Ductal Carcinoma in Situ. Small cell type, cribriform-micropapillary, smears show "intraductal proliferation" pattern: overstained balls and papillary or cribriform clusters, small hyperchromatic monomorphic nuclei (no myoepithelial cells), psammomatous calcifications in the clusters (seldom), background of old blood, macrophages (fig. 2.7, see color plate).

A definite distinction from papillomas is often not possible; histologic confirmation is required in all cases of "intraductal proliferation".

Large cell type, solid-comedo. Usually smears show clear evidence of malignancy and are reported as tumour positive.

In at least half of the cases a characteristic pattern is found (fig. 2.8, see color plate):
- background with necrotic debris, macrophages, calcifications
- frayed monolayers pleomorphic large cells
- apocrinoid cell features possible
- only few dissociated cells.

In these cases the presence of DCIS (either pure or as extensive component) can be suggested, especially if compatible with mammographic findings (branching calcifications).

Invasive Carcinoma

Papillary Carcinoma. Aspiration often yields thick brown fluid (fig. 2.9, see color plate). The smears show:
- overstained cell balls and papillary clusters
- columnar cell rows
- monomorphic round-oval nuclei
- background of old blood and macrophages.

Cytologically intracystic papillary carcinoma cannot be distinguished from invasive papillary carcinoma.

Mucinous Carcinoma. Aspiration yields thick gelatinous material, that has to be crushed between two glasses to obtain a smear.
The smear shows:
- pale pink-blue mucus with branching capillaries
- cell balls and monolayers or cuboidal cells
- monomorphic nuclei.

This smear pattern is very characteristic. Occasionally myxoid stroma from fibroadenomas may resemble mucus (fig. 2.10, see color plate).

Metastases of melanoma may imitate this tumour cytologically!

Medullary Carcinoma. At aspiration soft tumour. Large often sanguinolent cell yield smear pattern:
- very large, polymorphic cells
- clusters and dissociation
- very large nuclei, prominent nucleoli necrosis, macrophages, lymphocytes
- sometimes: squamous metaplasia.

These tumours may become cystic: underdiagnosis may occur if only cyst fluid is sent for examination (fig. 2.11, see color plate).

Adenoid Cystic Carcinoma. The smear pattern of this very rare breast tumour is highly characteristic:
- clusters with pink globular cores, surrounded by small monomorphous bipolar nuclei
- naked bipolar nuclei possible
- sometimes: monomorphous epithelial cells in small monolayers.

The stromal fragments of "collagenous spherulosis" look like ACC (fig. 2.12, see color plate).

Often underdiagnosed carcinomas

Tubular carcinoma/invasive cribriform carcinoma. The aspirate is often moderately cellular due to fibrosis. The smear contains:
- small clusters, less than 10 cells possible
- microacinar arrangement
- small nuclei, anisanucleosis, irregular nuclear membranes
- few bipolar nuclei
- sometimes psammomatous calcifications.

The smear pattern may at first glance resemble that of fibroadenoma and at second glance that of blunt duct adenosis (fig. 2.13, see color plate).

Invasive Lobular Carcinoma. The aspirate is usually moderately or poorly cellular due to fibrosis, and often contains benign epithelium, due to the growth pattern of this type of tumour.

Characteristic smears show (often retrospectively):
- small clusters, Indian files
- small cells, polygonal nuclei, molding, irregular nuclei with "noses"
- intracytoplasmatic vacuoles, signet ring cells, inclusions
- background with red stipling.

Interpretation of the smears is usually difficult due to mechanical artefacts and cell lysis.

FNA from (blunt duct) adenosis may imitate ILC (fig. 2.14, see color plate).

Apocrine Carcinoma. Smears from well differentiated apocrine carcinoma may look like apocrine metaplasia and hyperplasia in cystic change and be interpreted as such unless clinicians emphasize the solid character of the lesion (fig. 2.15, see color plate).

Smears show:
- monolayers and cords apocrin-cells
- sometimes: anisonuclelosis – irregular nucleoli
- necrosis, macrophages, naked atypical nuclei

Unusual Malignant Breast Tumours. These tumours are very rare and often unexpected findings. Almost always a biopsy is indicated for confirmation of the diagnosis and optimal classification.

Metaplastic Carcinomas. Squamous cell, spindle cell and giant cell metaplasia may occur in invasive ductal carcinomas, and may be encountered in smears. Squamous metaplasia is often imitated in breast tumours with large cells and necrosis (DCIS-comedo), and may also be found in medullary carcinoma. Spindle cell metaplasia may look like desmoplastic stroma changes, and should be distinguished from spindle cell sarcomas and from the stromal component of phyllodes tumours. Osteoclast-like giant cells can be found in smears from invasive ductal carcinomas with osteoclast-like stroma cells; these should be distinguished from the metaplastic giant cells in metaplastic carcinomas.

Sarcomas. FNA classification of soft tissue tumours is difficult. FNA is useful to exclude an epithelial origin, and to advice the clinicians to perform a biopsy for histologic classification (fig. 2.16, see color plate).

Non-Hodgkin Lymphomas. FNA diagnosis is usually easier than histology, in which small cell variants may imitate ILC, and large cell variants medullary carcinoma. In primary NHL of the breast, biopsy is indicated for immunopathologic classification and interpretation of growth pattern.

Smears are usually very cellular, with dissociated lymphoid cells, usually one cell type, with lymphoglandular bodies (cytoplasmic fragments) in the background (fig. 2.17, see color plate).

Metastases. In all "tumour positive" FNA's with unusual features (small undifferentiated cells, squamous cells, spindle cells, pigmentation) the possibility of a metastasis should be considered. Relevant clinical information may avoid overtreatment (fig. 2.18, see color plate).

General Criteria of Benignancy

Nearly all aspirates from benign lesions contain naked bipolar nuclei. These hyperchromatic, isomorphic, small (6–8 μm) nuclei can be found in the Background and in and around epithelial clusters. Lysis and, mechanical artefacts sometimes make recognition difficult.

Naked nuclei. Naked nuclei larger than 8 mm, varying in size, with nucleoli, and with degenerative changes may be found in cyst fluid (apocrine cell nuclei) and in pregnancy-lactation (secretory cells easily loose their vacuolated cytoplasm). These nuclei may be overdiagnosed, especially when laying in a proteinaceous granular "dirty" background.

 The cytologic diagnosis of malignancy should never be based on naked nuclei.

The presence of naked bipolar nuclei is the most important feature of benignancy. In smears with mixtures of benign and malignant cells naked bipolar cells may also be encountered.

Benign epithelial cell usually lie in large branching monolayers, with evenly spaced monomorphic nuclei. Monolayers may look like clusters in thick smears, and mechanically induced dissociation may occur in too forcefully prepared smears.

In fluid epithelial proliferations appear 3-mensional; intraductal papillary proliferations and intracystic apocrine hyperplasia may show overstained clusters, often with degenerative changes. Cytologically it may be very difficult to distinguish benign and malignant proliferations; we use the term "intraductal epithelial proliferation", which is an indication for biopsy and histologic study (fig. 2.19, see color plate).

Benign lesions usually yield less cellular aspirates than malignant. However fibroadenomas, especially in young women, may give yield to very cellular smears.

Well prepared smears will give no problems. However mechanically induced nuclear changes and pseudo-dissociation may cause overdiagnosis.

The criterium: benign lesions have small and monomorphous nuclei, malignant lesions large and polymorphic, is, of course, not absolute.

In all benign proliferative lesions (adenosis, fibroadenoma, gynaecomastia, pregnancy, lactation) nuclear enlargement and prominent nucleoli may be found, representing active cell metabolism. Usually nuclear margins are smooth, anisonucleosis within a monolayer is minimal, and nucleoli are small, solitary, and round.

Radiotherapy may induce atypia with conspicuous anisonucleosis within small cell clusters. However, the N/C ratio remains normal (fig. 2.20, see color plate).

Overstained clusters histiocytes, fibroblasts and epithelial cells with degenerative changes may be encountered in smears from cysts, ductitis and fat necrosis. These clusters look like clusters of atypical epithelial cells and may be overdiagnosed. However, the background usually contains leucocytes, which are hardly ever found in carcinomas (fig. 2.21, see color plate).

In general overdiagnosis can be avoided if the basic diagnostic criteria are strictly followed. Mechanically induced smearing artefacts and degenerative lytic changes should be recognised. Smear patterns usually can be easily recognised using a low power magnification. There is often no need to "screen" the whole smear with high power magnification to make a reliable diagnosis; it is very difficult to evaluate cytonuclear changes in overstained clusters and to interpret changes in each individual cell. One should be aware that differences in cytonuclear size are very much exaggerated in air dried Giemsa stained smears, and that only few pathologists use high power magnifications in the routine study of slides, more relying on tissue patterns than on cytonuclear details. The diagnostic category "atypia" should be restricted for cases of real uncertainty. Benign lesions cytologically Diagnose as "suspicious of malignancy" should be considered as false positive.

FNA patterns of benign breast lesions

Several benign lesions can be recognised in FNA of the breast.

Inflammation – Abscess. Aspiration yields purulent material (fig. 2.22, see color plate). The smear shows:
- proteinaceous debris, granulocytes
- macrophages, multinucleated giant cells
- often: overstained clusters of macrophages
- sometimes: microorganisms.

Some of the material may be used for bacteriological studies.

Cyst – Duct Ectasia. If clear cyst fluid is obtained at aspiration it can be thrown away, the

chance of finding malignancy being almost nil. If after draining a cyst a residual mass remains, FNA should be repeated (fig. 2.23, see color plate). Sediments of turbid fluids usually show:
- proteinaceous background, macrophages with hemosiderin
- naked nuclei (apocrine), degenerative cells
- apocrine metaplastic cells
- "cyst wall cells".

Cyst wall cells are clusters flattened apocrine metaplastic cells, macrophages and or fibroblasts, with degenerative cell changes (cytoplasmic vacuolisation, karyorrhexis, irregular hyperchromatic nuclei), which may be overdiagnosed by inexperienced observers.

Fat Necrosis – Suture Granuloma. Fat necrosis may mammographically and clinically imitate (recurrent) tumour. Although a firm lesion can be palpated, there is no resistance at aspiration (fig. 2.24, see color plate).
  The smear shows:
- dissociated fat cells
- lipophages, macrophages, multinucleated giant cells
- fibroblasts
- leucocytes.

Clustered macrophages and "active" fibroblasts may look like atypical epithelial cells. Relevant clinical information (previous surgery, trauma) will prevent overdiagnosis. In suture granulomas birefringent material can be found surrounded by foreign body giant cells.

Radiotherapy Induced Changes. FNA is increasingly performed in patients who underwent breast conserving treatment (BCT) for breast carcinoma. Lumps after BCT are difficult to evaluate clinically and mammographically, and may be caused by scarring, organising haematoma, radiotherapy induced fibrosis, fat necrosis or recurrent carcinoma. FNA is extremely useful to distinguish these lesions.
  However, radiotherapy induced atypia of normal, preexisting, glandular breast tissue may imitate malignancy, and should be recognised. The smear shows:
- poor to moderate cellularity

- clean background
- small epithelial clusters, microacinar
- conspicuous anisonucleosis, anisocytosis, normal N/C ratio
- sometimes: prominent nucleoli
- degenerative cell changes
- naked bipolar nuclei.

There will be no doubt about the benign character of these cells if smears from the primary tumour are available for comparison.

Benign Tumours

Fibroadenoma. Especially at young age the cell yield from FA is high (fig. 2.25, see color plate). Smears show:
- large, branching monolayers
- many naked bipolar nuclei
- pink stromal fragments.

During active growth the cytonuclear aspects mirror the proliferation: nuclear size may be impressive and nucleoli prominent. These changes should not be considered as atypical". Stromal fragments may occasionally be mucoid and imitate the Background of mucinous carcinoma. The juvenile fibroadenoma variant shows hyperplastic epithelium and hyperplastic stroma cells with enlarged nuclei. The smear pattern of gynecomastia resembles fibroadenoma, although the aspirate is less cellular. Proliferative changes in gynecomastia should not be overinterpreted.

Phyllodes Tumour. Aspirations are often sanguinolent and poorly cellular. The smears show:
- monolayers of hyperplastic epithelium
- cellular stromal fragments
- capillaries
- naked stromal cell nuclei, spindle cells.

This pattern may resemble that of fibroadenoma. The naked nuclei are larger than bipolar nuclei. Spindle cells (fibroblasts) are unusual in FA. Desmoplasia may imitate phyllodes stroma; the epithelium of phyllodes tumour, however, shows no signs of malignancy (fig. 2.26, see color plate).

Pregnancy – Lactation. Breast lumps during pregnancy and lactation are difficult to evaluate clinically and mammographically; there is often a delay in the diagnosis of malignancy. FNA may be extremely helpful, if pregnancy – lactation changes are recognised. FNA from normal breasts after approximately 4 months pregnancy and from lactating breasts show:
- moderate cellularity
- small monolayers and clusters hyperchromatic nuclei, no anisonucleosis, nucleoli vacuolated cytoplasm
- background with cytoplasm fragments, naked nuclei
- macrophages
- often: smearing artefacts.

Smears may be overdiagnosed if there is no clinical information of pregnancy/lactation (fig. 2.27, see color plate).

Granular Cell Tumour. This tumour may be occasionally be the target of FNA (fig. 2.28, see color plate). The smear shows:
- clusters and isolated large cells
- paracentral round nucleus
- pale granulated cytoplasm.

Paget's Disease of the Nipple. You may find cells from this lesion in FNA smears or imprint cytology or secretion from the nipple. The Paget cell is an intradermal spread from mostly an intraductal carcinoma (fig. 2.29, see color plate). You can find:
- more or less tumour cells intermixed sometimes with normal squamous cells
- large round or oval nuclei, sometimes with typical perinuclear halo (a sign of degeneration)
- abundant pale cytoplasm.

2.2.2
Fine Needle Aspiration and Mammary Secretion, Cytology and Core Biopsy[1]

U. SCHENCK

Cytology of breast secretions, aspiration cytology of the breast and core biopsy of the breast have been used for several decades [1, 2]. During this time the indication for the use of the methods underwent minor changes due to the development of other techniques. Special needles for core biopsy allow a wider application of this technique today. The present contribution focusses on symptomatic patients presenting with either lumps of the breast or mammary secretions.

Breast secretions, that are not associated with lactation or pregnancy may be caused by localised disease of the breast. Clinically it is not really possible to separate those secretions that might be caused by e.g. papilloma or intraductal carcinoma from those due to non neoplastic diseases. So there is no real alternative to the cytological examination of breast secretions. Most breast secretions have no malignant cause and only a limited number of breast carcinomas (below 5%) cause breast secretions. For this reason cytology does not play an eminent role in breast carcinoma diagnosis. Breast secretions that are due to breast carcinoma may also yield false negative cytology. Despite of this, cytology of breast secretions allows in some cases the early diagnosis of ductal carcinoma in situ and invasive ductal carcinoma which would go undetected with mammography alone. If cytology of breast secretions is widely applied, cytology will lead to the diagnosis of ductal carcinoma in situ or invasive ductal carcinoma in about 1% of the examinations. If mammary secretions are examined only in cases that seem suspicious, e. g. by bloody appearance of the secretion or high age of the patient, a much higher percentage of carcinomas will be diagnosed. Cytologically it may be difficult to separate papillomas and well differentiated ductal

---
[1] Talk held on the 16. Congress of the German Society of Senology, 12.–14. 9. 1996, Göttingen, Germany

Table 2.9: Breast Secretions, Munich Technical University and Bavarian Cancer Society, Cytological Examinations 1986–1995

	n	%
Unsatisfactory	69	1.3
Negative	3912	75.1
Repeat suggested	1106	21.2
Suspicious	109	2.1
Positive	10	0.2
Total	5206	100

carcinomas. So, in these cases histological examination and therapy has to be performed after adequate galactographic localisation of the lesions.

Table 2.9 shows the diagnostic groups of 5206 cytological examinations from 1986 to 1995. Our results seem to be comparable with those published by Mouriquand (1986) [3] and Wunderlich (1990) [4].

The number of cases in which we ask for repeat smear is quite high, since it includes all bloody secretions and those suggestive of benign epithelial proliferation which might correlate with hyperplasia in histology. Cases in which we ask for histology, mostly the cases in which we don't know if the cellular changes are due to papilloma or ductal carcinoma, are statistically grouped as suspicious. Positive is restricted to definitive cancer diagnosis.

Fine needle aspiration cytology has a tradition dating back to the twenties in the United States. Wide application started in Scandinavia and spread over Europe [1, 2]. Breast fine needle aspiration finds today a wide application also in the United States. Still its value has been questioned generally by those who are sticking to the concept, that each nodule of the breast has to be taken out and examined histologically. This concept was lately also challenged by a wider application of core biopsies. Presently it seems, that there is no consensus concerning the optimal choice of the methods. Those centers using fine needle aspiration cytology prefer to go on with this method, some of them will use the core biopsies additionally in a few cases. Table 2.10 shows a comparison of fine needle aspiration cytology with histology of core biopsies.

The application of fine needle aspiration cytology and core biopsy histology may be used for different reasons.

Reasons to perform Fine Needle:
- For preoperative confirmation of malignancy
- For preoperative confirmation of benignity
- To avoid frozen sections
- For better planning of operations
- For better patient information
- To avoid surgical biopsy
- For the diagnosis of neo adjuvant chemotherapy
- For the diagnosis and therapy of cysts

Today core biopsy histology is a useful method in the diagnosis of breast lesions and it can be presumed to yield good results, even if the sampler has little experience. It does not ask for a special training of the pathologist. Fine needle aspiration is much less complicated, more economical but requires more experience in needling the lesions, and reading the samples asks for an experienced cytopathologist. This is the reason, why fine needle aspiration is performed by the cytopathologists themselves in some countries, who can, if it is needed, have a quick cytological evaluation concerning adequacy of the sample.

Recent contributions by the Royal College of Pathologists [5] confirm the value of the triple diagnostic approach that has been used in some places for almost 30 years. Sneige (1996) [6] recently evaluated FNA and core biopsies for mammographically detectable nonpalpable breast lesions. The doctor dealing with breast lesions should be acquainted with the full spectrum of approaches. Often this experience cannot be offered at a single medical center but needs exchange of experience with other groups.

References: Page 190

Table 2.10: Differences among Fine Needle Aspiration and Histology of Core Biopsies

	Fine Needle Aspiration Cytology	Core Biopsy
Needle diameter	0,4–0,8mm	0.9–2.1mm
Needle type	Simple cannula	Special needle, e.g. "lance and cut"
Material	Aspirate, smear	Tissue cylinder
Fixation	Air drying or wet fixation	Formaldehyde
Staining	May Grünwald-Giemsa or Papanicolaou	HE (Hematoxilin-Eosin)
Patient information	Less/always explain the possibility of false-negatives	More/always explain the possibility of false-negatives
Desinfection	Little, like for blood analysis	Like for minor surgery
Local anesthesia	No	Yes
Skin incision	Not necessary	Often performed
"Feeling of tissue"	During needling	While positioning the needle
Needling direction	Mostly shortest way tangential for nodules close to the chest wall	Tangential to chestwall
Trauma	Little trauma	More trauma
Pressure dressing application	Not needed	Frequently used
Pain	Little pain	Local anesthesia
Processing of material	Faster	Takes more time
Invasive growth	Vague criteria	Mostly easy to recognize
Tumortyping	Possible, in most cases	Easier
Grading	Possible but not standardized	Standardized
Material for special methods	Very limited	Multiple sections and stains
DNA measurements	Possible on smears	Inaccurate on tissue sections
Hormone receptor analysis	More difficult	Easier
Sensitivity	About 90 %	About 90 %
Pos. predictive value	Above 99%	Above 99%
Sampling technique	Needs more practice	Needs little practice
Sample taker	Clinician/pathologist	Clinician
Evaluation of sample adequacy	Mostly needs microscopy	Macroscopic evaluation of tissue cylinder
Reduction of false-negatives	Fan-like aspiration, multiple aspirations	Multiple core biopsies
Evaluation of sample	Needs specially trained cytopathologist	No special training needed for anatomopathologist
Costs	Low	Higher
Time needed for procedure	Needs little time	Needs much more time

2.2.3
Guidelines for Cytology Procedures and Reporting in Breast Cancer Screening[1]

Cytology Sub-Group of the National Coordinating Committee for Breast Screening Pathology, National Health Service Breast Screening Programme (NHSBSP), Chairman: C. L. BROWN, UK

Introduction

In 1989 a Working Party of the Royal College of Pathologists produced guidance on breast cancer screening as it related to histopathology in two documents, *Guidelines for Pathologists* [1] and *Pathology Reporting in Breast Cancer Screening* [2].

In both of these documents fine needle aspiration cytology (FNAC) was referred to but at that time it was recognised that there were few pathologists with experience in fine needle aspiration of breast lesions. It was felt that the initial emphasis should be on training.

Three years into the NHS Breast Cancer Screening programme (NHSBSP) it has become obvious that many more centres than envisaged wish to include fine needle aspiration as an additional diagnostic test to provide a preoperative diagnosis of breast carcinoma and to reduce the number of operations for benign breast disease. This has major cost and morbidity saving implications for the management of breast disease, both in screening and symptomatic practice.

This wish has now become accommodated in the National Breast Screening Computer System, which is used by most of the regional services, including cytology as an integral part of assessment with additional imaging and clinical examination. Many centres now have stereotactic X-ray equipment and are using this for impalpable lesions, despite the statement in 1989 [2] that this was mainly a research tool and required further evaluation. Some early results have now been published but information on interval cancer rates post-aspiration will be the ultimate test and this is not yet available.

We are well aware however of the experience and training needed by both the radiological and pathological members of the team in order to produce meaningful results using image guided aspiration techniques.

With the background of this increasing use of FNAC it was felt necessary to produce guidelines in taking and interpreting cytology smears in a similar manner to the guidance given in the 1989 documents [1, 2] as it is generally recognised among units dealing with impalpable lesions that cytological assessment of these sometimes poses greater difficulty than palpable lesions.

While the techniques described in this manual are the recommended techniques for units embarking on aspiration for the first time and for units having problems with a high level of inadequate samples, it is recognised that there are other ways of achieving the same results and units may have developed other methods of operating which are equally valid and effective. This document is intended to provide guidelines only and is not meant to be prescriptive.

Use of Fine Needle Aspiration

Although some units in the NHSBSP appear to be achieving excellent benign to malignant ratios in the absence of FNAC, units which have embarked on the general use of FNAC for assessment of both palpable and impalpable abnormalities appear to be achieving much lower benign to malignant biopsy ratios. Recent results from one centre suggested that benign to malignant ratios could even be lowered as far as 1 to 7 after five years experience using FNAC as an integral part of the assessment procedure [3].

This is also recognised in the Quality Assurance Guidelines for Radiologists [4] where the following Outcome Objectives are suggested.

---

[1] Publication: Cytology Sub-Group of the National Coordinating Committee for Breast Screening Pathology (1993): *Guidelines for Cytology Procedures and Reporting in Breast Cancer Screening.* NHSBSP Publication* No. 22, 52 pages. (ISBN 1 87 1997 26 7) Copyright © 1993 by NHSBSP
 * NHSBSP Publications, National Breast Screening Programme, The Manor House, 260 Ecclesall Road South, Sheffield S11 9PS, UK
 Reprint by permission

Number of Benign Biopsies:
- With FNAC < 20 per 10 000
- Without FNAC < 40 per 10 000

Benign to Malignant Ratio:
- First year (all cases) 1:1
- Subsequent years
  - Prevalent screen with FNAC < 1:2
  - without FNAC < 3:1
  - Incident screen with FNAC < 1:4
  - without FNAC < 1:1

In addition FNAC can be used in combination with mammography and clinical examination findings to enable definitive surgery to be carried out at the patient's first operation avoiding the need for frozen section and reducing patient anxiety. The benefit of FNAC is influenced by the predictive value of mammography. In units where this predictive value is low then FNAC will have additional beneficial effects.

The highest levels of diagnostic accuracy in the pre-operative diagnosis of breast disease are achieved by using a triple approach [5]. This concept combines the results of imaging, clinical examination and FNAC. When all three modalities agree, the level of diagnostic accuracy exceeds 99 % [6]. It is of interest to note that similar levels of accuracy have been obtained for impalpable lesions where clinical examination was non-contributory [7].

If FNAC is negative in the face of strong clinical and radiological evidence of malignancy then it should be repeated, perhaps under imaging guidance, and, if still negative, an open biopsy or localisation biopsy should be performed.

 We strongly recommend that this combined approach is adhered to in the NHS Breast Screening Programme and that **under no circumstances should a cytological opinion of malignancy in the abscence of mammographic and/or clinical evidence of malignancy be taken as authority for therapeutic surgery.**

In cases where there is disagreement between modalities with a failure to achieve consensus after multi-disciplinary discussion, diagnostic histopathological biopsy is the appropriate procedure. As stated in the *Guidelines for Pathologists* [1], frozen section of these difficult lesions is inappropriate.

Benefits of FNAC Versus Drawbacks

As far back as 1933 Stewart [8] stated that for FNAC:
- It must not be inferred that diagnosis is always simple and that no errors have been made.
- Until the pathologist has familiarised himself with the various pitfalls, errors are certain to occur. These can be corrected only with knowledge gained from experience.

So far, however, the advantages of the method have far outweighed in importance the occasional error.

It is therefore clear from these and other more recent statements that there is a cost to be weighed against the benefits expected from FNAC and a cost-benefit table can be drawn up (table 2.11).

Taking the Aspirate

Palpable Lesions (See Appendix 1)

If the lesion is easily palpable then clinically guided FNAC by an experienced aspirator is the localisation method of choice as it is quick and accurate.

A syringe of appropriate size (usually 10 or 20mls) is used for fine needle aspiration in order to achieve adequate suction. For superficial lesions or in small breasts a 23G (blue) needle is sufficient and may produce less bleeding. In large breasts or in deeper lesions a 21G-(green)-needle may be necessary because of its extra length. Needles which have no dead space in the needle hub are best for FNAC (e.g. B & D Microlance). Finer gauge needles are used in some units with excellent results.

After cleansing the skin with a sterile swab the lesion should be immobilised so that an accurate aspirate can be taken. The needle is intro-

Table 2.11: Benefits and Drawbacks of FNAC

Benefits	Drawbacks
Diagnosis with simple test	Error in diagnosis may lead to overtreatment or delay in making the correct diagnosis
Cheap	Occasional complications (see below)
Avoids open biopsy in some cases and allows treatment of cancers at a planned operation	Requires skilled personnel
Can be performed on outpatients	Entails additional cost in terms of training and employment of skilled personnel
Avoids frozen section	
Reduces patient uncertainty and therefore anxiety	
Low complication rate compared with other diagnostic tests	

duced into the skin with no air in the syringe barrel. The needle is positioned at the anterior edge of the lump (which can usually be felt with the needle tip) and negative pressure is applied either with the thumb or, more easily, with a syringe holder. Several passes through the lesion, varying the angle of entry into the lesion and rotating the syringe slowly, are made, without withdrawing the needle from the skin, until a small drop of fluid is seen in the hub of the needle. Some aspirators advocate picking up the lesion, rotating the syringe during aspiration and varying the speed of passes to increase the yield. The negative pressure is released and then the needle is withdrawn from the skin. If a large amount of blood is obtained re-aspiration is advisable. The lesion may be felt with the needle tip (see below under sampling of lesions).

Breast lesions are often deeper than they appear. If there is doubt about whether the lesion has been sampled, then re-aspiration using a longer needle may be necessary. If there is no resistance to the needle from a lump which appears clinically not to be a lipoma then it is likely the lesion has been missed by the needle. Re-aspiration is advised, especially if the spread slide shows oily droplets throughout. Heavily bloodstained aspirates similarly may not be representative of the lesion and firm local pressure may be needed to limit haematoma formation.

If material appears in the hub of the needle, then using another needle it can be sucked out of the hub into the barrel of the new needle and expelled from there or retrieved by washing into transport medium.

Another method which uses a needle only and capillary action to draw the fluid into the hub has been described by Zajdela [9] but as far as is known this is not applicable to stereotaxis.

Impalpable Lesions

To obtain a representative sample from impalpable breast lesions FNAC must be carried out under image guidance. The imaging techniques best suited for guiding FNAC of impalpable lesions are:
- X-ray
  - Stereotaxis
  - Co-ordinate grid
  - Perforated plate
- Ultrasound

All of these procedures are best carried out by radiologists who are specialists in breast imaging or in a multidisciplinary team with a specialist radiologist present. Ultrasound guided FNAC is the technique of first choice for sampling impalpable breast lesions as it is easier to perform, more comfortable for the patient, and less time-consuming than the X-ray guided techniques. For impalpable lesions detected by mammography the radiologist must be certain that the abnormality seen on ultrasound is the same as the abnormality seen on mammography. Ultrasound can only be used when the radiologist is convinced that the abnormality is clearly visible using this technique. X-ray guided FNAC should be used where there is any doubt about the ultrasound appearances. In general ultrasound is suitable for mass sampling lesions (including stellate lesions) while X-ray guided FNAC is required for microcalcification and many parenchymal deformities which have no associated mass. If X-ray guided FNAC is necessary stereotactic equipment produces the greatest accuracy. There is no doubt that the co-ordinate grid method can produce excellent results in experienced hands but for units starting from scratch there appears to be a consensus that stereotaxis is the most accurate method. Only one screening unit to our knowledge in the UK uses the co-ordinate grid method in preference to stereotaxis.

 Cytology results from impalpable lesions should not be interpreted in isolation. Inevitably, inadequate and false-negative FNAC results are significantly higher for impalpable lesions. When the imaging findings are considered to be strongly suspicious of malignancy and FNAC is inadequate or benign then management should be based on the imaging findings or FNAC repeated under X-ray guidance.

Equipment

Ultrasound equipment which is suitable for routine breast examination is all that is required to perform ultrasound guided FNAC, but a needle guide attachment will ease the task of the aspirator.

All the X-ray guided techniques described above are similar in method and involve the localisation of a breast lesion under a modified compression plate similar to that used for plain mammography. Stereotaxis requires specialised equipment while the other two techniques can be carried out on the most basic mammography equipment. Both the perforated plate and co-ordinate grid techniques are inherently less accurate than stereotaxis as they involve manual measurements on a single image to localise the position of a lesion within the breast. Neither method allows for accurate calculation of a lesion's depth from the skin and the needle must be placed without the use of a needle-guide. Stereotactic equipment incorporates a needle-guide and allows for very accurate calculation from stereo images of a lesion's co-ordinates, including depth. However, in experienced hands comparable results for FNAC have been obtained with both the stereotactic and co-ordinate grid techniques.

Number of Aspirates

There are several reasons to explain why significantly greater inadequate sample rates are likely with FNAC of impalpable lesions when compared to FNAC of palpable abnormalities. The small size and fibrous content of some impalpable lesions makes fine needle sampling more difficult. An additional factor for X-ray guided stereotactic techniques is that it is not possible to vary the angle at which the needle passes through the lesion during sampling. For these reasons multiple sampling is recommended (often two or three but occasionally up to five separate punctures) as this will significantly increase the diagnostic yield. With experience it may be possible to reduce the number of punctures to two or three without affecting the inadequate rate. Two aspirates are usually sufficient for ultrasound guided procedures.

Needles and Syringes

22- or 23-gauge-needles of appropriate type and length are ideal for image guided FNAC. A needle with a trocar may be preferred as it is more rigid and is less likely to become blocked or contaminated during insertion. As with palpable lesions, a 10- or 20-ml-syringe is used to apply suction. A short extension tube between the needle and syringe is usually required for image guided procedures.

Personnel

The success of FNAC is directly related to the skill and experience of the operators. The number of staff involved should be restricted to the minimum possible. A core team of aspirators who perform all breast needling procedures should be established in each centre. Trainees must be closely supervised. An experienced radiographer is essential for X-ray guided procedures. For both X-ray and ultrasound guided FNAC it is recommended that an assistant skilled in specimen preparation, preferably an MLSO or a pathologist, is present. The procedure time is significantly shortened if an assistant deals with the specimens and smears the slides while the aspirator obtains further samples.

If a trained MLSO or pathologist is available to immediately assess the adequacy of the aspirate using a rapid staining technique, recall for repeat cytology can be avoided therefore reducing delay and distress.

Local Anaesthesia

As multiple sampling requires multiple skin punctures, the use of local anaesthesia may be used to anaesthetise the skin or ethyl chloride spray can be employed to freeze the skin. This may be particularly helpful for X-ray guided techniques with multiple samples which take significantly longer to perform. The use of local anaesthetic reduces the risk of pain-induced patient movement within the compression plate during the procedure. To avoid contamination of the aspirate the local anaesthetic should not be injected deep to the dermis. Many units, however, do not use local anaesthetic.

X-ray Guided Procedures

This description concentrates on the procedure of stereotactic guided aspiration but the procedures are broadly similar for all the X-ray guided techniques. (The co-ordinate grid and perforated plate techniques are well described in the literature [10, 11].) The oblique approach may be required for lesions in the axillary tail.

In the ideal situation the radiologist should:
- Check that the equipment and materials are correctly assembled before the patient arrives.
- Be present throughout the procedure and explain the process in full to the patient, particularly that several aspirates will be performed. The risk of syncope during the procedure is considerably reduced if the patient is reassured and relaxed by the clinician and other staff.
- Supervise the positioning of the patient and the applying of the compression plate. The shortest route from the skin to the lesion should be selected wherever possible. For lesions in the upper breast the cranio-caudal position is usually the most appropriate. For lesions in the lower breast lateral to medial or medial to lateral approaches should be chosen. The oblique approach is usually ideal for lesions in the axillary tail. A marker pen should be used to draw the outline of the window in the compression plate on the skin. Movement of the breast in the compression plate during the procedure will then be easy to detect.
- Supervise the X-ray tube movements required for obtaining the localisation images. It is often necessary to place the patient's head in an awkward and uncomfortable position when the X-ray tube is being tilted. Great care is required when this is carried out to avoid movement of the breast under the compression plate. After the localisation images have been obtained the position of the breast in relation to the pen marks should always be checked. If the breast has moved repeat films must be performed.
- Check carefully the localisation image and personally set up and calculate the localising co-ordinates. The breast should be repositioned and repeat films performed as often as is necessary to obtain an acceptable position of the lesion within the sampling field. For accurate depth calculation using stereotaxis it is essential that exactly the same part of the lesion is selected on both the stereo images.

Recommended Aspiration Procedure

Unless immediate assessment of adequacy of the specimen is available, multiple sampling increases the chance of obtaining a diagnostic yield and the inexperienced aspirator should attempt to obtain at least five separate samples at each stereotactic procedure. The centre of the lesion should be selected for the first needle pass (fig. 2.30: A). Subsequent needle passes should aim to sample the periphery of the lesion (fig. 2.30: B, C, D, E).

The "star" pattern of sampling is most appropriate for mass and stellate lesions. A less geometric sampling pattern may be more appropriate for lesions such as irregular clusters of microcalcification (fig. 2.31).

The needle (with trocar in place) should be rotated as it is advanced to prevent deviation caused by the angle of the bevel. The tip of the needle should initially be placed deep to the lesion being sampled by decreasing the Z-axis appropriately and a check-position film taken to confirm that the needle is in the correct position. The aspirations should proceed while this check-position film is being processed. Should the position be incorrect on the film then adjustments can be performed at this stage.

Suction is applied using a 10- or 20-ml-syringe attached to the needle via an extension

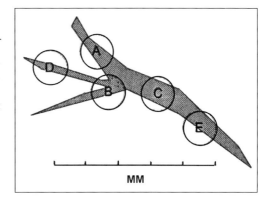

Figure 2.31, explanation see left

tube. Aspiration is preformed by passing the needle up and down vertically through the lesion, rotating the needle during each pass to use the needle bevel as a cutting edge. Only four to five passes are necessary with each needle. A characteristic "feel" as the lesion is transfixed is often appreciated (see below). With experience it is often possible to tell whether a good cellular specimen has been obtained from the appearance of the smear on the slide (see below).

 Suction must be released before the needle is withdrawn from the breast.

After each aspiration the syringe and needle is passed immediately to the MLSO, or other assistant who will prepare the specimen. Only two or three slides are necessary for each aspirate. While the MLSO prepares the slides the radiologist continues with the needle aspirations. The check film will be available at this stage and adjustments of position can be made if necessary. At least two, and up to five, separate aspirations should be performed using the pattern outlined in figure 2.30, pg. 75. The needle holder is repositioned appropriately for each pass using the check position film as a guide. A new needle is used for each aspirate.

Notes

If slides are smeared immediately and no check of adequacy of aspiration is available, then the

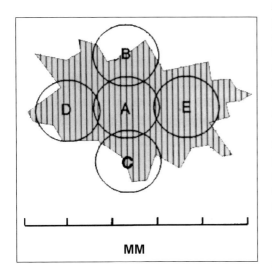

Figure 2.30, explanation see above

residue of each aspirate can be flushed into a transport medium. This sample can then be analysed after cyto-spinning if the slides fail to provide a diagnostic sample.

With bloody aspirates clotting occurs very rapidly in the needle making the slides difficult to prepare and interpret. A small amount of a bloody aspirate should be smeared on no more than two glass slides. The remainder of the aspirate can be washed into transport medium for later cytospin or cell block preparation.

If there is profuse bleeding (e. g. an arteriole has been inadvertently ruptured) FNAC should be abandoned and repeated after an interval of two to three weeks otherwise reactive changes may produce cytological difficulties (see pitfall organising haematoma, pg. 83).

If there is any doubt about whether the correct area has been sampled a small volume of non-ionic radio-opaque contrast medium may be injected down a new aspiration needle at the end of the procedure. The site of the contrast on mammography will indicate the area aspirated.

Ultrasound Guided Procedures

The technique required for ultrasound guided FNAC is very similar to that used for X-ray guided procedures but is inherently more flexible. As previously mentioned, ultrasound guided aspiration is much less time consuming and easier for both the patient and the aspirator. It is also very accurate as it allows direct real-time visualisation of the area being aspirated. The aspirator can be confident that the correct area has been sampled.

Equipment

A probe with a needle guide is helpful but by no means essential. Various probes are available depending on the manufacturer of the equipment resolution is optional with probes in the 7.5 to 10 MHz range. With experience most ultrasound aspirators will find that they require neither echogenic needles nor needle-guide attachments to achieve accurate sampling.

Make sure all the equipment is ready to use. Fully explain the procedure to the patient. Again, it should be emphasised that several aspirates may need to be performed.

Localise the lesion using the probe, set-up for the aspiration, and select the best approach. Avoid having to pass the needle through the nipple/areola area as this is often very painful. Use local anaesthetic if you or the patient feel that it is required.

Clean the ultrasound probe with an appropriate sterile solution. The same sterile solution is applied to the breast over the area through which the needles will pass. Alcohol-based sterile solutions are a convenient and effective means of both sterilising the skin and providing sterile acoustic coupling between the probe and skin. Ultrasound jelly may present a problem in interpretation for pathologists seeing it for the first time and should not be confused with calcium salts or necrosis.

 It should not be used during the aspiration procedure and, if used previously, should be carefully removed.

Advance the needle, under direct vision, into the breast until the tip lies just superficial to the lesion being samples. (Sound reflecting needles are commercially available to ease the identification of the tip of the needle within the breast but are not usually necessary.)

Once the needle is adjacent to the lesion being sampled, an extension tube and syringe are attached to the needle. As the aspirator must hold the ultrasound probe in one hand while manipulating the needle with the other, an assistant is needed to apply suction while the needle is passed up and down through the lesion. An alternative method is to use an aspiration syringe holder which is commercially available. This avoids the need for an extension tube or an assistant to apply suction, although an assistant is still necessary to deal with the specimen once obtained. Unlike stereotactic FNAC, the needle tack can be varied with each pass. The needle should be rotated as it is advanced. Continue to aspirate for 10 to 15 seconds or until material appears in the needle hub.

Suction must be released before the needle is withdrawn from the breast.

Sample preparation is the same as described above. If FNAC repeatedly fails to produce an adequate sample, ultrasound or X-ray guidance can also be used to obtain needle histology ("Tru-cut" or similar cutting biopsy needle).

Sampling of Lesions – Additional Information

Some breast lesions give a characteristic "feel" on the needle as it traverses the lesion. This can on occasion be a very helpful pointer as to whether the lesion has been truly sampled or not.

There are conveniently described as:
- No resistance = Fatty tissue
- Soft = Fibroadenoma, mucoid carcinoma, medullary carcinoma
- Rubber = Fibrocystic changes, lobular carcinoma, fibroadenoma
- Hard = Fibrous tissue, hyalinised fibroadenoma
- Gritty = Carcinoma, microcalcified tissue
- Cystic = Cyst in fibrocystic change.

Complications of FNAC

FNAC is remarkable complication-free, however certain rare problems should be considered.

Haematoma

All imaging investigations should be complete before FNAC is performed as haematoma formation, if it occurs, can cause confusion on subsequent mammography or ultrasound. Haematomas may cause problems especially if a larger vessel is punctured. In some cases the procedure may have to be abandoned and re-aspiration delayed until a later clinic visit as once a large haematoma has formed the lesion may no longer be localisable. Haematoma formation may not be painful for the patient at the time but often becomes so later and a recommendation for light analgesia e. g. Paracetamol may be appropriate.

Pneumothorax

This is a rare complication [12] found mainly in women with small breasts, in medial lesions, or when aspirating axillary nodes. It is not a problem with imaging aspiration such as stereotaxis or perforated plate and should not occur with an experienced ultrasound operator as the position of the needle can be seen. It is therefore more likely to occur with palpable lesions and with an experienced aspirator as the neophyte tends to be rather circumspect and, if anything, tends not to go deep enough. Large pneumothoraces should be obvious but the problem may go undetected if the pneumothorax is small. Subtle clues such as sharp pain, coughing or a hiss of air on withdrawing the needle without evidence of air in the syringe, may occur.

Fainting

This complication occasionally occurs during fine needle aspiration. It is of special significance during stereotaxis or perforated plate examinations where the patient has to be released from the machine and laid flat. The procedure usually has to be abandoned.

Preparing the Smears

Two or more slides are labelled in pencil with the patient's name and number before the aspirate is attempted and a spreader slide (which may be stained) is placed ready to spread the aspirate. The needle is removed from the syringe and air is drawn into the syringe barrel. Aspirated material is expelled slowly from the needle bore onto the labelled slides, a drop on each, near the labelled end. A variety of spreading methods may be used as illustrated in appendix 2, pg. 180. The action of spreading should be performed without undue downward pressure.

 The two slides should not be crushed together as this produces severe artefacts which preclude cytological diagnosis.

Fixing the Smears (See Appendix 3)

Fixation methods are critical and should be applied in consultation with the pathologist. There are two main fixation methods – air-drying and wet fixation – as described in appendix 3, pg. 181.

Fixation should be performed immediately after spreading as delay can lead to fixation artefacts precluding cytological interpretation.

The slide for wet-fixation is dropped immediately after spreading into a pot of alcohol or methanol, or can be sprayed with a fixative. Spraying must be performed carefully at a reasonable distance otherwise the material can all be washed to the edges of the slide and there become heaped up.

Air-dried smears should be spread thinly in a similar manner to allow rapid drying. Drying can be enhanced by wafting in air or using a hair drier on a cold setting.

Although not reliable the character of the spread slide may give a clue as to whether the sample is adequate (table 2.12).

The slides can then be sent to the laboratory, with a properly completed form, or stained immediately if there is a pathologist or MLSO present.

 The better the material and clinical information provided, the more reliable will be the cytological opinion.

The use of a transport medium (see section on equipment) into which the syringe and attached needle are washed out, and from which centrifuged or cytospin preparations are made, has several advantages. The preparative artefacts due to smearing can be avoided (see pg 181). The standardised method of preparation makes cytological interpretation and comparisons of cell size less subject to variations in smear technique. Multiple cytospin preparations can be made for further investigation by immunocytochemistry, for example for steroid receptor expression, and for teaching purposes.

Cyst fluids need only be looked at if bloodstained, turbid, or if a lump persists. A lump persisting after cyst drainage should be reaspirated. It is useful to send nipple discharges to the laboratory for cytological examination especially if these are bloodstained.

Using the Cytopathology Reporting Form

The cytopathology reporting form used may be the separate reporting form (figure 2.32) or the form generated specifically by the National Breast Screening System (see Appendix 2.2.3, pg. 164) which comes with the patient details already filled in by the computer. These both request essentially the same information although the computer generated form has spaces for radiographic information such as kV, mAs, side and type of localisation (palpable, ultrasound, stereotactic or other X-ray guided procedure) in the upper portion.

It may not be possible for the cytologist to enter certain details on the forms such as name of aspirator and type of procedure if they have not performed the aspirate themselves or have not been provided with the information on a request form.

Please note that due to a conversion error in the National Screening System some results recorded before January 1991 may be miscoded. See appendix 4, pg. 182, for further details.

Table 2.12, explanation see above

Oily drops	Fat (there may be occasional cells)
Clear fluid drying quickly into a granular appearance	Fibroadenoma, fibrocystic change, some carcinoma
Lightly or heavily blood stained with clumps of material	Carcinomas, inadvertent puncture of blood vessel with clotting
Thick viscous material difficult to expel from syringe	Inspissated cyst, mucoid carcinoma

			Figure 2.32: Computer Generated Form
Date performed:	Location:	Aspirator:	
Side:			
LOCALISATION TYPE	Comment (maximum 66 characters)		
kV:			
Total mAs:			
Total exposures:			
Total films:			
	Cyst aspiration without cytology:		
FNA CYTOLOGY			
Date reported:			
Specimen number:	Comment (maximum 132 characters)		
Specimen type:			
AS FNA (Solid) AC FNA (Cyst)			
ND Nipple discharge			
NS Nipple or skin scraping			
Cytological opinion			
C1 Unsatisfactory	C3 Atypia. probably benign	C5 Malignant	
C2 Benign	C4 Suspicious of malignancy		
OVERALL OPINION	Date:	Responsibility:	
Comment (max. 132 characters)			
	Opinion: R:	L:	
	Action:		
	(ES/EC)	Early recall interval:	
	(RF)	Referred to:	

Recording Basic Information

Centre/Location. Give the name of the assessment centre, clinic, department etc., where the specimen was obtained.

Side. Indicate right or left. For specimens from both sides use a separate form for each slide.

Specimen Type. Please choose one of the following terms:
- FNA (solid lesion): Fine needle aspiration of a solid lesion
- FNA (cyst): Fine needle aspiration of a cyst subjected to cytological examination
- Nipple discharge: Cytological preparation of a nipple discharge
- Nipple or skin: Cytological preparation of nipple or skin scrapings.

Localisation Technique. Please choose one of the following terms:

- Palpation: FNA guided by palpation
- Ultrasound guided: FNA guided by ultrasound
- X-ray guided: FNA guided by X-ray examination.

Please note that on the pre-printed form (figure 2.32) stereotaxis is included in this category while on the computer generated form there are two codes: S for stereotaxis and X for perforated plate or other X-ray guided method.

Pathologist. The name of the pathologist giving the cytological opinion, who must be registered at the screening office.

Aspirator. Enter the name of the person performing the fine needle aspiration.

Date. Enter the date of reporting the slides.

Case for Review. This is a field to indicate that a specimen has been sent for a further opinion or that the case is a particularly interesting example.

Recording the Cytology Opinion. See the section on reporting categories below. A comment field is included for extra information to be recorded. This is free text.

Reporting Categories

In the ideal circumstances one should aim towards a definitive diagnosis of malignancy or benignity. The proportion where this is possible will increase with the experience of both pathologist and aspirator.

C1 Inadequate. Indicates a scanty or acellular specimen or poor preparation. The designation of an aspirate as "inadequate" is to a certain extent a subjective matter and may depend on the experience of the aspirator and/or the interpreter.

Poor cellularity (usually less than five clumps of epithelial cells) is sufficient to declare an aspirate inadequate. Preparative artefacts or excessive blood may also be reasons for rejecting an aspirate as inadequate.

Preparative artefacts include:
- Crush, when too much pressure is used during smearing.
- Drying, when the dry smears are allowed to dry too slowly (dry smears should be dried quickly, wafting in the air can speed up drying) or when the wet-fixed smears have been allowed to dry out before fixation.
- Thickness of smear, when an overlay of blood, protein rich fluid or cells is obscuring the picture, making assessment impossible.

It is often helpful to make a comment as to the cause of inadequate specimens in the comment box on the form.

C2 Benign. Indicates an adequate sample showing no evidence of malignancy and, if representative, a negative report. The aspirate in this situation is often poorly to moderately cellular and tends to consist mainly of regular duct epithelial cells. These are generally arranged as monolayers and the cells have the characteristic benign cytological features. The background is usually composed of dispersed individual and paired naked nuclei. Should cystic structures be a component of the aspirated breast, then a mixture of foamy macrophages and regular apocrine cells may be part of the picture. Fragments of fibrofatty and/or fatty tissue are common findings.

A positive diagnosis of specific conditions, for example: fibroadenoma, fat necrosis, granulomatous mastitis, lymph node etc, may be suggested if sufficient features are present to establish the diagnosis with confidence.

C3 Atypia Probably Benign [13]. The aspirate here can have all the characteristics of a benign aspirate as described in the previous paragraph. There are however, in addition, certain features not commonly seen in benign aspirates. There could be any, or a combination of the following:
- Nuclear pleomorphism
- Some loss of cellular cohesiveness
- Nuclear and cytoplasmic changes resulting from e.g. hormonal (pregnancy, pill, HRT) or treatment influences (See diagnostic pitfalls). Increased cellularity may accompany the above features.

C4 Suspicious of Malignancy. The pathologist's opinion is that the material is not diagnostic of malignancy. This may be for three main reasons:
- The specimen is scanty, poorly preserved or poorly prepared, but some cells with features of malignancy are present.
- The sample may show some malignant features without overt malignant cells present. The degree of abnormality should be more severe than in the previous category.
- The sample has an overall benign pattern with large numbers of naked nuclei and/or cohesive sheets of cells, but with occasional cells showing distinct malignant features.

C5 Malignant. Indicates an adequate sample containing cells characteristic of carcinoma, or other malignancy. The interpreter should feel at ease in making such a diagnosis. Malignancy should not be diagnosed on the basis of a single criterion. Combination of the features listed in table 2.13, pg. 81, will be necessary to achieve this diagnosis. Some forms of calcification may not be visible on routine staining e.g. calcium oxalate, but may be visible using polarised light.

Calcification. It is very useful for the radiologist if the pathologist reports the presence of calcification within specimens taken from stereotactic or perforated plate guided FNAC when the abnormality is one of mammographic microcalcification. If calcification is present in these circumstances the radiologist or multidisciplinary team can be more certain that the lesion has been sampled accurately and that the likelihood of a false negative due to an aspiration miss is lower. This may allow the team to advise that the woman be returned to routine recall or early rescreen rather than biopsy with greater confidence.

Calcification alone does not discriminate between benign and malignant conditions.

General Diagnostic Patterns

The essential role of cytological diagnosis is to distinguish benign from malignant processes. The common general criteria used are illustrated in table 2.13. It is important to bear in mind that the morphological and histological patterns seen in both benign and malignant breast disease are quite varied, and this is reflected in the cytological appearances. For this reason, it is useful to have a working understanding of breast histology before approaching breast fine needle aspiration cytology. This knowledge can improve recognition of rare lesions and reduce numbers of false positive and negative diagnoses.

Table 2.13: General Diagnostic Criteria for the Recognition of Benign and Malignant Conditions

Criterion	Benign	Malignant
Cellularity	Usually poor or moderate	Usually high
Cell to cell cohesion	Good with large defined clusters of cells	Poor with cell separation resulting in dissociated cells with cytoplasm or small groups of intact cells
Cell arrangement	Even, usually in flat sheets (monolayers)	Irregular with overlapping and three-dimensional arrangement
Cell types	Mixtures of epithelial, myoepithelial and other cells with fragments of stroma	Usually uniform cell population
Bipolar (elliptical) bare nuclei	Present, often in high numbers	Not conspicuous
Background	Generally clean except in inflammatory conditions	Occasionally necrotic debris and sometimes inflammatory cells including macrophages
Nuclear characteristics		
Size (in relation to RBC diameter)	Small	Variable, often large depending on type of tumour
Pleomorphism	Rare	Common
Nuclear membranes (PAP stain)	Smooth	Irregular with indentions
Nucleoli (PAP stain)	Indistinct or small and single	Variable but may be prominent, large and multiple
Chromatin (PAP stain)	Smooth or fine	Clumped and may be irregular
Additional features	Apocrine metaplasia, foamy macrophages	Mucin, intracytoplasmic lumina

Diagnostic Pitfalls in Interpretation

Potentially false positive and suspicious diagnoses

Common Conditions

Lactational Changes. Even in the screening age group focal lactational changes can occur. This is uncommon but can produce occasional dissociated cells within an otherwise benign appearing smear. The dissociated cells may possess nucleoli and have larger nuclei than the surrounding benign cells. They do however have a moderate quantity of pale blue cytoplasm on Giemsa staining with lipid droplets in the cytoplasm. Caution in interpreting occasional dissociated cells in an otherwise benign pattern should be exercised even in the screening age range and the question "could these be lactational/secretory cells" should be specifically asked in these cases. Outside the screening age a history of pregnancy/lactation should always be sought and clinicians should always tell the pathologist of lactation or pregnancy.

Atypical Hyperplasia Within a Radial Scar or Papilloma/Adenoma.

This is a potential pitfall even with the triple approach to breast cancer. The lesion may appear mammographically worrisome and cytologically may product dissociated cells suspicious of malignancy. In general the smears, however, lack the cellularity of smears from carcinomas. The temptation to diagnose malignancy in poorly cellular smears is best avoided unless there is absolutely no doubt. A suspicious or atypical report or re-aspiration is preferable.

Apocrine Cells. Apocrine cells in smears may appear rather pleomorphic and may dissociate. Degenerate apocrine cells in cyst fluids may also have a rather worrisome appearance. Recognition of the dusty blue cytoplasm, with or without cytoplasmic granules with Giemsa stains or pink cytoplasm on Papanicolaou or Haematoxylin & Eosin stains coupled with the prominent central nucleolus is the key to identifying cells as apocrine. Awareness of the marked pleomorphism which may occur in degenerate apocrine cells and careful assessment of the cellularity and chromatin pattern should allow the distinction from the rare apocrine carcinoma. If there is doubt about the nature of apocrine cells it is better to err on the side of caution and give a suspicious or atypical report.

One particularly difficult lesion is atypical apocrine change in sclerosing adenosis [14], especially if this is associated, as it often is, with a complex sclerosing lesion or radical scar giving a mammographically worrying appearance. In this case the highly pleomorphic apocrine cells may not always appear obviously apocrine in smears. Features which may be helpful are the abundant cytoplasm with granules and the absence of necrosis. Spindling of cells in the centre of the clumps (myoepithelial cells from the sclerosing adenosis) surrounded by or intermingled with the atypical apocrine cells may be seen.

Fibroadenoma. Smears from fibroadenoma may give very worrisome appearance with marked pleomorphism and some dissociation. Fortunately this usually happens in actively growing lesions in teenage women rather than in the screening age range. The clue to the diagnosis is the presence of "stripped" bipolar nuclei. Smears containing these in significant numbers should not be diagnosed as malignant unless there are clear features of a benign epithelial lesion (with benign epithelial clumps) and also malignant clumps and dissociated malignant cells recognisable as a distinctly separate cell population. These smears, where the needle has passed through both a benign and a malignant lesion may be very difficult but the two distinct populations of epithelial cells should aid their recognition. Smears from some malignant tumours contain bare nuclei. These bare or stripped nuclei are not bipolar and have obvious malignant features identical to co-existing intact tumour cells. Often in fibroadenomas two cell types can be recognised in the cell clumps, even in the rather pleomorphic examples. Sometimes metachromatic stroma can be seen.

Radiotherapy Changes. These can lead to a false positive cytological diagnosis especially when the history of previous irradiation is not provided. The aspirate, however, is not very cellular and the interpretation of poorly cellular smears especially with a history or irradiation should be undertaken with caution as in item 3. Irradiation can cause marked nuclear pleomorphism and dissociation. Mammography may also be unhelpful or even false positive.

Organising Haematoma. This has been described as a pitfall by Oertel in her book [15] on Breast FNAC. Again the smears were not very cellular and the haemosiderin was interpreted as melanin leading to an erroneous diagnosis of metastatic melanoma. Problems can arise in aspirates taken shortly after a previous aspiration. This is due to the presence of activated macrophages and fibroblasts involved in the repair process. Re-aspiration should not be performed until two to three weeks after a previous aspirate in order to let this reaction settle.

Intra-Mammary Lymph Nodes. These should not cause a problem if the pathologist recognises the cells as lymphoid. Awareness that these can occur and can be aspirated should be enough to avoid an error. Lymphomas may be more difficult to distinguish from carcinoma but the lack of clumps should suggest the possibility and careful assessment including immunocytochemistry should distinguish the occasional carcinoma which shows almost complete dissociation with a rather plasmacytoid appearance. We have seen two examples of bone marrow in an aspirate of a lesion stated to be in the breast; the origin of this was unknown but assumed to be rib or myelolipoma. Neither of these lesions has been removed.

Atypical Lobular Hyperplasia [16]. If the needle enters an area of atypical lobular hyperplasia then cells with the characteristic appearance of lobular carcinoma cells may be obtained. These cells may have more rounded nuclei than the more usual squared nuclei with protrusions ("noses") seen in lobular carcinoma. (See also below: Columnar cell change)

 It should be borne in mind that, on cytological grounds alone, it is impossible to distinguish between atypical lobular hyperplasia and malignant lobular lesions.

Spreading Artefacts. Excessive pressure during the spreading of slides may produce dissociation of cells from benign clumps. If the cells within these clumps are also somewhat pleomorphic due to degenerative or atypical changes, then the dissociation may cause the cells to resemble dissociated malignant cells. The clue to this is often the finding of nuclear lysis and trails of chromatin due to the over-spreading artefact. Fibroadenomas are the most likely lesions to produce these problems when over-spread.

Columnar Cell Change Within Lobules ("Blunt Duct Adenosis"). This may produce dissociation and some authors have noted that the cells may resemble lobular carcinoma cells. Some of the cells are columnar in nature resembling bronchial epithelial cells. (See also above: Atypical lobular hyperplasia.)

Degenerate Cells in Cyst Fluids. Degeneration of cells within cysts can give pleomorphic appearances especially when these are larger apocrine cells. Cautious interpretation of cells within degenerate cysts is advised.

Uncommon Lesions

Granulomatous mastitis. Epithelioid macrophages in granulomatous mastitis can mimic carcinoma cells. They are associated with other inflammatory cells in the smear and numerous macrophages may be seen. The smear is also very cellular. In the presence of inflammation and a cellular smear the finding of multinucleate macrophages should alert the observer to the possibility of granulomatous mastitis. The rare cribriform carcinomas with multinucleate giant cells do not usually contain other inflammatory cells and are therefore distinguishable from granulomatous mastitis by their dimorphic picture of small malignant cells in clumps and singly and more basophilic "osteoclast-like" giant cells with larger nuclei and prominent nucleoli. Mononuclear forms of the multinucleate cells may also be present.

Granular Cell Tumour. This can present a worrisome appearance in smears. There is marked dissociation of cells which, although they have small nuclei, may contain occasional larger nuclei giving a pleomorphic appearance. The cells however do not look epithelial and benign epithelial clumps are seen between the dissociated cells of the tumour. The cells have eosinophilic granular cytoplasm on Papanicolaou or Haematoxylin & Eosin staining and a rather mottled pale mauve cytoplasm on Gismo stains looking rather similar to apocrine cells.

Adenomyoepithelial Lesions. These difficult and as yet incompletely understood lesions can show malignant cytological features because of dissociation of rather pleomorphic cells – which are in fact myo-epithelial. However obvious benign clumps and bipolar bare nuclei are present.

Collagenous Spherulosis [17, 18]. This lesion produces rounded globules staining a granular purple colour on Giemsa stains with surrounding spindle cells. There is a resemblance to adenoid cystic carcinoma with which the lesion can be confused. Biopsy in these rare conditions is advised.

Microglandular Adenosis [19]. This is reported due to tubulare formation as being a potential problem in diagnosis.

Adenoma of The Nipple. This has been stated to be a problem in some cases (Lindholm – personal communication).

Potentially false negative diagnosis

The most common cause of false negative cytological diagnosis is an aspiration miss. There are, however, types of carcinoma [20] which, by their nature, may produce a false negative diagnosis. The commonest of these are the following.

Tubular Carcinoma [21]. Tubular carcinoma cells often have much in common with benign breast epithelial cells, including uniformity, nuclear size and, often, absence of immediately obvious nuclear abnormalities. Knowledge of the mammographic findings, a lack of bare nuclei, individual cells with cytoplasm and occasional tubular profiles are pointers to the diagnosis. Paradoxically, the nuclei are often more regular and orderly than benign ductal epithelium and there is a single cell population in the clumps. Often it is not possible to give an unequivocal diagnosis but care should always be taken in interpreting smears from stellate opacities to avoid false negative results from this type of tumour. It should be noted that tubules can occasionally be obtained from benign lesions including radial scars [19, 21].

Lobular Carcinoma [16, 20]. Aspirates from this type of carcinoma are often difficult to interpret. The cellularity of these specimens is usually less than that seen in "ductal" carcinoma. A number of these patterns can be observed, ranging in cytological appearance from benign-looking uniform cells to atypical cells not dissimilar to those seen in invasive "ductal" carcinoma. The presence of small three-dimensional collections of cells with only slightly enlarged nuclei is helpful. A large number of cells with intracytoplasmic lumina (private acini) in association with the above features, is an indication of lobular carcinoma, although not specific. Nuclear irregularities and small protrusions from the nucleus ("noses") may also be seen. In some cases the nuclei are very small, less than 10 mm.

Apocrine Carcinoma. This rare type of carcinoma produces cellular smears. Difficulty in interpretation is related to the subtle appearance of the neoplastic apocrine cells and their resemblance to benign apocrine cells with degenerative changes. Clustering of cells and papillary formations are seen in benign as well as malignant lesions and are of little help. The key features of a malignant aspirate are the uniform cell population with nuclear atypia which one should not confuse with degenerative changes. Necrosis is also a helpful feature. Until one is aware of the marked atypical changes associated with apocrine cells in fibrocystic change the diagnosis of apocrine carcinoma should always be approached with caution.

Ductal Carcinoma In-Situ

 It should be noted that ductal carcinoma in-situ and invasive "ductal" carcinoma cannot be distinguished by cytology alone.

While some of the cases of ductal carcinoma in-situ are overtly malignant, the small cell type may present a diagnostic dilemma. The cellularity of these samples is moderate, never as cellular as frank carcinomas. One should be guided by the increased nuclear/cytoplasmic ratio in the presence of normal size cells. The abnormal nuclear chromatic pattern is a clue to the real nature of the lesion. The presence of some necrotic debris in the background should alert the interpreter to the possible malignant nature of the lesion. A clue in some cases can be obtained from the architectural pattern within the rather rigid and monomorphic clumps. In some cases a report of intraductal proliferation (atypical or suspicious) may be all that can be given and in such cases biopsy may be the only way to resolve the problem.

Carcinoma with Extensive Fibro-Elastosis. These tumours may give sparsely cellular smears which can lead to difficulties in diagnosis. Often it is not possible to be definitive and the need for caution in the interpretation of poorly cellular smears is again emphasised. Clear evidence of malignancy should be present in more than just a few cells.

Other Unusual Lesions

Silicone or Paraffin Granuloma. This may occasionally be problematic because of cell dissociation but the appearances are made easier with the recognition of multinucleate cells and oil or silicone droplets in the cytoplasm of the macrophages. Clinical data will be helpful here and clinicians should understand the need to supply the pathologist with proper clinical information on all breast lumps sampled by FNAC.

Benign Stromal Lesions. These lesions are occasionally aspirated when they produce an irregular mass on mammography or palpation. One of the more usual lesions to be mistaken for carcinoma radiologically is fibromatosis. On aspiration there are small numbers of stromal cells which are dissociated from each other. The cells are spindle in shape and have regular nuclear characteristics.

Phyllodes Tumours. The benign variants of phyllodes tumour may not be recognised as such on fine needle aspiration and may give a picture similar to fibroadenoma. Clues to the diagnosis include the presence of intact stromal cells, occasionally with nuclear abnormalities, and the finding of pieces of cellular mucoid connective tissue in the aspirate. Fibroadenomas can also show both these features however and the recognition of benign phyllodes tumours often depends on clinical and sonographic features. Occasionally phyllodes tumours can produce a false positive diagnosis of malignancy as can fibroadenomas. Malignant phyllodes tumours show a pattern of benign-appearing epithelial clumps with spindle cells showing obvious malignant nuclear features.

Metastatic Tumours. Metastatic tumours in the breast should always be considered in FNAC where a peculiar pattern unusual for breast tumours is seen. Melanoma and oat cell carcinoma are the most common. In melanoma, pigment and large intranuclear cytoplasmic inclusions may be visible. Ovarian metastases are often papillary with psammoma bodies (an uncommon feature of breast tumours), large clear cells full of glycogen may suggest a renal metastasis, squamous carcinoma cells may be from a primary breast lesion but may also be from a metastatic lesion etc. The triple approach may often resolve this problem also.

Lymphoma. The recognition of the lymphoid nature of an apparent primary breast tumour depends on the recognition of the spectrum of lymphoid cell types and the absence of clumps of cells. Immunocytochemistry may be necessary in some cases.

Malignant Stromal Tumours (Sarcoma). The commonest sarcoma to be aspirated in the breast is the angiosarcoma. This can show variable cytologic features but is often accompanied by a large amount of blood. Clumps of cells may occasionally be seen but the pattern is often that of malignant appearing or ovoid cells.

Malignant fibrous histiocytoma also gives a picture of dissociated malignant spindle cells. The major diagnostic dilemma is between metaplastic carcinoma and sarcoma and when this is a problem immunocytochemistry for epithelial markers may be necessary.

Prognostic Information

Currently breast FNAC samples are used predominantly for diagnostic purposes. In some centres, however, research studies have indicated that additional evaluation may be possible on this type of sample:
- Oestrogen and progesterone receptor immunocytochemical assays can be performed on direct smears or cytocentrifuge preparations [23, 24]. It must be borne in mind that these are labile soluble antigens and preparative methods are critical.
- Grading systems using microscopic or image cytometric methods can be applied to cytological samples [25, 26]. These studies have indicated that morphological characteristics of tumour cells can be used to provide information which is related to histological grade or to overall prognosis.
- While the histological type of tumours may be reflected in the cytological appearances, one must bear in mind that the stringent criteria used to define many histological types are based on purity of tumour and architectural features. For these reasons, although sometimes a type can be suggested, consistent typing of breast tumours is not, as yet, possible.
- Calculation of standard deviation of nuclear area has been evaluated as a method of increasing sensitivity of diagnosis [27] but is not generally used at present. It is thought by some workers to have prognostic significance.

Information on prognosis or receptors is used in some centres to determine optimum primary therapy where choices between surgery, primary chemotherapy and primary hormone therapy are being made. At present these types of investigation should be regarded as research applications and their efficacy in routine clinical practice is still to be determined.

Multidisciplinary Assessment and Decision-Making

The process of assessment of significant breast lesions involves the correlation of clinical, imaging and cytological/histological findings. This is best achieved in a multidisciplinary setting with the clinician, the radiologist and the pathologist discussing these findings together in open forum and reaching a consensus on the management of each case following predefined protocols. There are two schools of thought as to when this discussion should occur.

Some believe that, in the ideal situation, the decision-making process would be carried out in the clinic where the patient is first seen. The primary advantage is that the patient is made aware of the diagnosis, whether it be of malignancy or a benign process, with the minimum of delay at the time of the first presentation. The pathologist is also able to verify an adequate sample (including the presence of calcification in aspirates from microcalcification) and to suggest repeating the procedure where there is an inadequate or scanty yield of epithelial cells or when the cytological findings do not correlate with the radiology. This option requires that the pathologist, radiologist and surgeon must be freely available during the clinic and that, if malignant diagnoses are communicated to the woman, full support services, including nurse counselling, are provided. Women with benign disease can receive immediate reassurance avoiding a further clinic visit for results, with a resulting decrease in anxiety. It is not universally agreed that it is in the best interests of women with malignancy to receive the diagnosis immediately at a time when the support of relatives may not be available and it may be better to lead these women into the diagnosis gently by asking them to return to the clinic for a management plan at the next available clinic. These women can be told they will need the lesion removed and a full discussion can then occur at leisure between the clinicians to achieve the best management plan. This may be better than attempting to communicate the diagnosis immediately to the woman as many women require time to adjust to their circumstances before making rational decisions about treatment options with the surgeon and breast care nurse.

In the clinic situation it is essential that the pathologist is not put under undue pressure to provide an immediate definitive diagnosis in difficult or equivocal cases and, in these circumstances, a further aspiration will often yield more diagnostic material. The pathologist should resist any pressure to provide a diagnosis if he is uncertain.

It is often difficult to achieve the above and some believe that the decision-making process is best divorced from the clinic environment with the management of each case discussed at regular multidisciplinary meetings held in circumstances where all the relevant findings can be reviewed.

Who Should Take the Sample

The success of FNAC is directly related to the skill and experience of the aspirator [28] and there is strong evidence that the procedure is most successful when performed by a limited number of aspirators. In most circumstances FNAC can be successfully carried out when:
- Easily palpable breast abnormalities are sampled freehand by the designated experienced clinician who may be a pathologist.
- Clinically equivocal and impalpable abnormalities are sampled under image guidance by the radiologist. It may also be appropriate for the radiologist to sample lesions under image guidance when previous freehand aspiration has been unsuccessful.

The number of those performing FNAC in any one centre should be kept to a minimum and their performance audited as a matter of routine.

When resources allow it may be appropriate for the pathologist to become directly involved in the sampling procedure. This may be advantageous where there is no experienced clinical aspirator or where there are preparation problems, however it would be unusual for the pathologist to have sufficient knowledge of mammography and ultrasound to undertake image-guided biopsy procedures independently of the radiologist. The pathologist is most likely to become directly involved where the breast assessment team has decided to provide a same-day cytology service or where there are aspiration problems with a high percentage of inadequate specimens. It is probably not appropriate for FNAC to be carried out in a separate clinic set up solely for this purpose. This would only be cost-effective where the standard of aspiration would otherwise be poor and the pathologist has other symptomatic and non-breast aspirations referred to him.

Education and Training of Aspirators and Cytologists

Training and cytological diagnosis. National pathology training centres have been established in Edinburgh, Guildford and Nottingham as part of the National Health Service Breast Screening Programme initiative. The general activities of these centres have been summarised in previous screening Programme publications and Royal College reports [29].

The training and education sub-group of the National Co-ordinating Committee for Breast Screening Pathology has identified that breast screening pathology courses should include information about preoperative pathological investigations, particularly FNAC and that there is an urgent need for more specialist courses in breast FNAC which could involve collaboration with the British Society for Clinical Cytology (BSCC).

Courses in breast fine needle aspiration cytology are available in Edinburgh, Guildford, Nottingham and at the Royal Marsden Hospital, London. (See NHSBSP newsletter, *Network*, for details.) In addition the BSCC and other specialist centres now organise workshops or courses in fine needle aspiration cytology. (See BSCC and ACP course information literature.)

Centres involved in the screening programme in some regions also provide workshops for cytology QA which have a training and experience sharing function.

It is recognised that courses can only provide baseline knowledge and acceptable levels of performance in cytological diagnosis can only be realistically achieved by experience in routine practice. Ideally, experience should be gained through symptomatic breast work for a significant period before contemplating the reporting of impalpable lesions.

Experience can also be gained from aspiration of surgical specimens or imprint slides. Surgeons or radiologists should be encouraged to send specimens to training cytologists but the cytologist should only issue reports when adequate validation of the technique has been done. Under no circumstances should cytologists be pressured to report on breast FNAC until they themselves are happy with their level of training and experience.

Additional experience may be gained by secondment to neighbouring centres of expertise and by participating in regional External Quality Assurance (EQA) schemes.

Initiatives have been taken and the range of courses outlined above is considered at present to be appropriate for this need but will require evaluation on a regular basis.

Training and Aspiration Technique. The national training centres (see opposite) provide basic information on aspiration technique and some will provide personal hands-on experience as part of a secondment training. Some regional screening assessment centres also are willing to have observers at assessment clinics as a QA function for their region.

The Nottingham centre is planning to run regular courses on image guided FNAC technique from 1992.

Resource Implications

In the Forrest Report which was published in 1986 FNAC was not costed as an essential technique in breast cancer screening and indeed no detailed economic analysis has yet been performed on FNAC in screening in the UK. Time has demonstrated that a reduction in the number of benign biopsies and a reduction in second operations on cancer-bearing breasts can be achieved in centres which have a high level of expertise. This is borne out by the low benign biopsy figures reported by the Epping unit [3] as well as by the figures for benign to malignant ratios at open biopsy presented in the section on sensitivity and specificity.

The cost of outpatient investigation by cytology for symptomatic patients is of the order of one tenth of the cost of performing an open biopsy on a patient admitted to hospital (according to figures kindly provided by the John Radcliffe Hospital, Oxford). Other studies in the United States have discovered a similar reduction in costs of approximately 90% [30] and a recent good evaluation of the subject showing similar value in the UK can be seen in the recent article by Kocjan 1991 [31]. The FNA costs for stereotactic aspirations are higher (estimated at approximately double) but marker biopsy costs are also much higher. It is therefore apparent that the costs of FNAC, even if performed on several more patients than would otherwise have been subjected to open biopsy, is likely to be outweighed by the financial savings, even without taking into consideration the benefits in terms of reduced morbidity.

An estimate of the number of biopsies saved can be gained from the experience at Guildford looking specifically at stereotaxis [32]. The estimated benign to malignant ratio without stereotaxis in 250 cases of impalpable lesions based on the mammographic appearances alone would have been 1 to 0.94. The actual benign to malignant ratio achieved with stereotaxis was 1 to 2.5. In addition, seven extra cancers were discovered in the mammographic low risk group which would otherwise have not been biopsied at the first assessment.

The whole breast screening programme benefits from FNAC yet resources have not been redistributed to take account of this. Some laboratories have had to undertake extra work and extra training without extra funding. This is further compounded by the increasing use of FNAC in symptomatic services which, although not directly connected with the screening service, have improved in many centres as a consequence of the general raising of standards caused by the screening programme. District and Trust managers should be aware that FNAC can reduce surgical costs and should be aware of the need to transfer resources accordingly. This will be made easier as the large demands made on surgery during the start-up phases of screening programmes diminishes.

FNAC will be most effective within the framework of an integrated team approach to assessment and its quality must, like other aspects of the screening programme, be monitored.

Alternatives

The Forrest Committee and the National Co-ordinating Committee for Breast Screening Pathology are both of the firm opinion that there is no place for frozen section examination in the management of screen detected breast disease.

A number of groups have now shown that fine needle aspiration cytology can have an acceptable level of sensitivity and specificity in assessment and diagnosis of screen detected breast disease. In some assessment centres, the required level of cytology expertise may not be available; three main alternative approaches to assessment and diagnosis are available.

Pre-Operative Needle Biopsy. A number of needle biopsy instruments are now available which can obtain portions of breast tissue suitable for histological examination and diagnosis. In general these instruments are applicable to palpable abnormalities where the operator can fix the lesion manually and guide the cutting needle into it. The results of needle biopsy in symptomatic breast disease show a high level of sensitivity and specificity. There is currently little information on effectiveness in breast screening practice. Narrow bore cutting needles are available for image localisation needle biopsy, however these devices have not found wide acceptance as a high frequency of inadequate specimens have been experienced.

Some units use stereotactic and ultrasound guided core biopsy which may help to distinguish between in-situ and invasive lesions although one can never be sure that a representative area has been sampled.

Screw Needle or Fine Needle Aspiration Samples Processed to Histological Sections. Some centres have advocated processing of cytological screw needle tissue samples for histological examination. This approach is suitable for centres who wish to obtain pre-operative cellular samples but where there is insufficient cytological expertise available for interpretation of standard cytological preparations. Most assessment centres will have available routine histopathology services with the appropriate level of expertise for section preparation and diagnostic interpretation. Acceptable levels of sensitivity and specificity have been obtained in centres developing these techniques but at present there is little information from other centres choosing to adopt this methodology.

Diagnostic Surgical Biopsy. The Forrest model assessment process identified surgical biopsy of radiologically suspicious abnormalities as an appropriate technique. To ensure low levels of morbidity associated with biopsy it is essential that the volume of normal tissue removed around the suspicious abnormality is kept to a minimum and that there is a clear understanding that this is a diagnostic rather than a therapeutic procedure. Should a malignant process be identified through diagnostic biopsy, further therapeutic procedures can then be initiated. This method of diagnosis is recommended and adopted in many centres as the routine system or second line diagnostic system when fine needle aspiration cytology or needle biopsy histology have failed to obtain a satisfactory sample or given a non-contributory result.

Quality Assurance

Training. One of the major functions of quality assurance in breast cancer screening is the provision of training opportunities by discussion and circulation of slides. Some regions hold cytology sessions regularly where cases are seen and discussed in an informal meeting as a training exercise. There are also a number of courses run in breast cytology. Nottingham, Edinburgh and Guildford hold cytology courses as part of their national training function and there is a course run regularly at the Royal Marsden Hospital. National External Quality Assurance (EQA) schemes are in operation for cervical cytology but so far these have not been developed for breast cytology. EQA schemes are at present being developed on a regional basis.

Acceptable Levels of Sensitivity and Specificity. Many units have published figures of sensitivity and specificity of fine needle aspiration of palpable lesions in symptomatic practice and have clearly shown that there is a difference in both these measures depending on the experience and care of the aspirator. In units where the cytologist takes the aspirates and checks adequacy, sometimes giving an instant diagnosis, sensitivity and specificity are better with many fewer inadequate aspirates. Some units even use ultrasound or mammographically guided aspiration in palpable lesions where there is an inadequate aspirate to ensure that aspiration has been performed from the lesion.

Table 2.14, explanation see page 91

Absolute sensitivity (C5)	The number of carcinomas diagnosed as such (C5) expressed as a percentage of the total number of carcinomas aspirated.
Complete sensitivity	The number of carcinomas that were not definitely negative or inadequate on FNAC expressed as a percentage of the total number of carcinomas.
Specificity	The number of correctly identified benign lesions (the number of C2 results minus the number of false negatives) expressed as a percentage of the total number of benign lesions aspirated.
Positive predictive value of a C5 diagnosis	The number of correctly identified cancers (numbers of C5 results minus the number of false positive results) expressed as a percentage of the total number of positive results (C5).
Positive predictive value of a C4 diagnosis	The number of cancers identified as suspicious (number of C4 results minus the number of false suspicious results) expressed as a percentage of the total number of suspicious results (C4).
Positive predictive value of a C3 diagnosis	The number of cancers identified as atypia (number of C3 results minus the number of benign atypical results) expressed as a percentage of the total number of atypical results (C3).
False negative case	A case which subsequently turns out (over the next 3 years) to be carcinoma having had a negative cytology result (this will by necessity include some cases where a different area from the lesion was aspirated but who turn up with interval cancer).
False positive case	A case which was given a C5 cytology result who turns out at open surgery to have a benign lesion (including atypical hyperplasia).
False negative rate	The number of false negative results expressed as a percentage of the total number of carcinomas aspirated.
False positive rate	The number of false positive results expressed as a percentage of the total number of carcinomas aspirated.
Inadequate rate	The number of inadequate specimens expressed as a percentage of the total number of cases aspirated.

Cytology > Histology v	C5	C4	C3	C2	C1	Total
Total malignant	Box 1	Box 2	Box 3	Box 4	Box 5	Box 6
Invasive	Box 7	Box 8	Box 9	Box 10	Box 11	Box 12
Non-invasive	Box 13	Box 14	Box 15	Box 16	Box 17	Box 18
Total benign	Box 19	Box 20	Box 21	Box 22	Box 23	Box 24
No histology	Box 25	Box 26	Box 27	Box 28	Box 29	Box 30
Total C results	Box 31	Box 32	Box 33	Box 34	Box 35	Box 36
Total cases screened in period						
Total assessed						
Total FNAC performed						

Table 2.15, explanation see below

Definitions

The following calculations are intended to relate to the clinical evaluation of the effectiveness of FNAC rather than to evaluation of the laboratory component. Thus inadequate FNAC results are not excluded from the calculations as in some publications in the literature. Cytologists wishing to evaluate their statistics purely to see their own accuracy in diagnosis may wish to calculate the figures differently (table 2.14).

How to Calculate these Figures. It is intended that the computer system will be able to calculate these figures automatically from the data in the database cross-referencing with the histology or subsequent outcome and a report derived for quality assurance purposes (table 2.15):
- Cytology QA Standard Report
- Total cases screened in period
- Total assessed
- Total FNAC performed.

Each box (numbered 1 to 36) of the above table is calculated from the number of FNAC with a C code (C1, C2 etc) cross referenced with the worst histology diagnosis. The table and calculations (see below, table 2.16) should be produced for all FNAC tests (headed ALL TESTS) and also for all patients (headed ALL PATIENTS) where if two FNAC records are present the highest C number is taken. Only closed episodes should be used.

From the above table is then calculated the sensitivity and specificity in percentages for each of the categories in the cytology document. (Large numbers correspond to BOX NUMBERS in the above table.)

It is recognised that the specificities are approximate and will be more accurate the longer the date range of the analysis is from the date printed.

Suggested Minimum Values Where Therapy is Partially Based on FNAC.

- Absolute sensitivity (AS) > 60%
- Complete sensitivity (CS) > 80%
- Specificity (SPEC) > 60% (as calculated above; including non biopsied cases)
- Positive predictive value (+PV) > 95%
- False negative rate (F−) < 5%
- False positive rate (F+) < 1%
- Inadequate rate (INAD) < 25%
- Suspicious rate < 20%

These figures will obviously depend on aspiration techniques and the experience and care of the aspirator [27] and will vary widely between units. The figures are interrelated and strategy to improve one figure will affect others – thus if an attempt is made to reduce the inadequate rate this will often increase the number of suspicious reports, attempts to improve the specificity will increase the false negative rate and so on. Also attempts to reduce the benign biopsy rate by not biopsying the majority of lesions called benign cytology will reduce the specificity where this is based on benign histology results rather than on all aspirated cases.

A high proportion of impalpable cases aspirated in any series is likely to make the figures

Table 2.16: Symptomatic Cases

1 ABSOLUTE SENSITIVITY	=	$\dfrac{(1+25)}{6+25} \times 100$
(This assumes that all unbiopsied C5 results are carcinoma and are treated with primary chemotherapy or hormonal therapy.)		
2 COMPLETE SENSITIVITY	=	$\dfrac{1+2+3+25}{6+25} \times 100$
3 SPECIFICITY (biopsy cases only)	=	$\dfrac{22}{24} \times 100$
4 SPECIFICITY (full) (This assumes that all cases of atypia (C3) which are not biopsied are benign.)	=	$\dfrac{(22+28)}{24+27+28+29} \times 100$
5 POSITIVE PREDICTIVE VALUE (C5 diagnosis)	=	$\dfrac{31-19}{31} \times 100$
6 POSITIVE PREDICTIVE VALUE (C4 diagnosis)	=	$\dfrac{32-20-26}{32-26} \times 100$
7 POSITIVE PREDICTIVE VALUE (C3 diagnosis)	=	$\dfrac{3}{33} \times 100$
8 FALSE NEGATIVE RATE (This EXCLUDES inadequate results.)	=	$\dfrac{4}{6+25} \times 100$
9 FALSE POSITIVE RATE	=	$\dfrac{19}{6+25} \times 100$
10 INADEQUATE RATE	=	$\dfrac{35}{36} \times 100$
11 INADEQUATE RATE FROM CANCERS	=	$\dfrac{5}{6+25} \times 100$
12 SUSPICIOUS RATE	=	$\dfrac{32+33}{36} \times 100$

worse as there is more chance of missing a small area of microcalcification leading to a false negative or inadequate result and more likelihood of aspirating atypical hyperplasia, radial scars and tubular carcinomata, leading to a high level of suspicious or atypical reports. In screening with aspiration of impalpable lesions the results are likely to reveal lower values than those achieved in the symptomatic setting.

Some published date from the literature indicates what can be achieved with high quality cytology (table 2.17 and 2.18).

Table 2.17: Screening Cases – Data from Stereotaxis

No. of cases	Abs. sensit	Comp. sensit	Spec.	Positive pred. val	False negative rate	False positive rate	Inadequate rate	Aspir*	Ref. no.
1002	86.4%	97.3%	NS	100%	NS	0%	5.7%	Path	32
793	69%	80.7%	83.2%	100%	13.6%	0%	13%	Clin	33

NS = not stated; Aspir* = aspirator; Path = pathologists; Clin = clinician
NB: Despite the higher false negative rate in the first study [7] the addition of mammographic into the equation led to only one truly false negative case not biopsied. In two cases cancers developed in other quadrants subsequently and in five cases cancers developed contralaterally. The complete sensitivity of assessment in this multidisciplinary manner (including biopsy where mammography was sufficiently suspicious to override negative cytology) was therefore 99.7% – an excellent figure.

Table 2.18, explanation see page 92

No. of cases	Abs. sensit	Comp. sensit	Spec.	Positive pred. val	False negative rate	False positive rate	Inadequate rate	Type of lesion	Ref. no.
2594	55%	74.1%	56.5%	99.5%	19.5%	0.2%	8.6%*	Stereo	7
219	74.6%	93.6%	55.7%	100%	0%	0%	26%	Stereo	34
114	40%	93.3%	77.8%	100%	0%	0%	13.2%	Stereo	35
250	43.5%	69.4%	56.4%	100%	11.3%	0%	32%	Stereo	31

(Data have been recalculated from results given in the papers and represented as far as possible according to the definitions above.)
* as % of biopsied cases

In the last series [32] it is important to note that these are the figures obtainable on the early part of the learning curve. Other smaller series have been reported [37, 38] with varying results.

A breakdown into types of lesion in the studies above, where possible, illustrates a trend. Microcalcification was the least likely to yield a cellular sample and rounded opacities were most likely to be diagnosed correctly by cytology (table 2.19).

In screening it is important that good quality cytology is practised and if problems are encountered then corrective action is necessary. For example, in one screening unit the first 55 carcinomas detected were investigated with FNAC by clinical aspiration by multiple aspirators of varying experience.

Twenty-five of the 55 cases had FNAC and the results were poor due mainly to the smaller size of the lesions. Sixteen of the 54 benign cases biopsied were aspirated of which nine were inadequate specimens and only seven were diagnosed as benign in the same period. The total number of cases aspirated was 96. Impalpable lesions did not have cytology. Thirty-eight benign lesions were biopsied without having cytology:

- Absolute sensitivity: 32%
- Complete sensitivity: 52%
- Specificity (biopsied cases only): 43.8%
- False negative rate (as % of carcinomas): 8%
- Inadequate rate (biopsied cases only): 46.3%
- Positive predictive value: 100%
- Benign to malignant ratio at biopsy: 1.7:1.

Since then with X-ray, ultrasound and stereotactic guidance and clinical aspiration only by experienced staff these figures have been radically changed.

The next 89 carcinomas all had FNAC by one of the above methods including ductal carcinoma in-situ and impalpable lesions. Fifty-three benign cases were biopsied in the same period of which 13 were inadequate (C1). One false positive aspirate (C5) from a radical scar with apocrine atypia was seen in this period. Two highly suspicious diagnoses (C4) from atypical hyperplasia were seen. Eleven atypical (C3) aspirates (mainly from radical scars) were also present and 26 cases of benign (C2) cytology were biopsied for radiological or surgical

Table 2.19, explanation see above

No. of cases	Abs. sensit	Comp. sensit	Spec.	Positive pred. val	False negative rate	False positive rate	Inadequate rate	Type of lesion	Ref. no.
76	51.3%	87.9%	28%	100%	3.4%	0%	15.7%	Stellate	34+31
129	85.7%	100%	74.6%	100%	0%	0%	20.9%	Round	
237	48.1%	72.2%	49.7%	100%	0%	0%	32.6%	Microcalcif [12]	

reasons. The majority of cases with benign and some with inadequate cytology (fibrous tissue strands) were not biopsied (382 cases aspirated in this period). All lesions biopsied had FNAC by one or other of the localisation methods and most had immediate checking of adequacy of aspirates by "Diff-Quick" staining at assessment. The results were much improved:
- Absolute sensitivity: 70.8%
- Complete sensitivity: 92.1%
- Specificity (biopsied cases only): 48.1%
- False negative rate (as % of carcinomas): 4,5%
- Inadequate rate (biopsied cases only): 11.3%
- Positive predictive value: 98.4%
- Benign: malignant ratio at biopsy: 1:1.6.

Most of the cases returned to routine screening or early rescreen (243 cases) had benign cytology.

This shows there is little place for inexpert FNAC in breast screening but that with intensive use of FNAC including stereotaxis within assessment, good results similar to those in symptomatic cases is possible. This leads to substantial financial benefit but is expensive in terms of pathology time.

One study has shown that FNAC can still be cost-effective for tumour diagnosis even at a level of 37% absolute sensitivity.

Research

The research and development sub-group of the National Committee for Breast Screening Pathology have a role of identifying research and development areas.

Equipment manufacturers

- Syringe holders
  - Cameco Ltd. (Fits B&D plastic syringes 10cc) also available to fit either 10 or 20cc.
  - Nyegaard aspirator (Fits Sabre hard plastic syringes locc).
  - RH syringe holder (Fits B&D 10cc syringes) also available to fit 20cc syringes RH Medical Products. 11 504 College View Drive, Silver Spring, MD 20902–2501, USA.
- Screw needle instruments
  - Rotex Screew Needle Biopsy Instrument URSUS Konsult AB, Jungfrugatan 26, S11 444 Stockholm, Sweden.
- Transport medium
  - Cytospin Cell Fluid – Shandon Sciences Ltd. or Tissue culture medium.

References: Page 190

Membership of working group: see appendices 2.2.3, page 183

2.2.4
The Uniform Approach to Breast Fine Needle Aspiration Biopsy – A Synopsis[1,2]

Chairman: A. ABATI, USA

Introduction

The following is an outline-form synopsis of the guidelines for breast fine needle aspiration (FNA) biopsy developed and approved at a National Cancer Institute-sponsored conference in

---

[1] Publication: Developed and approved at a National Cancer Institute-sponsored conference, Bethesda, Maryland, USA (1996): The Uniform Approach to Breast Fine Needle Aspiration Biopsy – A Synopsis. Acta Cytologica 40(6): 1120–1126. Copyright © 1996 by the International Academy of Cytolog

[2] Developed and approved at a National Cancer Institute-sponsored conference, Bethesda, Maryland, USA, September 9–10, 1996, with representatives of the American Society of Cytopathology, Papanicolaou Society of Cytopathology, American College of Radiology, American College of Obstetricians and Gynecologists, American Academy of Familiy Physicians, Society of Surgical Oncology, College of American Pathologists, National Consortium of Breast Centers, International Academy of Cytology, American Society of Clinical Pathologists, American Cancer Society, American College of Surgeons and American Society for Cytotechnology. Reprint by permission
Address reprint requests to: Andrea Abati, M.D., Cytopathology Section, National Cancer Institute/ National Institutes of Health, Building 10, Room 2A19, 10 Center DR MSC 1500, Bethesda, Maryland 20892–1500

Bethesda, Maryland, USA, on September 9 and 10, 1996, with representatives of the American Society of Cytopathology, Papanicolaou Society of Cytopathology, American College of Radiology, American College of Obstetricians and Gynaecologists, Society of Surgical Oncology, American Academy of Family Physicians, College of American Pathologists, National Consortium of Breast Centers, International Academy of Cytology, American Society of Clinical Pathologists, American Cancer Society, American College of Surgeons and American Society for Cytotechnology. The guide-lines will be published in their entirety at a later date.

Indications

Indications for performance of FNA or core biopsies on palpable breast lesions

Sufficiently defined palpable breast masses of clinical or patient concern should be aspirated regardless of imaging findings where experienced FNA services are available.

Masses that can be clinically explained by normal anatomy and physiology, especially in young women, can be observed over the course of two menstrual cycles.

Any persistent or suspicious masses (asymmetry, fixed, not round, hard) or masses in patients with increased family risk factors should be biopsied regardless of the imaging findings.

Indications for performance of image-guided needle biopsy (FNA/core needle biopsy) on nonpalpable breast lesions

The recommendations for performing image-guided needle biopsy (IGNB) of a nonpalpable breast lesion detected by breast imaging are based on the availability of high-quality breast imaging performed by a physician qualified to interpret these images. The physician performing the biopsy should determine which type of needle biopsy and image guidance is most appropriate on a case-by-case basis.

Prior to IGNB of nonpalpable breast lesions, the following steps are indicated:
- A complete evaluation of the lesion with the appropriate imaging studies
- A careful physical examination of the breast, with special emphasis on the area detected by imaging, to ascertain if the lesion is, in fact, nonpalpable.

Lesions that may be subjected to IGNB include those that are highly suggestive of malignancy and suspicious for malignancy and some lesions at low risk for malignancy but for which the recommended follow-up with imaging is not feasible or accepted by the patient.

All imaging findings and key steps of the IGNB should be documented and recorded. A report of the procedure should be available.

The results of the imaging studies and (cyto)pathologic interpretation should be concordant. If not, further workup is needed (see Post-FNA recommendations), and the physician who performed the IGNB will make appropriate recommendation.

Communication between the physician who performed the IGNB and the referring physician and/or patient should be documented.

Follow-up of all IGNB should be done to record false positive and false negative results.

The accessibility of the lesion to stereotactic or ultrasound-guided biopsy is left to the judgement of the clinician performing the biopsy.

The decision to resort to an excisional, needle localization biopsy without a prior attempt at image-guided aspiration or core biopsy, and the determination of the need for an excisional biopsy in spite of a benign cytologic and/or histologic diagnosis by needle biopsy, are to be made by the clinician (see Post-FNA recommendations).

The presence of atypia on a cytologic or histologic preparation, the degree of which is to be determined by the pathologist, warrants an excisional biopsy.

FNA of both palpable and nonpalpable breast lesions may be an appropriate first diagnostic step since this procedure has been shown to be cost-effective.

The use of "blind" FNA on clinically normal-feeling breast tissue has been shown to be of no value in detecting occult breast carcinoma.

Pre-FNA evaluation should be recorded in a systematic manner.

The information required on the requisition form should include:
- Demographic data
- Clinical findings on the mass (size, location, circumscription, shape, fixation, changes in the overlying skin)
- History of prior chemotherapy, radiation or surgery
- History of the mass (all inclusive, including gynaecologic/lactational history)
- Imaging characteristics, including o'clock position and physical findings
- Family/personal history of breast carcinoma
- Hormonal history.

Obtaining written informed consent (IC) for FNA is considered an optional policy.

General guidelines in institutions/practices where obtaining written IC is required:
- Documentation of IC from each patient should be made.
- The content of the IC form may be tailored to the institutional/physician's practice/needs.
- The IC document should be retained permanently as part of the cytopathology files or patient's medical records.

Specific requirements to be contained on IC form:
- Patient's name
- Physician(s) performing procedure
- Patient's signature and date
- Statement of patient assent that the procedure, along with its risks and benefits, has been explained either verbally or through a descriptive brochure.
- Statement of patient assent that he/she is satisfied and that he/she has received sufficient information necessary to make an informed decision regarding the procedure.

The IC form may include statements regarding:
- Anaesthesia
- Signature of witness(es)
- Disclaimer on diagnostic accuracy
- Patient-oriented brochure or video for review prior to consent to the procedure
- Statements regarding the accuracy of the procedure (from medical literature, institution or individual physicians)
- Explanation to include information, including false negative and false positive diagnosis and complications.

Training and Credentialing

The FNA sampling procedure is highly operator dependent.

Factors contributing to successfully obtaining FNA specimens:
- Level of interest and training in FNA technique
- Volume of cases
- Immediate assessment of specimens by gross and microscopic evaluation
- Ongoing feedback regarding quality of specimens.

Recommendations for training requirements/prerequisites for physicians performing FNA of the breast

Sample acquisition. Physicians who perform breast FNA should include:
- appropriate selection of breast FNA subjects
- sample collection
- sample preparation.

Instruction and credentialing for sample collection should be "outcome based", not speciality based. Granting privileges to perform and report the results of breast FNA should be based on the comparison and concordance with surgical specimens from breast biopsies. Goal-based emphasis of instruction is on obtaining diagnostic material (i.e., cytohistologic correlation) in a reasonable number of cases. Merely defining a period of time spent on a cytopathology service, women's health or breast care service is an insufficient prerequisite of breast FNA credentialing.

Simulated sample specimens are recommended for initial training.

Outcome criteria for credentialing should consist of:
- The performance of a reasonable number of directly supervised breast FNAs without any resultant major morbidity, such as pneumothorax, yielding representative material sufficient for preparation in the great majority of the supervised procedures.
- After completion of a), the physician should prove competence in the successful preparation of a reasonable number of cytologic samples. Success would be considered the preparation of a sample that is deemed representative and interpretable by an experienced cytopathologist.
- If availability of an experienced teacher is limited, it is acceptable to initially use FNA in conjunction with open biopsy or very close clinical follow-up. After a reasonable and sufficient number of FNAs (at least 30) have been performed, evaluation of the cases done can be used for credentialing.

The first 20 FNAs after successful completion of formal, outcome-based training should be performed with available supervision.

Privilege maintenance

Insufficient sample rate of < 20%.
Sample interpretation:
- Credentialing for interpretation of breast FNA should be the responsibility of the pathology department and be outcome based.
- Quality assurance, quality control and continuing education are warranted on a regular basis.
- False positive rates should be minimized (<1%) in those institutions in which definitive therapy occurs following a positive result.
- False negative reports should be regularly assessed.
- Additional training should be documented when error rates exceed departmental thresholds.

FNA Biopsy Technique

The triple test: physical examination, imaging findings and cytologic examination should be used together for diagnosis.

The false negative rate of triple test diagnosis approaches that of surgical biopsy. The false positive rate of triple test diagnosis is comparable to that of frozen section.

Recommendations for defining the appropriate number of needle passes for FNA of palpable breast masses based on lesion size.

The average number of FNA passes recommended for adequate sampling of most palpable and nonpalpable breast masses is two to four. There are small, incremental diagnostic yields on additional passes, up to four, for palpable masses >1 cm. For smaller (<1 cm) masses, there is no incremental yield after three passes. With immediate specimen evaluation, fewer passes may be required for diagnosis. More than two to four passes may be needed in the following scenarios:
- If the lesion is difficult to stabilize or penetrate.
- If only scant material or a dry tap is obtained.
- If the lesion is larger than 4 cm and/or material is needed for special studies.
- If a carcinoma is suspected and the material obtained during the first two to four passes does not confirm the clinical suspicion.

Other considerations are:
- Confidence in needle placement.
- Size of the lesion (larger/smaller lesions may present sampling problems).
- The patient's level of tolerance for the procedure.

Guidelines for varying sampling technique for palpable breast masses based on lesion type, location and size (Recommendations assume aspirator proficiency in performing FNA)

General recommendations

- Aim needle for the central portion of the tumour

- Apply suction (2–10 ml). Amount of suction applied does not significantly alter specimen yield.

Small lesions

- Attempt optimal placement of needle through careful physical examination and consideration of needle angle and depth of penetration.
- Stabilize highly movable target by walking the lesion to an immobile position under the skin; sample with skin pulled taut.

Necrotic/fibrotic lesions

- Aim for rim of tumour
- Attempt to sample just inside the rim tangentially
- Feeling of increased resistance is usually encountered when the needle has entered the tumour's edge.

Tumour with small, solid core with radiation tendrils appearing as a large, palpable mass

- Attempt to sample from the core.
- Use needle as a probe, identifying core by sensing increased resistance.
- Sample widely in order to avoid missing neoplasm.

Nonaspiration technique

- Intensifies tactile sensations.
- Particularly useful for small, difficult-to-hit targets.
- Reduces blood in highly vascular lesions.
- Disadvantages are less abundant cellular yield and more common dry taps than when suction is used.

Lesions in upper inner quadrant

- Must be sampled carefully to avoid pneumothorax.
- Interrib lesions, if possible, should be moved on top of rib for sampling.

Choice of needles

- Generally, FNA utilizes 22–25-gauge needles.
- Larger needles work well on lesions with high density of epithelial cells and minimal stroma.
- Smaller-gauge needles are superior for highly fibrous lesions.
- Very small, 26–27-gauge needles are useful for intracutaneous lesions and, sometimes, for very small targets.
- The length of the needle is a function of the size and depth of the target. Generally, the needle should not be significantly longer than necessary to sample the target.

Preparation of cytologic sample for diagnosis and special studies

Preparation of the cytologic material for basic diagnosis:
- Direct smearing is the preferred method of preparation. Various smearing techniques are equivalent when performed correctly.
- Air-dried, Romanowsky-type stains and/or alcohol-fixed, Papanicolaou hematoxylin and eosin stains are optimal for basic diagnosis.
- Cell blocks in selected cases from separate, dedicated sample.

Preparation of the cytologic sample for ancillary studies. It is best to harvest additional material for ancillary studies at the time of initial sampling. Clinical presentation, as well as immediate assessment of sample, can be used to select cases requiring additional sampling. When additional material is not available, existing smears can be destained and used for some studies, including immunoperoxidase assays.

Special preparation for ancillary studies/prognostic markers. Cytospins or cell blocks are recommended for immunoperoxidase assays. Rinse cells directly into glutaraldehyde for electron microscopy. Estrogen/progesterone receptors (ER/PR) can be studied on smears, cytospins or cell block material after consulting with referral laboratory. Microbiologic studies when appropriate. Consult microbiology labo-

ratory for specimen handling. The following additional studies can be carried out on cytology specimens. Before collecting material, consult with local laboratory for preferences in specimen preparation:
- Image analysis: Feulgen (or other appropriate stain) immediately or on destained cytologic material
- Fluorescence in situ hybridization
- Polymerase chain reaction
- Immunoelectron microscopy
- Immunofluorenscence

Adequacy of FNA samples of solid nodules. An adequate specimen obtained by aspiration is one that leads to resolution of a problem presented by a lesion in a particular patient's breast. There is no specific requirement for a minimum number of ductal cells to be present for specimen adequacy. Adequacy is determined by two judgements:
- Opinion of the aspirator that the cytologic findings based on the report are consistent with the clinical findings and that the lesion was adequately sampled.
- Opinion of the pathologist examining the smears that the slides do not have significant distortion or artefacts and can be interpreted.

Specimen description should include quantity of epithelial cells:
- Few (occasional clusters)
- Moderate (clusters easy to find)
- Abundant (epithelial cells in almost every field)

Other cellular components should also be in specimen description.

Laboratories may choose to require a specific cell count as one of their own criteria for adequacy. There is no national standard that requires that a given number of cells be present for specimen adequacy.

Adequacy of FNA sample from a cyst. Adequacy of a benign cyst:
- When contents consist of thin, watery, green-grey fluid and there is no residual mass palpable following evacuation of the cyst contents, the fluid from such a lesion may be examined or discarded at the discretion of an experienced aspirator.
- Any residual, clinically significant mass requires further evaluation (FNA, biopsy).
- Any brown or red discoloration in the aspirate not considered to be traumatic warrants careful clinical and cytologic evaluation.

Diagnostic Terminology

The classification of FNAs will fall into one of five categories. Each category should be further described as appropriate, with an attempt made to place the findings into a specific pathologic entity such as that used in a surgical pathology diagnosis.

Benign. There is no evidence of malignancy. This should be followed with further description and classification as appropriate – e.g., findings are consistent with abscess or mastitis, fat necrosis, nonproliferative breast disease (cyst, apocrine metaplasia, etc.), proliferative breast disease without atypia, fibroadenoma, pregnancy-associated changes or treatment-induced changes, etc. (see Post-FNA recommendations).

Atypical/indeterminate. The cellular findings in this material are not diagnostic. This should be followed with further description and classification as appropriate, such as findings are suggestive of proliferative breast disease with atypia (atypical hyperplasia versus low grade carcinoma), papillary lesion (papilloma versus papillary carcinoma), fibroepithelial lesion (fibroadenoma versus phyllodes tumour), etc. Correlation of the cytologic findings with imaging characteristics and clinical impression (triple test) is warranted (see Post-FNA recommendations).

Suspicious/probably malignant. The cellular findings in this material are highly suggestive of malignancy. Tissue biopsy is recommended for a definitive diagnosis (see Post-FNA recommendations).

Malignant. The cellular findings are diagnostic of malignancy. This should be further characterized with the specific type of neoplasm when possible (see Post-FNA recommendations).

Unsatisfactory (due to):
- Scant cellularity
- Air-drying or distortion artefact
- Obscuring blood/inflammation
- Other

> *Tumour/nuclear grading of breast FNAs should be incorporated on all breast carcinomas whenever possible.*

The value of histologic grading of breast carcinoma is well established. Several grading systems have shown a correlation between cytologic and histologic grade. The following grading systems are applicable in the evaluation of FNA of breast carcinoma:
- Fisher's modification of Black's system (reversed grading system, with grade 1 representing the highest level of differentiation and grade 3 equivalent to anaplasia).
- Robinson's or Idvall's system (grades 1–3) corresponding to the Elston's modified Scarff-Bloom and Richardson system.
- Cytologic tumour/nuclear grading system should correspond to the grading system used for the evaluation of tissue.

Ancillary Studies/Prognostic and Predictive Markers

Indications for Assessment of Prognostic Factors (PFs) on Breast FNAs for Mammographically detected, nonpalpable breast lesions:
- Lesions that show malignant or atypical cells on FNA are removed by excisional biopsy. The evaluation of PFs is performed on the tissue specimen, and therefore, other than nuclear/tumour grade, it is not necessary to perform such studies on aspiration smears.
- T1 or T2 Breast Lesions
- Palpable T1 (≤ 2 cm in diameter) and T2 breast lesions (2 to ≤ 5 cm in diameter) with the diagnosis established by FNA are usually treated with lumpectomy or mastectomy, thereby making tissue available for the evaluation of PFs.

It is clinically very useful to ascertain tumour type, differentiation and tumour/nuclear grade on histologic sections, especially for stage I, node-negative cancers because adjuvant therapy recommendations are based, in part, on these parameters. In certain circumstances preoperative chemotherapy may be given to patients with lesions measuring ≥ 1.5 cm in order to increase the possibility of conservation.

PFs that may be assessed on aspirated cells in stage I, T1 and T2 tumours:
- tumour type
- cytologic tumour/nuclear grade
- ERs and PRs.

Optional markers to supplement tumour grading:
- proliferation markers (Ki-67, MIB 1 or %S + G_2M by flow cytometry)
- ploidy (Auer histogram type)
- T3 or T4 Breast Lesions

These patients generally receive preoperative chemotherapy. Aspirated cells or tissue biopsy may be the only tissue available for PFs.

PFs that may be assessed on aspirated cells in T3 or T4 lesions:
- tumour type
- cytologic tumour/nuclear grade
- ERs and PRs

Optional markers to supplement tumour grading:
- proliferation markers (Ki-67, MIB 1 or %S + G_2M by flow cytometry)
- ploidy (Auer histogram type)

Stage IV Breast Cancer. Assessment ERs and PRs in this setting is recommended on cytologic material. Metastatic breast cancer cells obtained by FNA for investigational markers are valuable in assessing a patient's eligibility for novel treatment protocols.

Post-FNA Recommendations

The cytologic diagnosis from FNA should be correlated with the clinical and imaging characteristics to formulate a final clinical, imaging (mammogram and/or ultrasound) and cytologic diagnostic triplet ("triple test") on which patient management is based.

Post-triple test recommendation:
- Benign triplets: Follow clinically with return visit within six months.
- Malignant triplets Refer for definitive therapy.
- Refer for definitive therapy following frozen section confirmation of diagnosis.
- Malignant cytologic diagnosis Refer for definitive therapy following frozen or permanent section confirmation of the diagnosis, at the discretion of the attending physician. Mixed or inconclusive triplets Perform excisional biopsy of the index nodule.

Whenever possible, the FNA report should closely replicate the form and content of a surgical pathology report. When this format is not used, the cytology report should include:
- A summary of the clinical findings
- Precise location of the aspirated lesion to include:
  - Laterality
  - Quadrant (o'clock position)
  - Distance from nipple
- The placement of cytologic findings into one of following five diagnostic categories:
  - Benign
  - Atypical/indeterminate
  - Suspicious/probably malignant
  - Malignant
  - Unsatisfactory
- Comments on specimen findings
- Comment on adequacy
- Recommendations for correlation of cytologic diagnosis with clinical and imaging findings and the need for clinical follow-up

2.2.5
Guidelines of the Papanicolaou Society of Cytopathology for Fine-Needle Aspiration Procedure and Reporting[1]

The Papanicolaou Society of Cytopathology Task Force on Standards of Practice, Chairman: K. C. SUEN

This guideline document was developed by the Standards of Practice Task Force of the Papanicolaou Society of Cytopathology, based on extensive literature reviews and the personal practical experience of task force members. The draft guidelines were then subjected to expert review. The task force made revisions to the drafts based on the responses received from the consultant members, who are recognized experts in fine-needle aspiration biopsy.

Fine-needle aspiration (FNA) is a simple, safe, and cost-effective procedure for the investigation of patients with a mass [1–3]. Clinicians, radiologists, and health care administrators have come to expect ready accessibility of this service, and with improvement of imaging equipment, even greater demands are to be expected. Although wider application is to he encouraged, casual performance of the technique may jeopardize its credibility and may be a potential source for medical liability. Furthermore, the practice of FNA has evolved into a speciality discipline with its own language, algorithms, and diagnostic criteria. To address these issues and to ensure a uniform standard of performance among laboratories, professional groups and societies should move to establish guidelines for training, practice, and reporting [4–8].

Conceptually, FNA can be viewed as a coordinated sequence of events:

---

[1] Publication: The Papanicolaou Society of Cytopathology Task Force on Standards of Practice (1997): Guidelines of the Papanicolaou Society of Cytopathology for Fine-Needle Aspiration Procedure and Reporting. Diagnostic Cytopathology 17 (4): 239–247. Copyright © 1997 by Wiley-Liss, Inc. Also simultaneously published in Modern Pathology. Reprint by permission

- collection of pertinent clinical data
- needle sampling of the abnormality
- specimen preparation and staining
- interpretation
- communication and reporting.

It is crucial that the pathologist, radiologist, and clinician work closely as a team. The referring clinician ultimately determines what management is most appropriate for the patient by integrating information obtained from the clinical data, imaging findings, and the cytopathologic report.

Fine-Needle Aspiration: Indications and Contraindications

FNA is the sampling of a target lesion by a fine-needle, 22-gauge or smaller. Virtually any mass that is either palpable or visualized by an imaging method can be sampled. FNA, however, should not be used indiscriminately. There should be a reasonable expectation of obtaining useful information from the procedure. Clinically insignificant small lymph nodes, vague induration or asymmetries, and other minor abnormalities are not true indications for FNA [9–11], although it is recognized that in apprehensive patients a negative report of an adequate sample can be quite reassuring [12]. FNA is a biopsy procedure and should be considered in the same light as a surgical biopsy [9]. It is a diagnostic tool and has no role in cancer screening, even in "at-risk" individuals. In certain clinical situations, FNA can effectively triage patients for further investigation, surgery, or other therapeutic options (e.g., thyroid and breast lesions) [6, 13, 14].

There are no absolute contraindications for FNA of superficial sites. An uncooperative patient may not be suitable for FNA. For deep-organ aspirations, patients with bleeding disorders or on anticoagulant therapy should receive appropriate medical consultation prior to FNA. Contraindications specifically applied to lung FNA include: advanced emphysema, severe pulmonary hypertension, marked hypoxemia uncorrected by oxygen therapy, and mechanical ventilatory assistance. Patients with suspected pheochromocytoma, carotid body tumour, echinococcal cyst, and highly vascular lesions should be aspirated with caution. Aspirations of ovarian malignancies are not recommended, unless the poor condition of patients precludes surgery or the lesion is a recurrence or metastasis of a previously diagnosed and treated cancer [15–17]. Aspiration of a clinically and radiologically benign ovarian cyst by an experienced clinician is considered reasonable, although this practice is not universally accepted because of the fear of rupturing a malignant cyst [18, 19]. FNA of primary testicular malignancies is also controversial and is not advocated [20, 21].

Complications

The fine-needle technique using 22-gauge or smaller needles is minimally invasive. Complications resulting from superficial aspiration are usually limited to an occasional small haematoma. Even in patients with hemostatic defects, bleeding can be controlled by applying local pressure [22]. Pneumothorax is a very rare complication of breast aspiration and aspiration of the supraclavicular or axillary region. Fatalities from superficial FNA are almost nonexistent; however, a death has been reported following FNA of a carotid body tumour [23]. For transthoracic FNA, the pneumothorax rate can be as high as 20–30%, but most are small and only 5–10% of pneumothoraces require intercostal tube decompression [24–26]. Rarely, deaths have been reported due to pulmonary haemorrhage or unrecognized tension-pneumothorax in emphysematous patients, but the majority of these deaths are associated with use of larger needles (18-gauge or larger). There was no death in one review of 5300 transthoracic fine-needle aspirations [27]. In abdominal FNA, major complications may occur but are rare. These include bile peritonitis, peritonitis, pancreatitis, haemorrhage, infection, needle tract implantation of malignancy (see below), and death. It has been reported that the mortality rate was 0.008–0.031%, the rate of major complications was 0.05–0.18%, and the rate of other complications was 0.16–0.49% [28–31].

The problem of seeding of the needle tract with tumour cells attracts much attention in the medical literature. The frequency of needle-tract seeding, using fine needles as defined above, is between 0.003–0.009% [10, 31–34]. Studies have not shown any difference in survival of patients with malignancy who were aspirated compared with those who were not [35–36].

Post-FNA tissue infarction is an uncommon problem but may interfere with subsequent histologic interpretation [37–40]. If the lesion has been previously aspirated, this information should be communicated to the surgical pathologist handling the surgical specimen.

Training and Education of Personnel

Pathologists who interpret FNA should have a sound knowledge of surgical pathology and a keen interest and demonstrable competence in cytopathology. The interpreting pathologist must ensure that his or her diagnostic accuracy is in keeping with that reported in the recent literature. Active participation in quality assurance and improvement programs is an excellent way to ensure professional competence. For pathologists who perform the FNA procedure (pathologist/clinician hybrid), basic skills in physical examination are important [11, 41–43].

Pathology residency programs and cytopathology societies must make a firm commitment to develop and improve the interpretive and associated skills of FNA at the resident and fellow level. Undoubtedly, it is individuals with solid fellowship training who are likely to have the greatest impact on the success and utility of FNA service in large centers. All pathology residents should have a meaningful, structured training, as this is the only way to ensure the success of the technique in smaller centers and rural areas. Residents should be exposed to cytologic practice with histopathologic correlation early in their residency program, and this involvement should continue throughout the training program with graded responsibility [44–48]. A collection of reference smears prepared directly from fresh surgical specimens is an excellent training resource for learning the range of cytological appearances of disease seen in various body sites and correlating between cytology and histology [49, 50]. There is no agreement as to the minimal number of FNA to be performed before an individual should be considered qualified to practice as an independent operator. Interpretive and procedural skills depend on individualized ability, motivation, and training. The training director should establish competency-based objectives for individual residents to be met at the end of the program.

Education of Clinicians

FNA is team work. As noted, pathologists' training is crucial, but educating referring clinicians and patients about the merits and potential pitfalls of FNA is equally important. Clinicians who are new to the procedure require education, by means of personal discussion prior to the procedure, timely feedback on results, discussion at tumour rounds and clinicopathologic conferences, and dissemination of inhouse manuals and relevant published articles. Currently, clinical residents' knowledge of FNA seems generally inadequate [51], and there is a need for FNA teaching in residency training programs or fellowship programs for family physicians, surgeons, oncologists, endocrinologists, and obstetricians/gynaecologists.

Pre-FNA Requirements

Discussion With Patients

Informed consent should be obtained from the patient. A written consent may be required, depending on local or institutional policies. Documentation of informed consent from each patient should be made and retained in the medical record. Patient education is an integral part of informed consent. It is necessary to inform and advise the patient that FNA is a sampling test and there is always a possibility of the specimen not being representative of the entire lesion. The true lesion could even be missed by the needle. Depending on the size, the nature, and the location of the lesion, the chances of failing to find a cancer when one is present are

1–5% [52, 53]. Therefore, after a benign FNA diagnosis, any enlarging or suspicious lump, noticed by the patient or the referring physician, will require close follow-up or further investigation. An information pamphlet may be provided to patients prior to FNA, so that they can become familiar with the details of the procedure, its advantages, limitations, and complications [54]. Written information, however, does not replace informed, direct discussion with patients to ensure that they understand the information provided to them.

Required Clinical Information

Clinical data should include the patient's name, identification number, sex, age, tumour location and size, physical and imaging characteristics of the lesion (solid or cystic, single or multiple), presenting symptoms and duration, and working clinical diagnosis. Any relevant past or present history of infectious disease, malignancy, and use of chemotherapy or radiotherapy must be recorded. Complicated cases may require specimen triage for special studies. In these situations, discussion between the pathologist and the clinician prior to the aspiration will facilitate specimen-handling decisions. Many mistakes and loss of opportunities for the most appropriate workup of the case can be avoided if direct communication between pathologist and clinician is established.

Technical Considerations

Procurement of FNA Specimens

FNA may be performed by the pathologist, clinician, or radiologist. For superficial lesions, the trained cytopathologist is often the person best suited to perform the procedure. It has been repeatedly demonstrated that the best FNA result is obtained if the person who interprets the smears is the same person who has procured the aspirate material [48, 55–57]. On the other hand, good results can be obtained if the aspirator and interpreter are proficient but not the same person [48, 58]. For deep-seated targets that require imaging localization, experienced interventional radiologists are best suited to perform the biopsy. Exceptions to this tenet are pulmonologists well-trained in the technique of transbronchial and transthoracic FNA.

Regardless of operator, it is important that the practitioner has been adequately trained in the procedure and does it frequently enough to maintain proficiency. Suffice it to say that single-pass sampling performed by individuals poorly schooled in the technique and submitted to the laboratory on one or two slides suffering from multiple preparatory deficiencies does not generally provide diagnostic material. The percentage of unsatisfactory or inadequate specimens for each individual aspirator is a useful indicator of operative skill. Aspirators who persistently exceed acceptable rates should be identified and offered remedial training. An acceptable rate for inadequate specimens is 10–15% (Ljung BM, personal communication) [59]. However, this varies widely in different clinical settings and in various anatomic sites.

The details of the actual biopsy procedure can be found in many excellent references [8, 10, 42, 52, 54, 60, 61]. Generally, 22- to 25-gauge needles are used. For densely fibrotic lesions and highly vascular lesions, the smaller caliber (25-gauge) needles perform better. For very small cutaneous lesions, 26- or 27-gauge needles are useful. Except for aspiration of deep-seated lesions, the use of local anaesthesia is optional. The rules for universal precautions must be observed when handling specimens [62]. Immediate examination of the aspirates for adequacy, while the patient remains in the biopsy suite, reduces the number of inadequate samples and decreases the number of needle passes performed. In addition, the "quick-read" identifies cases benefiting from triage of the current or additional passes for ancillary studies.

Although FNA specimens are traditionally obtained by suction, the recently described technique of needle sampling without suctioning is a good alternative for many types of cases [63–66]. It provides the operator a better tactile sensation as the needle enters the lesion, and is ideal for small lesions. When sampling a vascular organ, such as the thyroid, the technique produces a less bloody sample. When the nonsuction technique fails to yield an adequate sample, the conventional aspiration may be used, and vice versa. Even for the aspiration of deep-seated lesions, the nonsuction technique has been successfully applied by some workers [67–69].

Specimen Preparation and Staining

The simultaneous use of both wet-fixed and air-dried smears is recommended, although the exclusive use of either method is acceptable. These two methods of preparation complement each other, and their concomitant use facilitates interpretation. Air-dried smears are Romanowsky-stained: many centers use a modified Wright-Giemsa stain (e. g., Diff-Quik). An ultrafast Papanicolaou staining technique has been developed recently and is used successfully for rapid staining of air-dried smears [70]. Wet-fixation is achieved by immediate immersion of slides in 95% ethanol or by spray fixation followed by alcohol immersion. Alcohol-fixed slides are stained by the Papanicolaou or hematoxylin-eosin method.

Smeared large tissue fragments stain poorly and add little useful information. They should be picked up gently with a pipette or needle to avoid crush and placed directly in formalin for cell block preparation.

To maximize cell recovery, the needle may be rinsed in 1–2 ml of balanced salt solution or RPMI medium. The rinse is held in reserve to be used for cytospin, cell block preparation, or flow cytometry at the discretion of the cytopathologist.

Recently some centers have reported success with the use of thin-layer preparations for cervical/vaginal and nongynecologic exfoliative specimens [71, 72], but their exclusive use for general diagnostic purposes in FNA specimens remains to be established [73, 74]. The use of "thin preps" is an attractive alternative to direct smears in situations in which the aspirated material is procured by clinicians lacking expertise in slide preparation [74]. Most experienced cytopathologists, however, prefer direct smears to smears prepared from material rinsed in a fixative. At present, the quantitative and qualitative criteria for FNA diagnosis are based on conventional smear preparatory methods. The extent to which these can be recapitulated in "thin prep" materials remains to be investigated. There is concern that the architectural pattern of the smear and extracellular matrix components important to many diagnoses may not be fully preserved. Furthermore, these methods deprive one of the opportunity to prepare air-dried smears.

Ancillary Studies

Standard histochemical and immunochemical techniques can be performed on cytospin preparations, cell blocks, or direct smears. When performing immunocytochemical analyses, antibodies in general perform better on cytospins or cell block preparations than on smeared material. Cell blocks also allow for a more expanded panel of antibodies to be used. While smeared material can be used, the results must be interpreted with caution. Immunostaining of smeared material often suffers from poor staining, excessive background staining, and lack of true similarly processed controls. Other ancillary special studies, including microbiological culture, electron microscopy, flow cytometry, image analysis, evaluation of estrogen receptor/progesterone receptor status, cytogenetics, and molecular diagnostics utilizing polymerase chain reaction (PCR), fluorescence in situ hybridization (FISH), and Southern blotting techniques can all be performed on FNA material [75–80]. The cytopathologist and cytotechnologist must be familiar with the preparatory requirements specific to each of these special procedures. These special tests should be used selectively. While some of these ancillary tests are complex and costly, they are generally available in referral or university centers. Novel sources of material and evolving diseases require that the cytopathologist and cytotechnologist be alert to and conversant with the applications of new technology and new uses of standard techniques.

Interpretation

Objective

FNA interpretation involves assessment of cell morphology, cell-to-cell interaction, tissue fragment architecture (microbiopsy), and the extracellular matrix, integrated with clinical and imaging data [81]. The interpretation may equal a specific histologic diagnosis (e. g., squamous cell carcinoma), a differential diagnosis (e. g., follicular thyroid neoplasm, adenoma vs. carcinoma), or a descriptive diagnosis describing components of a disease process (e. g., metaplastic apocrine cells and histiocytes consistent with fibrocystic change). It may also exclude a specific clinical diagnosis (e. g., a FNA showing a benign adrenocortical nodule rules out a metastasis in a patient with a lung malignancy). The objective of FNA is to provide the referring physician information on the nature of the sampled tissue in order to focus appropriate diagnostic and therapeutic decisions, all at minimal risk to the patient.

Diagnostic Categories

Inadequate/Unsatisfactory

Inadequate or unsatisfactory FNA reports should be treated as "non-results" with further investigation required. Under no circumstances should the cytopathologist be reluctant to report that an FNA is inadequate so as not to lull the clinician and the patient into thinking that the sample is diagnostic of a benign process. A statement in the report on the reason for the unsatisfactory nature of a given aspirate can be helpful for quality assurance and quality improvement purposes, as well as for instruction of the physician taking the sample.

A smear may be inadequate or unsatisfactory for a variety of reasons, including:
- 1) acellularity/hypocellularity
- 2) poor fixation
- 3) poor preparation (crush artefact)
- 4) poor staining
- 5) excessive blood obscuring cellular details
- 6) excessive necrosis or debris.

Other factors that may adversely affect specimen adequacy include irreparably broken slides, inadequate patient identification, inadequate clinical data, and lack of identification of the type and source of specimen.

A major cause of inadequate specimen reports is a scanty or acellular sample. However, the required minimal number of cells present that defines specimen adequacy is variable, influenced by the intrinsic nature of the lesion and operator skill. When the cytopathologist receives insufficient clinical data, he or she must rely on smear cellularity as the dominant criterion for specimen adequacy, otherwise assessment of specimen adequacy should incorporate clinical findings [12, 82].

Clearly, when there is a strong clinical or radiologic suspicion of malignancy, a hypocellular sample containing no malignant cells is not adequate. In other cases, however, such a sample may be adequate [83]. For instance, FNA of a poorly defined, fibrotic induration of the breast (e.g., fibrocystic lesion) is typically hypocellular. What is considered adequate for evaluation of such a lesion may not be an adequate sampling of a well defined solid lesion, especially if it is suspicious clinically or mammographically ("triple test" approach) [84, 85].

Operator skill and experience play a role in determining specimen adequacy. Hypocellular specimens obtained from clinically and radiographically benign fibrotic breast lesions by expert aspirators may well be representative of a benign lesion and hence sufficient. Similar aspirates obtained by aspirators with little training and experience are most likely insufficient and should be so designated [82]. Similarly, an aspirate of an enlarged salivary gland showing only normal tissue would suggest the diagnosis of sialosis, if the lesion after careful examination was sampled by an experienced aspirator [86]. A similar aspirate taken awkwardly by a novice is considered inadequate, since it is not certain if the target has been properly sampled.

Benign

This is an adequate sample showing no evidence of malignancy. This diagnostic category can be further divided into two subgroups:

- Aspirates in which a specific diagnosis can be rendered because the benign cells show characteristic cytologic features enabling the pathologist to arrive at a specific diagnosis, such as Hashimoto's thyroiditis, pulmonary hamartoma, and tuberculosis or fungal disease, among many others.
- Aspirates in which only a negative, narrative diagnosis is possible. For instance, a description of the presence of metaplastic apocrine cells and histiocytes would be consistent with fibrocystic disease. Note that to issue a statement that simply says "no malignancy is identified" can be misleading. It implies that the cytopathologist sees no malignant cells. However, it does not mean that a malignant tumour can be absolutely excluded. To ensure that the clinician understands the implication, the use of the longer statement "no malignancy is identified in this sample" is preferred. A report of "no malignancy" is a valuable piece of information to the clinician, if it is based on adequate sampling from different parts of the lesion and correlated with clinical/imaging findings.

The frequency, nature, and clinical significance of these types of interpretation vary widely for different body sites and for various patient presentations.

Atypical Cells Present

This interpretation is applied to an adequate sample containing mostly benign cells but including a few that are atypical in appearance where malignancy is an unlikely possibility. An interpretation of "atypical cell present" should not be a "stand-alone" diagnosis, but should be accompanied by a recommendation for clinical correlation, follow-up, and/or further investigation for confirmation of the process. (The acceptance of the "atypical" category is not unanimous among expert consultants. A minority express the view that the use of this category may cause diagnostic confusion, and that the "atypical" category should not be separated from the "suspicious" category. Cytopathologists should make a decision as to whether cellular features are benign, suspicious, or malignant.)

Suspicious for Malignancy

This interpretation is applied to a sample on which a definite diagnosis of malignancy cannot be rendered because:
- The sample contains a few malignant-appearing cells which are poorly preserved, or too few cells for confident diagnosis, or is obscured by inflammation, blood, or cell debris.
- The sample is adequate and there are some features of malignancy, but it lacks overtly malignant cells.
- The clinical history suggests caution despite a few malignant-appearing cells present (e.g., cavitating TB or bronchiectasis, viral cytopathic effect, and chemotherapy or radiotherapy effect).
- The smear background suggests tumour necrosis, although well-preserved malignant cells are not identified.
- The cytologic criteria of malignancy overlap with benign lesions. Clinical data and physical findings are critical for interpretation (e.g., low-grade lymphoma, soft-tissue spindle cell lesions, breast lesions with atypical change, and some endocrine neoplasms).

A "suspicious" diagnosis should not be a "stand-alone" diagnosis, but should be accompanied by a recommendation for confirmation of the disease process.

Malignant

This category is used for adequate samples containing cells diagnostic of malignancy. In most cases, the type and primary site of the malignancy can be determined on routine microscopic examination aided by clinical and/or imaging findings. The extent to which special stains and other special laboratory techniques are used to pursue the histogenesis and functional characteristics of a poorly differentiated tumour is dictated by the clinical situation and therapeutic options.

Reporting and Communication

Reports of FNA should be precise and clinically relevant, should use consistent terminology readily understood by clinicians, and should be generated in a timely fashion [87, 88]. The ability to clearly communicate complex and varied findings to the referring physician is crucial. Since the FNA report may be read and interpreted in the future by different clinicians who may not be familiar with the technique, it is important that the report should stand on its own as a complete document. The report should clearly state the name of the aspirator, number of lesions that have been aspirated, the exact location of each lesion, and the number of punctures performed for each lesion.

The report may follow a surgical pathology format, using the terminology of surgical pathology. A section containing a microscopic description of the aspirate may be included if the pathologist thinks it is indicated. Specific diagnoses or descriptive diagnoses could be given, depending on the confidence of the cytopathologist and the complexity of the case. If a definitive diagnosis is not possible, a statement indicating the differential diagnostic possibilities and their relative likelihood may be included. Comments may be included in the microscopic description section or as a separate section. It is appropriate for the cytopathologist to make recommendations for surgical excision, clinical follow-up, or any other tests. If a cytologic diagnosis requires histologic or frozen-section confirmation prior to institution of definitive therapy, this instruction should be clearly stated in the final diagnosis or comment. Microscopic description and recommendation need not be a part of every report if the diagnosis is obvious or uncomplicated. Histologic type, degree of differentiation, and the suggested primary site of the tumour can all be given in the final diagnosis.

Turnaround Time (TAT)

Rapid reporting is one of the major assets of FNA. Timely communication of results relieves patient anxiety, obviates further unnecessary investigations, shortens or eliminates the hospital stay, and ensures prompt therapeutic action. It is recommended that the TAT be of the same order as for a high-priority surgical biopsy. When an on-site cytopathologist is present and "quick-read" of aspirates is the usual practice, an immediate preliminary diagnosis can be provided [89, 91]. When an interpretation is truly "preliminary" and subject to substantial amendment or revision later, this should be clearly communicated. Like frozen sections, difficult cases should be deferred. In the majority of cases it is possible to issue a final report within 24 hr of the receipt of the aspirate specimen. If delay is expected, an oral report can be given by the cytopathologist, with the understanding that the final written report might have to be modified in light of the information later provided by special stains and/or other ancillary studies. All such verbal communications should be documented in written form.

Quality Assurance and Improvement

Quality assurance (QA) and quality improvement (QI) programs are an integral part of FNA practice. The laboratory must comply with relevant federal, state, and local legislation. In the US, each cytology laboratory must satisfy the regulations and standards of the Clinical Laboratory Improvement Amendments of 1988 (CLIA '88) [92] or equivalent standards developed by professional societies that have received deemed status. Useful information and guidance for implementing QA/QI programs are described in the College of American Pathologists' *Quality Improvement Manual in Anatomic Pathology* [93] and other publications [94, 95]. Each laboratory should document its performance and compare with the results reported in the literature.

Cytology/Histology Correlation and Clinical Follow-up

Clinical follow-up of cases with cytology-histology correlation is one of the best monitors for evaluation of outcome [96].

This quality control measure is greatly facilitated by computerization of the laboratory. Surgical pathology and autopsy files are searched at regular intervals, and in some cases a letter may be sent to the clinician for follow-up information. Discrepant cytologic/histologic cases are excellent resources for self-assessment, quality improvement, and minimizing future errors. These cases must be carefully reviewed and the cause of a discrepancy resolved and documented in quality assurance records.

Summary

- As medical care moves toward outpatient and managed care, FNA becomes an indispensable biopsy procedure that can replace many surgical biopsies.
- The reliability of the procedure is maximized by rapid assessment of the aspirates and by the team approach (the cytopathologist, radiologist, and clinician working closely together).
- Proper training and maintenance of competency are central to success.
- QA and QI programs are excellent means to monitor competency and improve performance.
- Aspirators who persistently produce a high rate of unsatisfactory aspirates (>15%) should be identified and given remedial training.
- Clear, precise communication and rapid turnaround time for reporting are critical.

References: Page 192

Standards of Practise Task Force Members: see Appendix 2.2.5, page 185

2.3 Molecular Genetic and Molecular Biological Parameters

2.3.1 The prognostic significance of genetic parameters in breast cancer

C. ROHEN, P. ROGALLA, J. BULLERDIEK

Breast cancer is an increasingly important cause of illness and death among women in Western countries. For estimating the development and progression of these tumours several prognostic markers are helpful such as tumour size, histopathological classification, estrogen-receptor status etc. (Elledge et al., 1992; McGuire and Clark, 1992; Wong et al., 1992). However, a long list of new potentially prognostic factors has been suggested mainly including genetic parameters (Deville and Cornelisse, 1990; Wolman et al., 1991; Gasparini et al., 1993; Klijn et al., 1993). These genetic markers include molecular genetic alterations e.g. mutations or amplifications of specific gene regions, DNA content analysis by flow cytometry or cellular proliferation markers. In the last few years, large series of cytogenetic investigations were also performed (Heim and Mitelman, 1995). So far, there is no definitive correlation between subtypes of karyotypic deviations and tumour behaviour, but different recurrent chromosomal aberrations have been described as e.g. trisomies 7, 8, and 18 (Bullerdiek et al., 1993; Rohen et al., 1994; Pandis et al., 1995). Therefore, chromosome aberrations may helpful in diagnosis and/or prognosis in the near future as well.

Cytogenetic investigations in breast cancer

Cytogenetic studies have been revealed on direct preparations of breast cancer cells (Rodgers et al., 1984; Gebhart et al., 1986) as well as on short-term cultures from primary material (Geleick et al., 1986; Hainsworth et al., 1991; Pandis et al., 1993; Thompson et al., 1993; Rohen et al., 1994) or from breast cancer cell lines (Jones-Cruciger et al., 1976; Barker and Hsu, 1978). The cytogenetic results revealed both apparently diploid cells (Zhang et al., 1989; Geleick et al., 1990) and complex karyotypes (Hill et al., 1987; Hainsworth et al., 1991) depending on the type of preparation techniques. Another method has been developed to support the classical cytogenetics, i.e. the interphase cytogenetics by FISH (fluorescence in situ hybridization) technique. Using this method, it is possible to overcome the problem that specific cell populations have a different proliferative potential in vivo or a different ability to divide in cell culture. Therefore, analysis of all parts of the tumour is possible independent of their growth potential in vitro.

Classical cytogenetic investigations in primary breast cancer revealed a wide spectrum of chromosomal aberrations. As numerical deviations trisomies of the chromosomes 7, 8, 18, and 20 have been described as the sole chromosomal abnormality (Bullerdiek et al., 1993; Rohen et al., 1994; Pandis et al., 1995). Among the structural anomalies described in the last few years were rearrangements of chromosomal regions 1p22, 1p36, 1q10–11, 3p11–13, 4q21, 6p11–13, 6q21–27, 7p11–q11, 7q31–32, 8p11–q11, 11q21–25, 16p10, 16q21–24, 17p11, and 19q13 (Geleick et al., 1990; Hainsworth et al., 1991; Bullerdiek et al., 1993, Thompson et al., 1993; Rohen et al., 1994; Pandis et al., 1995; Steinarsdóttir et al., 1995).

Correlation between the tumour karyotype and the clinicopathologic characteristics in breast cancer samples has been done by few groups. In 1992, Zafrani et al. have evaluated the clinicopathologic significance of homogeneously staining regions (HSR) corresponding to loci of gene amplification. No significant correlation of HSRs was observed in the tumours of patients with unfavourable prognostic factors (high histologic grade, metastatic axillary nodes, loss of hormonal receptors) with the exception of the factor "young age". However, based on their own unpublished data they demonstrate that the presence of HSRs correlates with the rate of chromosomal aberrations and that these rearrangements also correlate with poor prognostic factors. Both chromosome rearrangements and gene amplifications can be regarded as biologic markers of tumour progression. Hainsworth et al. (1992) showed that rearrangements of chromosome 1p correlate with poor prognostic parameters. Clonal chromosome aberrations involving 1p was found in 14 of 25 (56%) breast cancer samples. Comparison with clinicopathological parameters revealed that the presence of those deviations was significantly associated with unfavourable prognostic factors as absence of ER or high histological grade. No significant association was found between the presence of 1p rearrangements and nodal status, tumour size, PR status, and age of women. In a cytogenetic study by Steinarsdóttir et al. (1995) no association between karyotypic changes in general and the presence of lymph node metastases or hormone receptor status could be identified but a possible correlation between an altered chromosome 1 and lymph node metastases has been proposed. In 1996, Pandis et al. presented a comparison of clinicopathologic features with cytogenetic results in 125 breast cancer samples. For correlation analysis different parameters were compared, e.g. age of women with the modal chromosome number or histologic type with number of aberrations. The results showed that the level of karyotypic deviations correlates with the tumour biology e.g. lobular carcinomas yielded normal or near-diploid karyotypes whereas ductal carcinomas, especially grade-III tumours revealed more than 3 aberrations and sometimes near-triploid or near-tetraploid karyotypes. Regarding the aggressiveness of both tumour types, lobular carcinomas were more low-grade tumours than ductal carcinomas.

In summary, the available cytogenetic results might suggest the possibility of clinical-cytogenetic correlations. Therefore, further cytogenetic investigations including molecular-cytogenetic techniques seem to be necessary for understanding the biological behaviour of breast cancer.

Proliferation rate in breast carcinomas

An important prognostic factor in breast cancer is the proliferation activity of the tumour cells which can be determined by different methods (Goodson et al., 1993; Weidner et al., 1993; Gasparini et al., 1994; Keshgegian and Cnaan, 1995):

- Counting of mitotic figures in histologic sections
- Measurement of DNA content (DNA ploidy) and proliferative activity (S-phase fraction (SPF)) using flow cytometry or image analysis
- Detection of proliferation-associated antigens by immunochemistry i.e. Ki-67 and the proliferating cell nuclear antigen (PCNA)
- Tumour labeling indices by thymidine or bromodeoxyuridine (BrdU) labeling.

A classical method for determination the proliferation activity in tumours is the counting of mitotic figures in routine histopathologic sections (Baak, 1990). However, there is still a matter of debate about the reproducibility of this method. Although mitotic figure counting is the simplest and most widely applicable method there is criticism based on different interpretation of mitosis by different pathologists, technical factors, and use of different methods to perform mitotic figure counts (i.e. counting of mitotic figures per 10 high power fields (HPF) or determination of the percentage of mitoses (usually based on 1000 tumour cells) (Weidner et al., 1993; Keshgegian et al., 1995). Weidner et al. (1993) reported that when correctly evaluated the percentage of mitoses correlates with the BrdU labeling index (BLI). Counting of mitosis in 10 high power fields showed less correlation with BLI. Keshgegian et al. (1995) correlates different proliferation markers with other standard prognostic factors in breast cancer. Their study confirms that mitotic figure counting either as a percent of tumour cells or in 10 high power fields strongly correlates with different prognostic parameters. They concluded that the "simplest and best method for determining the proliferative fraction of a breast carcinoma is the mitotic figure count...".

Another proliferation marker is the DNA content analysis (DNA ploidy) and proliferative activity (S-phase fraction (SPF)) by flow cytometry on fresh/frozen tissue specimens or paraffin-embedded material. There is evidence that abnormal DNA content of tumour cells correlates with tumour aggressiveness and may, therefore provide prognostic information (Hedley et al., 1987; Cornelisse et al., 1987; Kallioniemi et al., 1988; Beerman et al., 1990). Although this is a widely used method at present different equipment, different protocols for performing analysis, and for interpretation of the data exist (e.g. heterogeneity of tumour sample) (Hedley et al., 1993). Furthermore, flow cytometry requires a reasonable large amount of tumour tissue whereas computerized image analysis appears to be a more and more practical tool for DNA measuring (Ghali et al., 1992; Luzi et al., 1994).

However, by flow cytometry some studies have shown that patients with aneuploid tumours (i.e. abnormal amount of DNA) have a worse prognosis than patients with diploid tumour cells (normal amount of DNA). The S-phase fraction, i.e. the fraction of cells with a DNA content comparable to that of DNA synthesizing cells has shown to be an important prognostic factor in primary breast cancer (Cornelisse et al., 1987; Hedley et al., 1987; Ewers et al., 1991; McGuire and Clark, 1992). In a study by Ewers et al. in 1991, the SPF and ploidy status were determined in 580 primary breast tumours by flow cytometry. The aim of that study was to evaluate the SPF as a prognostic marker, both as a single factor and in combination with ploidy status. For classification the patients were grouped according to the degree of axillary lymph node involvement. Correlations of flow-cytometry-derived ploidy status and the SPF value to clinical and pathologic variables and prognosis have been reported and it could be shown that the values of SPF are lower in diploid than in non-diploid breast carcinomas. Ploidy status was of prognostic value in node-negative cases whereas SPF was of prognostic value in node-negative as well as node-positive cases (in the latter only 1–3 axillary lymph nodes were involved). The predictive value of flow cytometric DNA analysis was further improved when ploidy status was combined with SPF. It has been shown that both variables had a more predictive strength than the SPF alone, e.g. node-negative patients with non-diploid tumours and an SPF $\geq 12\%$ had the worst prognosis, and manifested the highest rate of early distant recurrence. In a study by Stål et al. (1992) interrelations between DNA content, SPF, hormone receptor status, and age of patient have been examined in 1342 frozen breast cancer samples. Comparison of DNA ploidy and S-phase fraction showed that the corresponding median values of S-phase fraction in the subgroups of DNA diploid and non-diploid tumours were 4,2% and 10,3%, respectively, underlining the fact that in this study was also a correlation between ploidy status and SPF value. Relation of the hormone receptor status showed that both the ER-positive and PR-positive tumours showed lower mean S-phase levels that receptor negative tumours. These relations, high S-phase fraction with DNA aneuploidy and absence of receptors is also well documented in other studies (Dressler et al., 1988; Stål et al., 1989). Altogether there are many studies indicating that flow cytometric studies on DNA content can provide prognostic information in node-negative breast cancer patients (Meyer and Province, 1994; Witzig et al., 1994). DNA-ploidy and SPF were often correlated with relapse-free survival and overall survival and seemed to be a possible predictor for prognosis.

However, for standardization of flow-cytometric DNA analysis as prognostic indicator "a recognized qualification in flow cytometry, strict intra-laboratory and inter-laboratory quality control programs, standard quality control parameters, definitions for ploidy status, evaluation criteria, and parameters for S-phase modelling need to be clearly established before widespread use of the technique" (Spyratos, 1993).

Another practical tool for measuring DNA content in tumour cells seems to be the image analysis. In the studies by Ghali et al. (1992) and Luzi et al. (1994) DNA-ploidy of 115 and 66, respectively, fresh/frozen breast carcinomas were compared by image analysis versus flow cytometry. It has been shown that image analysis has significant advantages over conventional flow cytometry, including e.g. equipment, examination of very small amounts of tumour samples, capability of detecting rare cells with higher degree of ploidy, and capacity to classify cellular populations according to specific morphologic.

The detection of proliferation-associated nuclear antigens by immunohistochemistry is currently an area of great interest. The most widely studied marker for proliferation activity of tumour cells is the monoclonal antibody Ki-67. Ki-67 detects proliferating cells in the S, G_2, M, and G_1 phases of the cell cycle, but not resting cells in the G_0 phase (Rudas et al., 1994). The major advantage is that it is a simple immunohistochemical non-radioactive procedure (Rudas et al., 1994). The disadvantage with the Ki-67 antibody, however, is that it is reactive only with frozen tissue (Keshgegian and Cnaan, 1995). Recently, other Ki-67-equivalent monoclonal antibodies have been developed, i.e. Mib-1–3 and Ki-S1, which are work with paraffin-embedded histologic sections as well (Cattoretti et al., 1992; Key et al., 1993; Kreipe et al., 1993). Positive correlations of the Ki-67 antibody with other clinicopathological parameters have been shown in some studies. e.g. studies by Sahin et al. (1991), Gasparini et al. (1992), Gasparini et al. (1994) and Mirecka et al. (1993) indicating that a high proportion of cell nuclei staining for Ki-67 correlates with a poor prognosis. In a study by Rudas et al. (1994) including the examination of 184 primary breast cancers no statistical significance was observed between clinical outcome and Ki-67 expression (overall survival and recurrence free survival). Therefore, the application of Ki-67 as prognostic marker is still controversial and needs further investigation.

Another proliferation marker is the proliferating-cell nuclear antigen (PCNA) which is a 36-kDa non-histone nuclear protein and a cofactor for DNA polymerase δ. The advantage of PCNA is the possible detection in paraffin-embedded material allowing to use archival sections. Proliferating cell nuclear antigen increases during the late G_1-phase, peaks in the S-phase of the cell cycle and decreases in G_2/M (Bravo et al., 1987a). Recently, antibodies that recognize PCNA in tumour sections have been developed (Ogata et al., 1987) and the most applied antibody is PC 10 (Waseem and Lane, 1990). Gasparini et al. (1994) compared in a study of 168 breast cancer samples the prognostic value of the S-phase fraction and that of the antibodies to Ki-67 and PCNA and found that PCNA had no prognostic value for relapse-free survival and overall survival. Furthermore, no prognostic interaction was found between the S-phase fraction and PCNA. The study by Keshgegian and Cnaan (1995) also compared proliferation markers, i.e. mitotic figure count, S-phase fraction, PCNA, Ki-67, and Mib-1 in 135 breast carcinomas. This study revealed an association between PCNA positive values with high histologic tumour grade and DNA aneuploidy, but no correlation with between PCNA and patient age, tumour size, lymph node involvement, and hormone receptor status. Therefore, also for proliferating cell nuclear antigen the results are controversial and there are also technical differences in fixation and processing conditions and difficulties in interpretation (Wada et al., 1994; Sarli et al., 1995).

The tumour labeling index is another proliferation marker and is based on the incorporation of DNA precursors during S-phase. In many studies for cell cycle analysis the thymidine labeling index (TLI) was used, a radioactive method using 3H-thymidine. A non-radioactive alternative in comparison to the TLI is the 5-bromodeoxyuridine labeling index (BLI) (Weidner et al., 1993). Bromodeoxyuridine is a thymidine analogue which overcomes some technical problems that can occur when determining the TLI. In a study by Weidner et al. (1993) a positive correlation of mitotic figure counting with BLI was done in 55 breast carcinomas. Preoperative in vivo infusion of BrdUrd was used to label 109 breast carcinomas in an investigation by Goodson et al. (1993). Furthermore they were able to examine axillary lymph nodes of 30 women of the same series. Labeling index was determined as the fraction of labeled nuclei per 2000 tumour nuclei. Their results demonstrated a strong correlation between the labeling index of both the primary breast cancer and the corresponding axillary lymph nodes of the 30 patients and may, therefore, indicate the predictive value of this parameter.

Analysis of loss of heterozygosity (LOH)

Cytogenetic and molecular genetic analysis of breast carcinomas have shown high frequencies of loss of heterozygosity, i.e. allelic losses. Usually LOH studies are based on restriction fragment length polymorphism (RFLP) of certain alleles. Using the method of RFLP analysis different losses of alleles have been described so far in breast cancer. Involved sites of LOH have been found in chromosome arms 1p, 1q (Chen et al., 1989), 3p (Andersen et al., 1992; Chen et al., 1994; Buchhagen et al., 1994), 6q, 7q, 8p, 11q (Hamptom et al., 1994), 11p (Ali et al., 1987), 13q (Thorlacius et al., 1991; Andersen et al., 1992; Cleton-Jansen et al., 1995), 16q (Tsuda et al., 1994; Tsuda and Hirohashi, 1995), 17q (Andersen et al., 1992; Futreal et al., 1992; Callahan et al., 1993; Negrini et al., 1994), 17p (Andersen et al., 1992; Matsumara et al., 1992), 18q, and 22q.

For the most of these regions the involved genes are unknown. However, in some cases than the by screening identification of tumour suppressor genes were successful representing the most likely targets of these LOH. Tumour suppressor genes are another classes of cancer genes which act in a recessive way i.e. tumour is related to inactivation of both alleles e.g. by point mutations or chromosomal deletions. One of them is the p53 tumour suppressor gene of which the normal allel encodes for the 53-kD nuclear phosphoprotein TP53 and maps to chromosomal band 17p13.1. The p53 protein was first identified as a phosphoprotein that bound to the large T-antigen of SV40 virus transformed cells (Lane and Crawford, 1979). **p53** functions as a negative regulator of cell growth and inhibits transformation (Finley et al., 1989). It has been implicated in control of the G1 checkpoint, leading to the speculation that p53 protects the genome by detecting DNA damage and allowing time for DNA repair. If DNA damage is irreparable cells are committed to apoptosis. If the normal function of the p53 gene is deviated maintenance of these essential functions is no longer guaranteed resulting in replication of defective cells, more rapid cell proliferation, and cell transformation. Therefore, mutant p53 acts rather as an oncogene than a tumour suppressor gene (Stainbridge, 1990; Cox et al., 1994; Elledge and Allred, 1994). However, it is the most commonly mutated gene yet identified in human cancer including breast carcinomas (Hollstein et al., 1991; Cox et al., 1994).

So far, comprehensive immunohistochemical and molecular analysis have been done to detect p53 allele losses, p53 mutations, and p53 expression (at the mRNA and protein level) in breast cancer. Using different amplification techniques, especially the polymerase chain reaction-single strand conformation polymorphism analysis (PCR-SSCP) of exon 5–9 of the p53 gene and direct sequencing of mutated specimens, changes indicative for mutations have been found in many studies. Mutation analysis of touch preparations, formalinfixed paraffin-embedded or frozen tissues of primary breast tumours revealed mutations in exons 5 to 9 of the p53 gene in 17% to 46% of the tumours investigated. The most frequent type of mutations are point mutations like transversions (e.g. G-T transversions at CpG dinucleotides) or transitions (e.g. $G:C \rightarrow A:T$ transitions) but also microdeletions appear to cluster in the highly conserved regions of the gene in exons 5–8 (Osborne et al., 1991; Runnebaum et al., 1991; Sommer et al., 1992; Thompson et al., 1992; Andersen et al., 1993; Eeles et al., 1993; Umekita et al., 1994).

Expression studies of p53 is based on the observation that in normal cells p53 is generally undetectable by immunohistochemistry. Missense mutations in the p53 gene produce nuclear immunoreactivity with several anti-p53 antibodies, as might be expected from an increase in half-life of the altered protein in comparison to the wild-type protein (Sommer et al., 1992). Immunohistochemical staining detects this abnormal accumulation of p53 and is therefore an indirect indication of a mutation (Elledge and Allred, 1994). Northern blot analysis or immunohistochemical techniques on cytologic specimens, paraffin-embedded sections, frozen tissue or touch preparations using polyclonal as well as different monoclonal antibodies (e.g. CM-1, PAb 421, PAb 1801) revealed positive staining in 22–62% of the cells (Bártek et al., 1991; Koutselini et al., 1991; Poller et al., 1992; Thompson et al., 1992; Thor et al., 1992; Andersen et al., 1993: Bhargava et al., 1994; Umekita et al., 1994a; Umekita et al., 1994b).

The rate of p53 alterations detected depends on the type of mutation analysis. There are some studies comparing different methods, i.e. expression studies versus molecular analysis, indicating a correlation between p53 accumulation and p53 gene mutation (Thor et al., 1992; Andersen et al., 1993). However, it has also been shown that the presence of mutations does not always result in positive nuclear staining and vice versa (Thompson et al., 1992). Under different conditions (e.g. ultraviolet light) positive staining is also present in "normal" cells (Eeles et al., 1993). The varying frequency of nuclear staining also depends on technical parameters, e.g. choice of tumour material or quality of the antibodies used. However, there is a strong association between the presence of p53 gene mutations and presence of nuclear p53 protein accumulation (Andersen et al., 1993).

The prognostic significance of p53 alterations in breast cancer has been shown in different studies in which mutation of p53 and nuclear accumulation of p53, respectively, were compared with pathobiological features (hormone receptor status, histologic grade, stage, lymph node metastases, age at diagnosis, tumour size, erbB2-amplification, proliferative fraction). Thor et al. (1992) showed that immunohistochemically detected "accumulation of the p53 protein has independent prognostic significance in both lymph node-positive and lymph node-negative patient subsets and correlates with absence of the estrogen receptor and with high nuclear tumour grade". In a study by Andersen et al. (1993) p53 alterations (mutation and/or nuclear protein accumulation) were significantly associated with positive node status, T-status >1, negative estrogen/progesterone receptor status, presence of erbB2 gene amplification, and invasive ductal histology. Furthermore, p53 alterations have been also shown to be an independent marker of shortened survival in this study.

However, p53 mutation and/or p53 protein accumulation is associated with negative estrogen/progesterone receptor status (Thor et al., 1992; Thompson et al., 1992; Andersen et al., 1993; Thoralcius et al., 1993; Bhargava et al., 1994), erbB2 overexpression (Poller et al., 1992; Andersen et al., 1993), high histologic grade (Poller et al., 1992; Thor et al., 1992; Bhargava et al., 1994; Umekita et al., 1994b), proliferative fraction (Bhargava et al., 1994; Umikita et al., 1994b), and shortened survival (Thor et al., 1992; Andersen et al., 1993; Thoralcius et al., 1993).

Furthermore, germ-line mutations of p53 play a role in the predisposition to familial breast cancer. The so-called Li-Fraumeni syndrome is a rare autosomal dominant cancer syndrome involving cancers of the breast, brain and a number of other cancers. When analysing p53 mutations in Li-Fraumeni syndrome families Malkin et al. (1990) found defective alleles in all of them.

BRCA1/BRCA2

The great majority of malignant breast tumours are due to acquired mutations. Only about 5–14% of breast cancer patients have inherited mutations leading to these tumours (Børresen, 1992; King, 1992). These mutations have been shown in the tumour suppressor gene p53 leading to the Li-Fraumeni syndrome, the gene causing ataxia teleangiectasia, and the genes responsible for early onset familial breast and ovary cancer, e.g. the breast cancer susceptibility genes BRCA1 (Børresen et al., 1992; Easton et al., 1993).

In 1990, Hall et al. reported linkage of BRCA1 to chromosome 17q12–q21. In 1994, Miki et al. were able to identify the BRCA1 gene by positional cloning methods. The BRCA1 gene is expressed in different tissues including breast and ovarian epithelium, and encodes a predicted protein of 1863 amino acids containing a zinc-finger motif suggesting that it could be a transcription factor. BRCA1 appears to encode a tumour suppressor, i.e. functions as a negative regulator of cell growth suggesting that the functional BRCA1 protein is present in normal breast and ovarian epithelium tissue and is mutated, reduced, or absent in some breast and ovarian tumours (Miki et al., 1994). This is supported by a microcell-mediated chromosome transfer (MMCT) method by Casey et al. (1993) which demonstrated in vitro growth suppression of the p53 wild-type MCF 7 breast cancer cell line by normal chromosome 17 transfer.

As for its molecular structure the BRCA1 gene spans a large genomic DNA region of about 100 kb containing 22 Exons (Miki et al., 1994). The mRNA transcript is 7.8 kbp long with a coding region of 5592 bp (Miki et al., 1994). A wide spectrum of mutations of the BRCA1 gene in samples from patients with breast and ovarian cancer has been described. Analysis of approximately 200 families showing a higher incidence of breast cancer revealed over 120 distinct germline mutations (Futreal et al., 1994; Shattuck-Eidens et al., 1995; Collins, 1996; Grade et al., 1996). Most of these mutations have been only identified in one or two families. Only a few mutations were found repeatedly as for example the 185delAG mutation in exon 2 and the 5382insC in exon 20 (Collins, 1996). 55% of all mutations are localized in the relatively large exon 11, 5,5% in exon 2 and 4,7% in exon 16 (Grade et al., 1996). Approximately 90% of mutations are frame-shift, nonsense, or splice mutations leading to an expression of a truncated protein product (Shattuck-Eidens, 1995). At present, the number of BRCA1 mutations and polymorphic variants reflecting no predisposition to breast cancer is still rising. For example, recently Sobczak et al. (1997) were able to show some new BRCA1 mutations and variants in Polish women.

Women possessing a germline BRCA1 gene mutation have a very high risk (approximately 85%) of developing malignant breast tumours (and a risk of 50% to get ovarian cancer) (Collins et al., 1996). In contrast to sporadic breast cancers BRCA1 related tumours are characterized by early age at onset of the disease. The average age of patients with BRCA1 related breast cancers is 43 years whereas patients with sporadic breast cancers show an average age of 63 years (Marcus et al., 1996). In addition, BRCA1 related breast cancers presented lower mean aneuploid DNA indices, lower TNM stages, a prevalence for a higher histological grade, and higher proliferation rates in comparison to non-hereditary breast cancers (Marcus et al., 1996; Eisinger et al., 1996). Carcinomas with medullary or atypical medullary features are frequently observed in the group of BRCA1 related breast cancer patients (Marcus et al., 1996; Eisinger et al., 1998).

The second breast cancer susceptibility gene i.e. BRCA2 has been cloned by Wooster et al. (1995). It has been localized to chromosomal region 13q12–q13 (Wooster et al., 1994). The BRCA2 gene is composed of 27 exons and spans a genomic DNA region of over roughly 70 kb (Tavtigian et al., 1996). The mRNA transcript is 11–12 kp long. The highest level of expression has been detected in breast and thymus (Tavtigian et al., 1996). The encoded protein consists of 3410 amino acids (Tavtigian et al., 1996) and has transcriptional activation function (Bertwistle and Ashworth, 1998). Recently, Siddique et al. (1998) were able to show that the amino-terminal region of BRCA2 has a histone acetyl transferase activity.

The distribution of BRCA2 mutations appeared to be uniform whereas the mutation profile has been assumed to differ from that of BRCA1 (Tavtigian et al., 1995). The first fifteen BRCA2 sequence alterations which have been described so far have been identified in 6 of the 26 coding exons reflecting a normal spreading of mutations (Tavtigian et al.; 1995; Wooster et al., 1995). Most of these mutations were deletions altering the reading frame leading to truncated proteins (Wooster et al., 1994; Tavtigian et al., 1995). Beyond these predominantly existing deletions other mutations e.g. insertions and point mutations have been described as well (Schubert et al., 1997; Serova et al., 1997).

BRCA2 related patients show an earlier age of onset of disease than non-inherited breast cancer patients (Marcus et al., 1996). In comparison to BRCA1 mutations patients with BRCA2 mutations are older at onset of the disease (Schubert et al., 1997). At the clinical level BRCA2 related tumours presented a lower TNM stage (Marcus et al., 1996). In contrast to other breast cancer patients those with BRCA2 related breast cancer had more tubular-lobular group carcinomas (Marcus et al., 1996). Unlike BRCA1 the BRCA2 gene is not involved in a higher risk for ovarian cancer because ovarian cancer occurred only in a few BRCA2 associated families (Schubert et al. 1997). BRCA2 is involved in female as well as in male breast cancer development. Over the entire lifetime BRCA2 mutation carriers have a 80% risk of developing breast cancer (Schubert et al., 1997).

An early detection of breast cancer is leading to improved surgical cure rates. Therefore, the detection of a predispositional mutation may be of importance because more efforts can be made for diagnosis of cancer. Due to the wide spectrum of mutations it can be necessary to sequence the whole gene if within a family at risk an analysis for BRCA1 or BRCA2 mutations has to be performed for the first time. However, a cancer predisposition test for BRCA1 or BRCA2 mutations should be embedded in the context of genetic counselling (Lynch et al., 1997) and should be restricted to women of so-called high risk families. The strongest risk factors are the early age at onset of disease of family members and the family history of breast cancer. Recommendations for cancer predisposition testing including both these risk factors have be made for example by the American Society of Clinical Oncology (1996).

However, at present the existence of all mutations and normal variants of the BRCA1 and BRCA2 genes is not known, leading to some false-positive and false-negative test results. In addition, some false negative results may also occur due to other cancer susceptibility genes the existence of which have been suggested based on a couple of statistical data (Schubert et al., 1997; Serova et al., 1997). Therefore, efforts will be focussed both on the detection of all BRCA1 and BRCA2 mutations and variants and on the cloning and mutation analysis of other BRCA genes.

In 1995, Shattuck-Eidens et al. reported a mutation analysis in 1086 women with either breast or ovarian cancer and with or without familial history. The results revealed that "thirty-eight distinct mutations were found among 63 mutations identified through a complete screen of the BRCA1 gene. Three specific mutations appeared relatively common..." (Shattuck-Eidens et al., 1995). By complete screening of the coding sequence of the BRCA1 gene 86% were frameshift, nonsense, splice, or regulatory mutations often seen in exon 11 of the gene. The authors conclude that more screening is necessary for determining recurrent mutations and for developing a simple diagnostic test for BRCA1 mutations.

References: Page 196

2.3.2
DNA Grading and DNA Typing of Mammary Carcinomas – A Method for an Objective Assessment of the Morphological Status of the Cell Nucleus

R. BOLLMANN, U. BOSSE

The prognosis of a mammary carcinoma is mainly determined by means of the classical clinical-morphological parameters such as tumour stage, histological type, histopathological grading and receptor status [1]. These data form a basis for the therapy planning. The requirements of modern tumour diagnostics in treatment of breast cancer thus demands pathologist's statement concerning the complete morphological-functional variation range of neoplastic growth [2]. It is a well-known fact that statements in many cases are subjective assessments, not easily reproducible. Frequently they do not permit reliable statements concerning the tumour biology in general. Some carcinomas, which according to the classical factors listed above ought to have a favourable prognosis, turn out to have an early relapse rate and lead to patients death within 5–10 years. Thus, some 20–40% of patients in stage I ($T_1 N_0$) experience a relapse after 5–10 years or fail to survive for this period of time [3]. In those cases the subjective morphology has given a deceptively favourable picture of the tumour biology, and is responsible for the failure to employ adjuvant therapy.

In this difficult situation, DNA cytometry can offer more objective assistance as well as supplying data which can be compared in a scientific manner.

In most malignant neoplastic lesion, numeric chromosomal aberrations (aneuploidy) can be detected. This also occurs in cancers of the breast [4, 5, 6]. Cytogenetic investigations showed that aneuploidy is present in both more aggressive breast cancers in an advanced stage (e.g. nodally positive, poorly differentiated, invasive or large tumours), as well as in cancers which according to the classical conventional parameters really ought to have a favourable prognosis. Tumours of this kind clearly represent a high-risk group, so that the cytogenetic evidence of aneuploidy correspondingly acquires a prognostic significance [5]. Cytogenetic investigations, however, are complicated and expensive; this means that at present they have no practical significance at routine diagnosis. Statements about the net DNA content of a tumour-cell population and therefore about the chromosomal status of mammary carcinoma are also possible by means of DNA cytometry, since a close correlation between DNA values as measured by DNA cytometry and the status as revealed by means of cytogenetic investigations has been established [4]. DNA-aneuploidy represents the cytometric equivalent of chromosomal aneuploidy.

DNA measurements are performed by flow cytometry and static or interactive cytometry.

At flow cytometry, a suspension of single tumour cells is investigated. It is possible within a relatively short period of time to measure a large number of tumour cells; a morphological identification of the cells measured, however, is not possible. In flow cytometry, both tumour cells and stroma cells are measured simultaneously with the result that incorrect measurements may follow.

The results of flow-cytometric measurements of DNA ploidy of mammary carcinomas published so far are contradictory, whereby this problem is largely one of methodology [7].

Thus, for example, in the case of scirrhous tumours with a high stroma content, incorrect results will be obtained, since in flow cytometry it is normally not possible to distinguish between stroma cells and carcinoma cells.

In the not-too-distant future, multi-channel parameter measurements will improve flow cytometric measurements, which will be comparable to those of interactive cytometry [8]. The additional cytometric determination of the proliferative fraction in diploid carcinomas is also of great importance [9].

In interactive cytometry, only carcinoma cells which have been verified as such by microscopic examination are actually measured. This leads to more accurate results, with a higher rate of aneuploidy.

The value of interactive DNA cytometry in the prognostic evaluation of breast cancers has been demonstrated in other studies [7, 10, 11, 12].

The Practice of DNA Cytometry

In routine diagnosis we prefer cytological imprints from the freshly cut surface of the tumour. In order to exclude as far as possible a heterogeneous DNA distribution, the preparations are taken from various sections of the tumour.

Paraffin-embedded material can also be measured when the cells have been brought into a single cell suspension (Hedley method).

The DNA content of the nuclei in the imprints is determined with the aid of interactive image analysis. We used the newly developed CYDOK (manufactured by Hilgers, Königswinter), which fulfils the systematic requirements for precise DNA photocytometry [13, 14].

After hydrolysis with 4N HCl at 28 °C for 45 minutes, the imprints were stained with Schiff's reagent according to Feulgen's method [13].

The principle of measurement is based on the digitized picture of the microscopic preparations. The integrated optical density of Feulgen-stained internal standard cells with a DNA content of 2c (e.g. lymphocytes or granulocytes) is compared with that of the cells to be measured. In this way the relative DNA content can be determined.

Nonneoplastic stromal cells are used as an internal standard.

The cells to be measured can be selected by means of an interactive mode. The measurement of the integrated optical density is performed automatically.

At least 20 reference cells are measured along with at least 250 tumour cells, selected at random. Pycnotic or incomplete nuclei are not taken into account during measurement.

The computer calculates the DNA parameters which will be described later. These then can be printed together with the DNA histogram.

Since a spontaneous polyploidy has been observed in apocrine-metaplastic mammary epithelia [15], the single-cell interpretation of aneuploidy by the so-called 5c method is problematic in breast cancers. In our investigations we therefore usually use the stem line interpretation of aneuploidy [13, 14]. This classic interpretation of aneuploidy is based on the modal value of a cell population, in other words on the most frequently occurring value (= peak). Aneuploidy is diagnosed if this value differs significantly from that of the reference cells when the Kolmogorov-Smirnov test is applied.

The ability to distinguish between aneuploid and diploid tumours produces important prognostic factors, especially in nodally negative tumours [11]. Present knowledge indicates, however, that a more precise interpretation of the DNA data is both possible and desirable. Certain DNA parameters can be deduced from cytometric measurements, e.g. the DNA Index (DI), the DNA Malignancy Grade (MG) and the Proliferative Fraction. These values have been examined on several occasions to ascertain their clinical validity. They make possible an objective DNA grading. Further parameters, e.g. entropy of DNA distribution, currently are being tested.

DNA Grading as a Basis for an Objective Grading of Breast Cancers

The histopathological grading of breast cancers developed by Bloom and Richardson is one of the classical morphological prognostic factors. It consists of a points system where the assessment is based on the number of tubular structures and morphology of the nucleus [2].

The classical histopathological grading system bears a close correlation to the probability of the patient's survival and to such clinical parameters as e.g. the involvement of the lymph nodes, metastases and success or failure of treatment. However, the reproducibility is very poor [10]. Statistically speaking, prognostic relevance of histopathological grading is undisputed; nonetheless, in individual cases it does not permit a satisfactory degree of certainty regarding the assessment of the prognosis. The pTNM system does not overcome these uncertainties despite recent improvements.

Our experience and results of other studies let us recommend a combined DNA grading which takes into account the DI and the DNA-MG as well as the fraction of proliferation.

DNA Index (DI)

When demonstrated by means of DNA cytometry, aneuploidy is an expression of a chromosomal aberration; the extent of the aneuploidy is reflected in the DNA Index. The DI is the relationship between the modal value of the measured cell population and the reference cells. It thus defines the position of the so-called stem line. A DI of 1 therefore corresponds to a stem line of 2c; a DI of 2.5 corresponds to a stem line of 5c. The occurrence of additional subsidiary peaks is attributed to a heterogeneous stem line. It reflects an increasing cytogenetic instability.

Our own investigations of 401 breast cancers [16] confirm the results of Dutrillaux, who was able to demonstrate that cytogenetically and cytometrically determined DI values correspond exactly and that both distribution curves are bimodal [4]. In our series, too, the distribution histogram of the DI corresponds exactly with the cytometrically measured chromosome counts, whereby here, too, the distribution is bimodal. A group is distributed fairly evenly around diploid values (DI 0.91–1.2); the second group permits a somewhat diffuse distribution to be recognised, with a peak around DI 1.51 and 1.9.

According to the cytogenetic results, three groups of breast cancers should be regarded as representing an advanced stage of progression with the following chromosome counts or DI: fewer than 40 chromosomes, corresponding to a DI 0.9; chromosome counts between 52 and 65 chromosomes, corresponding to a DI of 1.3–1.5; and more than 90 chromosomes and a corresponding DI of 1.9 [4].

DNA Malignancy Grade (DNA-MG) According to Böcking

The prognosis of a tumour depends among other things on its genetic instability – in other words, on its variance around the normal 2c value, the so-called 2c Deviation Index (2c-DI). The logarithmic conversion of this 2c-DI gives the DNA Malignancy Grade according to Böcking on a linear scale from 0–3 [10, 14].

By splitting the groups of breast tumours to these three categories according to the DNA-Malignancy Grade, Böcking and his colleagues were able to differentiate between significantly different chances of survival. The DNA Malignancy Grade also bears a significant correlation to the lymph node status; its reproducibility is superior to that of subjective classifications and seems more suitable as the subjective differentiation suggested by Auer, who divided histograms into four classes [10, 17]. The DNA Malignancy Grade permits an assessment of the risk of early relapse [18].

The results of our investigations confirm that there is a statistically significant relationship between histopathological grade or lymph node status and the DNA parameters DI and DNA-MG [16] so that both parameters can build the basis for an objective DNA grading system, since they are both reproducible.

Proliferative Fraction

The determination of the proliferative activity as an additional parameter has proved to be of value particularly in the case of diploid tumours. This can be calculated on the one hand through the determination of the S-phase fraction. This has proved to be statistically significant for the risk of relapse, but so far no relationship to the chances of survival has been established. On the other hand, the S-phase fraction is relevant for the so-called Proliferative Fraction (% S + % G2M), whereby the limit should be set at 12,5 [9]. Diploid tumours with a cytometrically determined fraction of proliferation >12,5% belong to the high-risk group. This fraction of proliferation can be determined, at least approximately, by means of interactive DNA cytometry. A comparison with immunohistochemical marker investigations is also possible.

DNA Histograms as a Basis for DNA Typing

In the day-to-day histological diagnostic routine, importance is attached to the so-called typing, in other words to determination of the histological tumour type (ductal, lobular and special types). Here the same problems of poor reproducibility occur as in the grading of the tumours. The poor reproducibility of the typing also explains the widely varying frequency rates for various groups of tumour in published reports. Typing is further complicated by the existence of mixed types of tumour.

The differing clinical behaviour of ductal and lobular carcinomas is obviously explained by genetic differences; both types of tumour show significantly different values for DI and DNA-MG. The lobular carcinomas demonstrate in all stages considerably lower values than ductal ones [16]. This fact points to a higher genetic stability of lobular carcinomas; however, to date there are no corresponding cytogenetic investigations to support this hypothesis. There is, however, clinical evidence to support the theory of biological differences between the two histological types of carcinoma [19].

The majority of invasive lobular carcinomas reveal a diploid histogram with low DI and DNA-MG. For histology this case belongs to the so-called classic type. In the case of pleomorphous types of lobular carcinomas, however, the relationships are different, and these tumours also are more malignant [20]. Thus it would be possible to distinguish between ploidy distribution of the two types of invasive lobular carcinoma by means of the DNA histogram. In the case of pleomorphic variant the measured values are considerably higher than for the classic type [16, 21]. Tubular and atypical tubular carcinomas also demonstrate a similar behaviour.

The histological phenotype of a tumour is thus mirrored by an objective value in the DNA histogram.

DNA histograms reflect the chromosomal situation of a tumour and permit to some extent a quasi-genetic classification of neoplasia. DNA measurements allow an insight into tumour biology and an objective characterisation of morphological patterns. The DNA distribution of the measured cells can be clearly presented and interpreted by means of histograms. Since during the course of the progression of the tumour there will be constitutional changes in the number of chromosomes, a tumour will produce different histograms depending on the stage it has reached. The various types of histogram are related to the tumour biology and permit a genetic classification of the growth.

A first attempt at a systematic classification of breast cancers by means of a DNA histogram was produced by the Stockholm DNA working group. It describes four types [11]. This Auer scheme has been internationally accepted, although it cannot always be reproduced [10, 17].

Schenck and colleagues [22] recently proposed a histogram classification which also takes into account the share of the fraction of proliferation, apart from the position of the stem line (figure 2.33). This scheme can be used as a basis for a genetic classification of breast cancers in the sense of a DNA typing as studies of our group have shown [16]. Investigations are being carried-out to test whether this new classification could be done automatically with the computer to overcome the subjective moment of the histogramm interpretation. Own preliminary results show that this might be possible with the new technology of laser-scanning (CompuCyte) cytometry. This method is to be seen as combining all positive aspects of flow and image cytometry without the negative aspects of both these methods.

Using the data described, a combined DNA grading and typing can be determined (table 2.20), which permits a binary decision particularly with regard to the risk factor.

Summary

Based on results of the DNA measurements of 401 breast cancers and the details of previous studies, we would like to propose a combined DNA grading and DNA typing in addition to the subjective morphology of breast cancer (table 2.20).

Using this method can facilitate clinical decisions regarding therapeutic measures to be taken (table 2.21):
- In nodally negative DNA high-risk carcinomas, additional chemotherapy should be considered [23].

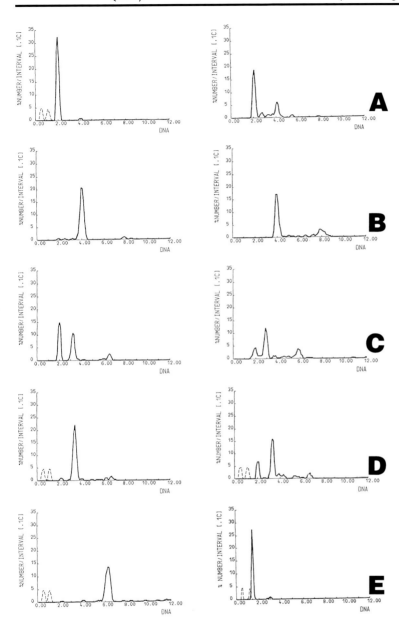

Figure 2.33: Typical DNA distributions in breast carcinoma. (A) DNA diploid. (B) Tetraploid. (C) Triploid. (D) Stemline at 3.5c. (E) Hypertetraploid and hypodiploid (right side). (A–D) Left side nonproliferating and right side proliferating histogram. Reprint by permission of Dr. Schenck and Dr. Wied.

	DNA-low-risk	DNA-high-risk
DNA Index (DI) [4] and	≥ 0.9 < 1.3 or > 1.5 < 1.91	< 0,9 > 1.9 or > 1.29 < 1.51
DNA Malignancy Grade (DNA-MG) [10] and	≤ 1	> 1
Fraction of proliferation [9]	< 12.5 %	> 12.5 %
Histogramm type [16.22]	A, E	B, C, D, F

Table 2.20: Combined DNA Grading and Typing of Mammary Carcinomas

Table 2.21: Clinical Significance of the Combined DNA Grading and Typing of Mammary Carcinomas

	Chemotherapy in nodally negative carcinoma	Abandonment of axillary revision	
		In T_{1a} carcinomas	In carcinomas of all T classes in older patients
DNA-Low-risk	No [23]	Should be considered [24]	Should be considered [24]
DNA-High-risk	Yes [23]	No	No

- In T1a carcinomas with a low DNA risk, an axillary lymphadenectomy may be avoided, as is currently under discussion [24]. In older patients with DNA low-risk carcinomas, an axillary lymphadenectomy may be avoided independently of the T classification. This, too, is under current discussion [25].
- In DNA high-risk carcinomas, radical operations should be reconsidered in view of the probability of early relapse.
- DNA cytometry permits an objective grading of the histopathology of breast cancers.
- DNA analyses can be undertaken before surgery using cytological puncture material.

References: Page 202

2.3.3
Quality Assurance in Mammary Cytology by Means of DNA Cytometry

R. BOLLMANN

International opinion today is unanimous that, when undertaken by an experienced operator in critical cases, the puncture cytology of mammary lesions is a reliable method, especially when quality standards are taken into account [1].

As a diagnostic method, mammary puncture cytology has many advantages for both patient and physician: speed, effectiveness (compared with an open biopsy), minimal irritation and no resulting scar. If a tumour is discovered the patient can prepare herself emotionally, and therapeutic decisions can be discussed before the operation is performed. Using the cytological results, the physician can decide whether a further biopsy can be carried out as an outpatient procedure, or which patients should be admitted to hospital.

Bearing this in mind, the frequent reluctance application of this method seems incomprehensible. Ignoring possible historical reasons, it may be attributable to the poor comparability of data concerning sensitivity and specificity of mammary puncture cytology. This is caused on one hand by the variety of methods employed, on the other hand it raises from differences in the forensic implications of cytological puncture based diagnoses. Furthermore, most of the studies are retrospective [2]. In a literature review it can be found that the sensitivity of mammary cytology lies in the range of 72–99% with a mean value of 87%. Specificity is found between 89% and 100% [4].

Fine-needle aspirations of the breast are more sensitive than punch biopsies [3]. Nowadays, puncture cytology of lesions detected by means of mammography is used to lower the number of false-positive mammographical diagnoses. For this reason it is particularly important to avoid false-positive cytological results, that is to say, to improve the specificity of the cytology.

Cytologically doubtful results are obtained in up to 20% of all mammary punctures [4]. These doubtful cytological results can be explained as follows:

Compared with ductal mammary epithelia, some carcinomas show very few cytological abnormal criteria. In contrast to this some benign lesions (e.g. fibro-adenomas) often have a large number of nuclear abnormalities. Under hormonal or pharmaceutical stimulation of the mammary parenchyma, a considerable num-

Table 2.22: DNA Cytometry of 92 Mammary Aspirates with Cytologically Doubtful Results [4]

Histological results	aneuploid	non aneuploid
58 carcinomas	56	2*
8 ADH	8	–
26 mastopathies	–	26

ADH = Atypical ductal hyperplasia
Positive correctness for manifest malignancy = 97 %;
Specifity = 100 %; Negative correctness = 93 %
* But with high proliferative fraction

ber of nuclear abnormalities may in certain circumstances occur and can be difficult to differentiate from malignant changes.

In such borderline diagnostic situations, DNA cytometry[1] offers valuable assistance.

DNA analysis by static cytometry of mammary aspirates increase the diagnostic ability and can result in an increased sensitivity and specificity by evaluation of DNA-ploidy [5, 6, 7]. In the author's own investigations [4] of 92 mammary aspirates with cytologically doubtful results, this procedure resulted in a positive confirmation or correlation for manifest malignancy of 97 % and a negative correlation of 93 % (table 2.22).

The sensitivity could be increased by taking into account the fraction of proliferation [7]. In our series this raised the sensitivity to 100 %.

We recommend the following procedure (figure 2.34).

Aspirates which are difficult to classify but which demonstrate DNA aneuploidy should be clarified histologically (figure 2.35), since carcinomas are very frequently aneuploid. Benign aneuploid lesions may possibly represent pre-malignant changes [8], so that their extirpation is justified even in those cases which subsequent histological analysis reveals to be benign.

In the case of a euploid, cytologically atypical population without an increased fraction of proliferation, malignancy is less likely (figure 2.36). The course of action to be followed is determined according to triple diagnostic criteria.

DNA cytometry of doubtful mammary aspirates represents a means of maintaining stan-

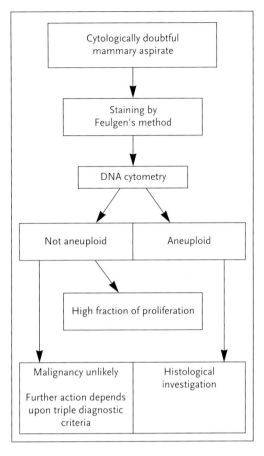

Figure 2.34, explanation see left

dards, since it can recognise neoplastic cells and lead to the clarification of doubtful results. Cytological „bad day errors" have thus become avoidable.

Quality Assurance in Mammary Cytology through DNA Cytometry:
- Detection of neoplastic cells
- Clarification of uncertain results
- Avoidance of "bad days errors"
- Establishment of comparable data bases
- Pre-operative determination of the DANN typing and grading
- DNA regressive grading through down staging after chemotherapy

The procedure also permits an objective down staging (grading of DNA regression) following chemotherapy [9].

---

[1] refer to Bollmann und Bosse in the book

References: Page 204

Figure 2.35: Difficult-to-classify aspirate with atypical epithelia. DNA-cytometrically aneuploid. Histology: Highly differentiated papillary mammary carcinoma pT1c G1 N 0/21.

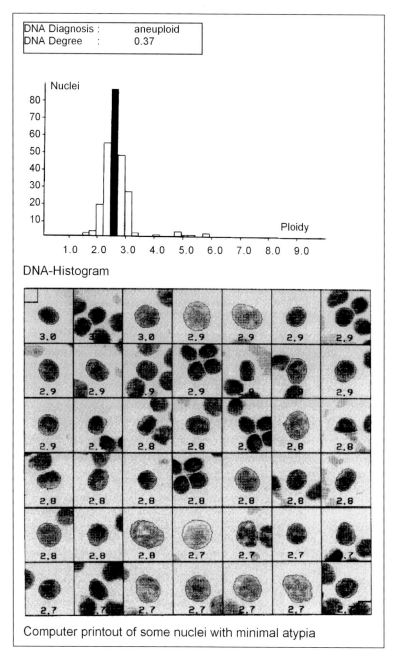

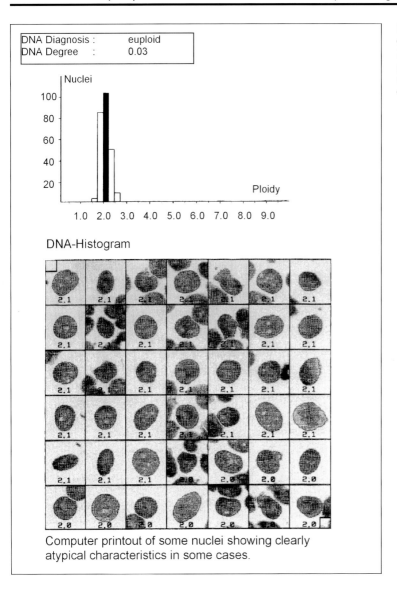

Figure 2.36: Difficult-to-classify atypical aspirate. DNA-cytometrically euploid. Histology: Ectopic mammary tissue with ductal hyperplasia.

2.3.4
Chromatin Arrangement as a Prognostic Marker in Node Negative Breast Cancer Patients, measured in Different Thick Tissue Sections

R. ALBERT, J. G. MÜLLER, P. KRISTEN, H. HARMS

Introduction

In principle breast cancer patients without nodal involvement have a good prognosis compared to those patients who are node positive. Despite this cold fact up to 30% of the node negative patients ultimately die of their disease. Another fact is that every year the number of node negative patients within the group of all breast cancers increases – at the moment about 50% of newly diagnosed breast cancer patients have primary tumours without nodal involvement – and this trend is not at its end [1]. Although studies in the last years have shown that not all patients will benefit from adjuvant therapies like combination cytotoxic and/or hormonal therapy [2], it is possible to define subsets of axillary node negative patients with prolonged disease free (DFS) and overall survival (OS) [3, 4].

Until now the clinical usage of prognostic markers, including those which correlate to DFS and OS in different studies, can not give a recurrence risk estimation for each individual patient. At present, grading systems from the Armed Forces Institute of Pathology [5] and World Health Organization [6] are the basis for most decisions concerning use of adjuvant therapy in lymph node negative breast cancer patients [7].

In June 1990 National Institutes of Health (NIH) recommended at their Consensus Development Conference that nuclear grading is a highly significant prognostic marker, when evaluated by experienced pathologists and investigations with great node negative patient collectives and long follow up times support this statement [8, 9]. But existing nuclear grading systems, judging chromatin structure visually, suffer from subjectivity and poor reproducibility [3, 29].

The interobserver reproducibility of the Bloom and Richardson Histological Grading Scheme [10] and its Nottingham modification [11], which at present seems to be the most clearly defined, was tested in different studies. In nearly all these attempts reproducibility results in the three grading components tubule formation, nuclear pleomorphism, and mitotic rate was worst for nuclear pleomorphism [12, 13]. This was one reason for the mostly high interobserver variations for histological grading of the tumours, even when the observers were trained by the same tutors [14]. Only precise grading guidelines and experience combined with optimal fixation techniques will improve interobserver agreement [15, 16]. Therefore, until now such systems are only practicable for some specialists and not applicable in daily routine diagnostics.

High resolution image analysis is a perfect tool to objectify nuclear grading and studies in the last years have shown, that image analytical texture features correlate significantly with DFS and OS of node negative breast cancer patients. Cooccurrence and run length features [17]. Markovian features [18], or number, localization and optical density of chromatin regions [19] were distinct attempts for finding prognostic relevant nuclear characteristics. Thus it is about time for an objective and reproducible nuclear grading system to estimate prognosis immediately after excision of the primary tumour.

Our aim was the development of a risk profile system, based on the chromatin distribution within the tumour cell nuclei of the primary tumour. With image analytical algorithms nucleus features were extracted, giving a mathematical description of the chromatin structure.

Tumour cell nuclei of relapse and nonrelapse patients were differentiated for the definition of two nuclei types: High risk tumour cell nuclei (HRTuC) and low risk tumour cell nuclei (LRTuC). With a binary classification tree, constructed by the commercial classification program CART (Classification And Regression Trees) [20], tumour cell nuclei of relapse and nonrelapse patients were separated. The distribution of tumour cell nuclei from each individual patient in the two groups HRTuC and LRTuC was determined as the measure to obtain prognostic information.

With this approach it should be possible, to make a statement for any patient about her individual prognosis. The ratio HRTuC: LRTuC could give a relapse risk estimation to the attending physicians for optimizing treatment decision.

Materials and Methods

Archival hematoxylin and eosin (HE) stained paraffin embedded tissue sections from 145 different primary tumours of node negative breast cancer patients were investigated. Patients were treated by ablatio mammae with axilla dissection without administration of any adjuvant therapy. Surgeries of primary tumours were between January 1980 and December 1986. Relapses (n = 57) occurred between 3 and 79 months after surgery. Mean follow up time of the nonrelapse patients (n = 88) was 111

Table 2.23, explanation see below

Characteristics		Patient group			
		2D	2D3D	3D	all
Section thickness (μm)		2–4 μm	5–7 μm	8–12 μm	2–12 μm
Patients	Relapse	13	30	14	57
	Nonrelapse	33	40	15	88
	All	46	70	29	145
Follow up*	Mean	98	112	119	111
Nuclei	Absolute	8,528	12,248	4,661	25,437
	Mean per case	185	175	161	174
Histology	IDC	34	61	19	114
	IDIS	5	6	3	14
	ILC	7	3	7	17
MSBR	Grade I	18	29	9	56
	Grade II	16	21	9	46
	Grade III	9	17	7	33

* mean follow up time of the nonrelapse patients in months
IDC: invasive ductal carcinoma
IDIS: invasive ductal carcinoma with a predominant intraductal component
ILC: invasive lobular carcinoma
MSBR: Modified Scarff-Bloom-Richardson grading (available from 135 patients)

months. For comparison of different image analytical techniques (2-dimensional 2D, 3-dimensional 3D, and mixed 2D3D), our data set was separated in three subgroups, dependent on the thickness of the tissue sections (table 2.23).

Light microscopic images of the 2–4 μm sections were scanned in one focus level whereas the thicker sections were analyzed in 5–9 consecutive focus settings. Between 15 and 25 independent image scenes per tissue sample were taken in each case. With this method we obtained – after deletion of artefacts and nuclei which were cut by the image border, damaged or clumped – a total of 25 437 tumour cell nucleus images.

Cytophotometric Equipment

Scanning of cell scenes was performed in an Axiomat or Axioplan microscope (Zeiss, Oberkochen, Germany). A color frame grabber (DT2871, Data Translation, Marlboro, MA, USA) digitized the red, green, and blue channel output signals (R, G, B) of the 3° chip CCD camera (DXC-750P camera, Sony, Tokyo, Japan). The absolute sampling density was 8,2 pixels/μm of the tissue section. For the analysis of the thicker sections the focus was reproducibly adjustable in steps of 0,1 μm. Image segmentation and feature extraction were realized by especially developed software, programmed in FORTRAN on a workstation (DECstation 5000/240, Digital Equipment Corporation, Maynard, MA, USA).

Cytophotometric Measurement

To remain independent of special preparation techniques we used archival standard HE stained tissue sections from patients with surgery of a primary tumour 10 or more years ago. Three protocols were developed:

- 3D-protocol for sections with a thickness of 8–12 μm. This sections were scanned in 5–9 settings (distance 1 μm) and analysis was made in a compressed image containing the information of the three median planes of each nuclei, which satisfied quality judgement [21]. Additionally this image was deconvoluted with the outside focus images.
- 2D3D-protocol for sections with a thickness of 5–7 μm. Scanning procedure was done also in 5–9 focus settings, but for each nucleus the focus level with highest contrast was used for further investigation. Each

nucleus was analyzed only in the selected focus position without using the information from images of other levels. Scanning time and storage requirements are identical to 3D analysis. The advantage of the 2D3D protocol is the decrease in computation time.

- 2D-protocol for sections with a thickness of 2–4 µm. In thin sections cell scenes were scanned in one focus setting, which seems to have highest contrast for all visible nuclei to get as much information as possible for nuclei image segmentation and feature extraction. The advantage is a high decrease in scanning time, computation time, and storage requirements, but there is a great loss in respect to the information content of the tissue sections.

Cell Image Segmentation

The segmentation of cell images in the components cell nuclei, cytoplasm and background is the first and important step in image analysis. In tissue sections, where cells are mostly cut to more or less thick slices, the automatic image segmentation is not a trivial procedure.

In HE stained tissue sections, which were scanned in 5 to 9 focus settings in steps of 1 µm, the three mean images were used to construct a binary mask of the cell nuclei images. The maximal difference of the blue and red channels were taken as a coarse threshold for segmentation of this three images. The three single mask images were combined to one preliminary binary mask. Touched cells were separated by a gradient filter algorithm. With further geometric operations according to a cell model as described in [22] the real binary masks for the nuclei are determined.

Image Information Compression

The image of each focus setting contains only a part of the whole information of the cell, because in a light microscope the depth of the focus is limited. Each single image is blurred by the outside higher and lower focal planes of the section. To increase the information content the lowest values of the mean images of the RGB channels were taken and the images of the level 2 and n-1 were deconvoluted by the outside focus images which were filtered by the Defocus Optical Transfer Function of the near focus settings [23]. In the resulting color image the information of 3 or 5 focus planes was compressed and the chromatin structure was emphasized. An example of this increase in information is shown in figure 2.37.

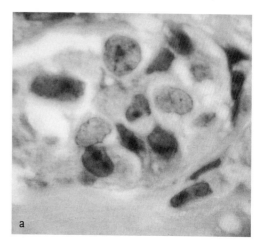
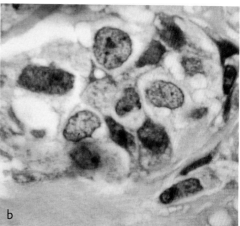

Figure 2.37: a) The image shows one focis level of a cell scene. Although it would be possible to analyze some of the nuclei, it is obvious that taking measurements from all nuclei in this single plane is not possible because most are out of focus. Extracted feature values would be uncharacteristic. b) This image shows the new constructed image with the compressed information of the whole series of focus levels. Extracted features can give a characteristic description of chromatin structure and distribution.

Feature Extraction

The chromatin distribution features were extracted from the red channel of the compressed image since the red channel contains highest contrast in HE stained cells. The chromatin structure was analyzed with texture line analysis [24], where lines from the maximum of the gradient filtered image were taken and statistical evaluated. This is a well proven measure for homogeneity or irregularity of chromatin architecture. The chromatin distribution according to the center or the border of the nucleus were determined by lines with equal distance to the border of the nucleus. The mean gray values of the red channel and the standard deviation were calculated within each distance line. The variation coefficient and other features were determined as described in [21].

In this investigation features measuring the regularity and the distribution of the chromatin (more to center or border standing) are the most significant for distinction of HRTuC and LRTuC.

Classification

Extracted feature values of all cells were the input data of the learning samples for CART. With CART we constructed one binary classification tree for each of the three protocols: 3D analysis (Tree3D), 2D3D analysis (Tree2D3D), and 2D analysis (Tree2D).

For estimation to control accuracy of the constructed trees we used 10-fold cross-validation, because the whole data set is permitted for generating the classifier [25, 26]. For the purposes of the accuracy test, the data are split into a learning and a test sample.

Because of the different nuclei quantities, tumour cell nuclei of relapse and nonrelapse patients were equally weighted (50%) by CART for the classification process. Thus the more frequent class was not preferred.

Nuclei with similar chromatin structure are located in the same endnode of a classification tree. Obviously tumour cell nuclei of relapse patients represent a greater malignancy than tumour cell nuclei of nonrelapse patients. Therefore in the selected classification trees all nuclei in endnodes with more nuclei from relapse patients were called high-risk tumour cell nuclei (HRTuC), because these nuclei represent the higher malignant potential. The nuclei of the remaining endnodes with a higher portion of tumour cell nuclei of nonrelapse patients were called low-risk tumour cell nuclei (LRTuC), because of the lower malignant potential. The final step in the classification procedure was to determine whether the majority of tumour cell nuclei of each patient was classified as HRTuC or LRTuC.

Ultimately we compared the classification results. As much relapse patients as possible should have the majority of tumour cell nuclei in the high-risk group, the nonrelapse patients in the low-risk group.

Results

A highly expressive nuclear grading system can be developed by using thick tissue sections with great information content. The information in thicker sections contains important additive components, in respect to chromatin structure and distribution.

Segmentation

The automatic image segmentation was correct for the 5–9 µm sections in more than 93% of the cells. For sections of 2–4 µm thickness the correctness decreased to 70%. The reason for this is the incompleteness of the cells as result of the cutting.

Individual Prognosis

Separation between tumour nuclei of relapse and nonrelapse patients was made by CART with three different classification trees, one for each patient group. All results are listed in table 2.24.

Independent on the image analytical technique the tumour cell nuclei of the primary tumour of relapse and nonrelapse patients show clearly quantifiable differences in respect to chromatin structure. This is obvious even in 2–4 µm sections, but evaluation of the chromatin structure is much better in thicker sections and therefore correct classification rates

Table 2.24, explanation see page 129

Characteristics of the binary classification trees		Patient group		
		2D	2D3D	3D
Number of endnodes		20	27	9
Number of features		12	12	8
Correct classification rate for the nuclei (%)	LS	62.5	71.8	64.5
	CV	61.1	68.7	59.0
Correct classification rate for the patients (%)	Relapse	100	92.5	100
	Nonrelapse	63.6	93.3	93.3
	All	73.9	92.9	96.6
Portion of HRTuC (mean ± standard deviation in %)	Relapse	69.5±10.8	69.2±13.8	83.3±8.4
	Nonrelapse	40.0±26.0	28.0±16.4	50.9±14.6

LS: learning sample
CV: cross validation

for the assignment of patients was significantly higher in analyses with thicker sections. In 3D-analysis the classification result could be improved by shifting the threshold for distinction of the patient groups from 50% to 65%. The distributions of relapse and nonrelapse patients by percentage of HRTuC, using different image analytical methods, dependent on the section thickness, are shown in the figures 2.38–2.40.

In 3D-analysis the classification tree constructed by CART utilized 8 features for the differentiation between nuclei of relapse and nonrelapse patients, 4 features were measures of the chromatin distribution and 4 for chromatin structure or texture. No single feature alone was significant for the classification. Only the combination of two or more features yielded to a subgroup of HRTuC or LRTuC. The chromatin distribution in the calculated nucleus lines and their variation coefficient and standard devia-

tion were the most important features followed by the localization of the chromatin, more centered or at the border. If there were bigger holes or chromatin concentrations in the nucleus it tended to be a LRTuC. If the chromatin structure was uniform coarse, the probability for a HRTuC increased. This combination of chromatin features is difficult to understand with the human eye. In 2D- and 2D3D-analysis the described facts were very similar.

Discussion

At the moment all defined groups of so called high-risk-patients within the collective of node negative breast cancers include only about 10–15% of patients and the relapse risk is only about 30–40% [17, 27, 28, 29]. Thus even in such subgroups for more than 60% of patients an adjuvant therapy, generally burdened with

Figure 2.38: Learning sample 3D (n = 29)

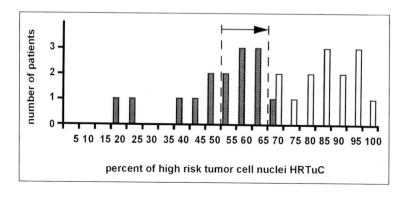

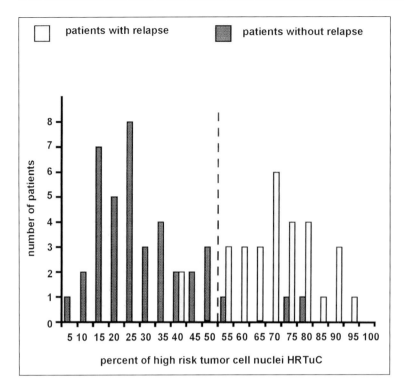

Figure 2.39: Learning sample 2D3D (n = 70)

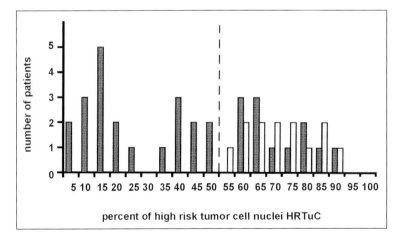

Figure 2.40: Learning sample 2D (n = 46)

considerable side effects, would be without any therapeutic sense. The main aim of the developed nuclear grading method is the definition of three prognostic groups with poor, uncertain, and good prognosis, with an uncertain group as small as possible. For example high risk patients could be treated with adjuvant therapies, patients with uncertain prognosis would be kept under intensive observation, and low risk patients would be controlled in normal follow up periods. Using the data of our investigations it seems to be possible to define subgroups with less than 20 % of patients in the uncertain prognosis group and correct classification rates of about 95 % for patients with poor or good prognosis.

References: Page 204

2.3.5
Cytometric Results of DNA Imaging and Established Prognostic Factors in Primary Breast Cancer

C. M. SCHLOTTER, S. KROPP, U. BOSSE,
U. VOGT, A. BOSSE, K. WASSMANN

Summary

Seven parameters measured by means of cytometric DNA imaging (DNA average, DNA index, 2c deviation index, 5c and 9c exceeding events, variation coefficient of tumour cells and degree of DNA malignancy) in 125 consecutively occurring breast cancers were compared with the classic prognostic factors used in the assessment of breast cancer (size of tumour, nodal status, number of affected lymph nodes, histology, grading, hormone receptor status, age, menopausal status) in order to discover possible correlations.

Of the tumours assessed, 24.8 percent were classed as diploid and 75.2 percent as aneuploid. A differentiated subdivision of the tumours into the categories diploid, hyperdiploid, tetraploid and hypertetraploid according to their DNA index resulted in an accumulation in the hyperdiploid index group (48%). 56.5 percent of the breast cancers lay within the unfavourable malignancy range (≥ 1). It was possible to demonstrate statistically significant correlations between individual DNA parameters and established prognostic factors such as N stage, menopausal status, progesterone-receptor status, histology and grading. In each case the DNA values which varied most strongly from the diploid 2c value correlated with unfavourable "high-risk" breast cancer factors. The T stage and the estrogen-receptor status were revealed as being largely independent of the ploidy of the tumour preparations. A classification of breast cancers with the help of objective, easily reproduced parameters is an addition to conventional histomorphological methods of tumour grading, which are dependent upon subjective judgements by the investigator and which demonstrate a lack of reproducibility.

Approach to Problems

The established classical prognostic factors in breast cancer are used to divide the patients into different prognostic groups. They also serve to assist in the planning of appropriate post-operative therapy. One example of the traditional prognostic factors is histomorphological grading. When this is used to assess the biology of the tumour, it represents a subjective prognostic parameter which is dependent upon the experience of the investigator. It also demonstrates a lack of reproducibility and consistency [1–8].

For this reason, a search has been made for new, objective parameters which will enable a differentiated classification of breast cancers and permit a characterisation according to tumour biological criteria. In combination with traditional prognostic factors, these new prognostic parameters are intended to facilitate the classification of breast cancers and decisions regarding post-operative therapy, especially in the case of nodally negative carcinomas.

It is the aim of this investigation to demonstrate possible correlations between classical prognostic factors associated with breast cancers and the results of DNA cytometry in order to gain information regarding the prognostic validity and importance of DNA parameters.

Investigative Material and Methods

Relevant data from 125 patients who presented consecutively with breast cancer were evaluated. The patients had undergone operative treatment for a primary unilateral mammary cancer during the period 1992–1995.

With regard to the cytometric DNA imaging, in order to prepare for the measurements, surface biopsy preparations (imprint cytology) of fresh breast cancer samples were prepared immediately after excision. In order to safeguard internal standards, a biopsy of bleeding tissue was also prepared from the incision material. After prefixing with Merco-Fix, the preparations were stained according to Feulgen's method. The cytometric DNA measurements were undertaken with a DNA cytophotometer CYDOK manufactured by Hilgers of Königswinter, Germany. Further equipment included a commercial microscope manufactured by Leitz Diaplan with a black-and-white video camera attachment, a NEC Multi-sync 3D screen and computer connected to a Hewlett Packard ink jet printer.

When the slide preparations were examined under the microscope, the cell nuclei of the breast cancer samples had been stained to differing degrees and could be seen on the screen. As an internal standard, at least 20 reference cells were used as a comparison in each case (normal body cells such as lymphocytes, granulocytes, connective tissue cells or ripe epithelial cells). Finally, at least 150 tumour cells were examined and measured on the computer screen. The system recognises the cell nuclei and determines their integrated optical density.

When this method is used, various easily operated menu functions permit the measurement to be carried out in an uncomplicated manner. A cell which appears morphologically suspicious is marked by a click of the mouse, and the measured DNA content appears on the screen beside the cell in question. In addition, cells which have already been measured can be stored or cells which are lying too close together can be separated by using the mouse, thus permitting the individual assessment of each cell in turn. By the selection of cells which seem morphologically suspicious and visual control by an experienced investigator it is possible to avoid the concurrent measurement of stroma or other normal body cells.

All histological and cytometric investigations were carried out by a pathologist (U. B.).

By means of a questionnaire, general information concerning the patients was collected. This included such classical prognostic parameters as pathological TNM classification, histological type, histological grading, steroid receptor status and seven DNA parameters gained as a result of cytometric imaging (DNA average value, DNA index, 2c deviation index, exceeding events, variation coefficient, DNA grade of malignancy according to Böcking, table 2.25).

A comparison was made between all DNA parameters and the prognostic parameters of the breast cancers in order to reveal possible correlations. In addition, averages of the DNA parameters in the various tumour stages, histological groups and steroid receptor classes were compared with each other.

The age of the patients at diagnosis lay between 27 and 86 years, with an average of 59 years and a distinct peak in the 51–65-year age group.

Upon examination of the menopausal status of the patients, 32 (26%) were found to be pre-menopausal and 93 (74%) were post-menopausal.

The weight of the patients examined averaged 71 kg with a minimum of 47 kg and a max-

Table 2.25: Definitions of DNA Parameters

DNA-Parameters	Definitions
Modal value	Position of the base line
DNA Average value	Average DNA content of the measured tumour cells
DNA Index	$\dfrac{\text{DNA content of the tumour cells}}{\text{DNA content of the reference cells}}$
2c Deviation index	Variation of the DNA values around the 2c-value
5c Exceeding events	Absolute total of cells with a DNA content of $\geq 5c$
9c Exceeding events	Absolute total of cells with a DNA content of $\geq 9c$
Coefficient of variation (diagnostic cells)	$VC = \dfrac{\text{Standard deviation}}{\text{Arithmetric mean}} \times 100\%$
Degree of malignancy of DNA	Logarithmic calculation of the 2c deviation index; degree of the extent of the scattering of value around the diploid 2c value

imum of 103 kg. The peak in the distribution of weight lay between 60 kg and 69 kg.

Amongst the 125 patients, 16 were nulliparous (13%). The number of births in the case of the remaining women ranged from 1 to 6 with a peak of 2 births (29%).

In the case of 18 women (15%), the family anamnesis revealed a case of breast cancer amongst female relatives.

Taking into account the tumour stage, all patients underwent either a modified radical mastectomy (59 cases) or a breast-conserving segmental mastectomy (wide excision, 58 cases) or a reduction mastectomy (8 cases).

As a further operative procedure, in the case of 121 patients an axillary lymphodectomy was performed; an average of 14 lymph nodes were removed and examined histologically. A total of 71 (57%) nodally negative patients was determined compared with 54 (43%) nodally positive ones, who revealed between one and 28 affected lymph nodes. 50 (40%) of the patients, predominantly in the nodally positive category, received in addition a course of chemotherapy according to the CMF, EC or FEC scheme (30.4%, 5.6%, 4.0%).

In 71 cases hormone therapy with the antiestrogen Tamoxifen (69 cases) or the aromatase blocker Aminoglutethimide (2 cases) was also carried out.

In addition, 63 (51%) of the patients also underwent a course of radiotherapy of the tumour site. In most cases this was the obligatory irradiation following breast-conserving surgery.

With regard to the site of the tumour, 62 carcinomas (50%) were located in the left and 63 carcinomas (51%) in the right breast. More than 60% of the tumours were situated in the upper outer quadrant. It was ascertained that the right upper outer quadrant was the most common site of the tumour, with a total of 41 cases (33%), whereas the left upper outer quadrant was the site of 38 tumours.

With regard to the histological typing, 66 carcinomas (53%) were ductal and 38 (30%) were lobular. In addition, the tumours investigated included two medullary, six mucinous, two papillary and eight mixed lobular-ductal carcinomas.

By taking the TNM stage into account, it was possible to categorise 57 cases (46%) as Stage T1, 60 cases (48%) as Stage T2, one case (0.8%) as Stage T3 and seven cases as Stage T4. When the Stage T1 cases were further subdivided into T1a, T1b and T1c, 50 of the 57 cases fell into the category T1c, corresponding to a tumour size of > 1–2 cm.

The average tumour size was 2.14 cm with a minimum of 0,4 cm and a maximum of 6 cm. As regards the lymph node status, 71 patients (56.8%) were found to present with an N0 stage, 52 (41.6%) with an N1 stage and 2 patients (1.6%) with an N2 stage.

In only one case could a distant metastasis in the bone area be detected at the time of the investigation.

The histological grading classified three tumours (2.4%) as Grade 1, 19 (15.2%) as Grade 2, 39 (31.2%) as Grade 2–3 and 64 tumours (51.2%) as Grade 3. Thus, a total of 22 carcinomas (17.6%) could be classified as "low grade" (G1/G2) and 103 cases (82.4%) were classified as "high grade" (G2–3/G3).

When the biochemical estrogen and progesterone-receptors were determined, all measurements < 20 fmol/mg were interpreted as negative and all values ≥ 20 fmol/mg were interpreted as definitely positive. In the case of two carcinomas it was not possible to determine the receptors, with the result that the figures for 123 patients were available for evaluation. In the case of 43 patients (35%) the estrogen-receptor (ER) was shown to be negative and in the case of 80 patients (65%) it was ER-positive. Negative progesterone-receptor (PR) values were found in 48 women (39%) and positive PR values in 75 women (61%). When the results for the receptor status were combined, 51 women (41.5%) were classified as ER+ve/PR+ve, 29 cases (23.6%) were ER+ve/PR–ve. In the category ER–ve/PR+ve there were 24 women (19.5%) and in the ER–ve/PR–ve category there were only 19 cases (15.4%).

All statistical calculations and data analysis were carried out using the SPSS for Windows program, version 5.0. In order to establish possible correlations the Pearsons Chi-Square test for contingency tables was applied. In addition, significance tests were carried out by means of variations analysis tables in order to check group-specific average differences. A probability of $p \leq 0,05$ was considered to be statistically significant.

Results

DNA cytometry results

Table 2.26 shows a summary of statistical data of the DNA parameters of the 125 breast cancer patients.

The values of the DNA index range from 0.90 to 3,79 with an average value of 1.62 and an accumulation of values in the hyperdiploid range (1.101–1.89). If the DNA index is divided into groups 0.9–1.1 and >1.1 corresponding to a subdivision into diploid and aneuploid categories, a total of 31 cases (24.8%) were observed to fall within the diploid group in contrast to 94 cases (75.2%) in the aneuploid group. Taking into account the differentiated subdivision of the DNA index into diploid (0.9–1.1), hyperdiploid (1.101–1.89), tetraploid (1.9–2.1) and hypertetraploid (>2.1) categories, a total of 31 diploid (24.8%), 60 hyperdiploid (48%), 12 tetraploid (9.6%) and 22 hypertetraploid (17.6%) carcinomas were diagnosed. There were no cases of hypodiploid carcinoma (DNA index <0.9).

Correlation of the DNA Parameters with Classic Prognostic Factors

In a comparison of the menopausal status with the cytometric results, statistically relevant correlations were discovered in the case of the 2c deviation index and the 9c exceeding events. Observation of the 2c deviation index revealed a clear trend in the group of pre-menopausal patients to higher index values. The postmenopausal status correlated with the lack of 9c exceeding events.

No statistically significant relationship could be established between the DNA parameters and the T Stage or the size of the tumour.

The nodal stage correlated with the DNA index, the 5c and 9c exceeding events and the DNA degree of malignancy. No relevance could be found in the division of the DNA index into diploid and aneuploid categories. However, if the subdivision into diploid, hyperdiploid, tetraploid and hypertetraploid tumours was taken into account, it was observed that the tetraploid tumours correlated with stage N0, since in only one of the 12 cases of tetraploid tumours were the lymph nodes also affected. A converse trend applied in the group of hypertetraploid carcinomas, which were most commonly found in stages N1/N2 ($p = 0.02$). The nodally positive stages N1/N2 correlated with a higher number of 5c and also 9c exceeding events. In the case of nodally negative patients, significantly lower degrees of malignancy were observed than in the case of the nodally positive patients.

If the number of affected lymph nodes was also taken into account, however, no further significant correlation with the DNA parameters could be observed.

The comparison of the histological carcinoma types (lobular, ductal and other types of carcinoma) with the cytometric values produced a

DNA-Parameter	Minimum	Maximum	Average	Median
DNA Average value	2.05 c	9.34 c	3.71 c	3.52 c
DNA Index	0.90	3.79	1.62	1.41
2c Deviation index	0.10	71.20	6.89	3.82
5c Exceeding events	0	99	10.25	5
9c Exceeding events	0	18	1.52	0
Variation coefficient	4.96%	62.07%	29.99%	30.50%
Degree of malignancy of DNA	0.01	3.27	1.16	1,24

Table 2.26, explanation see page 135

large number of significant results. The group of lobular carcinomas tended to display lower DNA average values and 2c deviation indices than the ductal carcinomas. Furthermore, almost two thirds of the lobular tumours displayed between zero and two 5c exceeding events, whilst 71% of the ductal carcinomas displayed three or more 5c exceeding events. Similar results can also be demonstrated in the relationship between histology and DNA degree of malignancy. 65.8% of the lobular breast cancers displayed a degree of malignancy < 1, whilst 68% of the ductal tumours displayed a degree of malignancy > 1.

When the gradings were examined, significant correlations could be demonstrated with the DNA average value, the 2c deviation index, the 5c exceeding events and the DNA degree of malignancy. If the gradings were subdivided into three classes (G1/G2, G2–3, G3), there was a proliferation of low DNA average values in the G1/G2 group, whilst the majority of G3 carcinomas were characterised by a DNA average value ≥4. In addition, a correlation was established between G1, G2 and G2–3 gradings and lower 2c deviation indices, 5c exceeding events and DNA degree of malignancy. Thus, 16 of a total of 22 G1/G2 tumours demonstrated a degree of malignancy < 1, whilst most G3 carcinomas (70%) had a degree of malignancy > 1.

The comparison of the estrogen- and progesterone-receptor status with the DNA parameters revealed only a correlation between the progesterone-receptor status and the DNA index. The subdivision of the index into diploid and aneuploid tumours (DNA index 1) compared with the groups of positive and negative progesterone-receptors revealed a significant increase of progesterone-negative cases in the aneuploid range (DNA index > 1.10). Of 31 carcinomas in the diploid index category, only seven (22.6%) were revealed to have negative progesterone-receptors.

When comparisons were made using the differentiated classification of the DNA index into diploid, hyperdiploid, tetraploid and hypertetraploid (DNA index 2), it could be observed that significantly more progesterone-positive receptor carcinomas lay in the diploid and tetraploid groups. In contrast with this, the tumours with progesterone-negative receptors were to be found in the hyperdiploid and hypertetraploid region of the index.

After further classification into estrogen-receptor/and progesterone-receptor groups (ER/PR), no significant correlations could be detected with the DNA parameters. The observation of the DNA index revealed only a tendency for the groups ER+ve/PR+ve and ER−ve/ PR+ve to occur in the diploid index class (0.9–1.1). The

Table 2.27, explanation see page 137

Prognostic factors	DNA-AV	DNA Index 1	DNA Index 2	2c DI	5c EE	9c EE	CV	DNA-DM
Menopausal status	–	–	–	0.005	–	0.05	–	–
T Stage	–	–	–	–	–	–	–	–
N Stage	–	–	0.02	–	0.03	0.02	–	0.04
No. of affected lymph nodes	–	–	–	–	–	–	–	–
Histology	0.0003	–	–	0.0007	0.003	–	–	0.009
Grading	0.001	–	–	0.001	0.003	–	–	0.006
ER	–	–	–	–	–	–	–	–
PR	–	0.03	0.02	–	–	–	–	–
ER/PR	–	–	–	–	–	–	–	–

Abbreviations: DNA-AV = DNA Average value; DNA Index 1 = diploid/aneuploid; DNA Index 2 = diploid/hyperdiploid/tetraploid/hypertetraploid; 2c DI = 2c Deviation index; 5c EE = 5c Exceeding events; 9c EE = 9c Exceeding events; CV = Coefficient of variation; DNA-DM= DNA Degree of malignancy groups ER+ve/PR–ve- and ER–ve/PR–ve tended to show a DNA index > 1,1 (p = 0.08).

Table 2.27 shows a summary of the significant correlations of the DNA parameters with the conventional prognostic factors relating to breast cancer (Chi Squares tests for contingency tables, $p \leq 0.05$).

Comparisons of Average Values

By means of variation analysis tables, significance tests were undertaken to investigate the differences in average values in the various classes of conventional prognostic factors. In addition, the average values of age, size of tumour, and estrogen and progesterone-receptors in the various classified DNA parameter groups were also compared.

The calculation of the DNA parameter average values in the tumour stages T1, T2, T3/T4 revealed a sharp increase of average values in 5c exceeding events.

The comparison of the average values in the lymph node stages N0 and N1/N2 revealed significant differences in the case of category 9c exceeding events and the coefficient of variation of tumour cells.

Upon investigation of the differences in the number of affected lymph nodes (0, 1–3, > 3), statistically significant differences in the averages of the coefficient of variation were discovered.

With regard to the grading of the tumours, significant differences in the DNA index, the 5c exceeding events, the coefficient of variation and the DNA degree of malignancy were established.

In a comparison of the average values of the DNA parameters for lobular, ductal and other carcinomas, a large number of significant differences were established. There was in each case an increase in the average value in the case of the ductal carcinomas compared with those in the lobular category. Significant changes were deduced with regard to the DNA average value, 2c deviation index, 5c and 9c exceeding events, coefficient of variation and DNA degree of malignancy.

In a comparison of the individual DNA parameters in the pre- and post-menopausal group, statistically significant differences were discovered in the 2c deviation index, the coefficient of variation and the DNA degree of malignancy. In each case, higher values were found in the pre-menopausal group.

The investigation of differences in average values in the DNA parameters in the various hormone receptor groups produced no statistically significant results. However, in the

Table 2.28, explanation see page 138

Prognostic factors	DNA-AV	DNA-Index	2c DI	5c EE	9c EE	CV	DNA-DM
Pre-/postmenopausal	–	–	0.01	–	–	0.001	0.03
T1/T2/T3–4	–	–	–	0.02	–	–	–
N0/N1–2	–	–	–	–	0.03	0.01	–
0/1/> 3 affected lymph nodes	–	–	–	–	–	0.03	–
Lobular/ductal/other	0.01	–	0.04	0.03	0.01	0.04	0.003
G1–2/G2–3/G3	–	0.01	–	0.03	–	0.01	0.01
ER+ve/PR+ve	–	–	–	–	–	–	–
ER+ve/PR–ve	–	–	–	–	–	–	–
ER–ve/PR+ve	–	–	–	–	–	–	–
ER–ve/PR–ve	–	–	–	–	–	–	–

Abbreviations: DNA-AV = DNA Average value, 2c DI = 2c Deviation index, 5c EE = 5 c Exceeding events, 9c EE = 9c Exceeding events, CV = Coefficient of variation, DNA-DM = DNA Degree of malignancy

Table 2.29, explanation see below

Prognostic factors	DNA-AV	DNA-Index	2c DI	5c EE	9c EE	CV	DNA-DM
T Stage							
T1	3.51c	1.60	4.96	8.32	1.04	27.96%	1.05
T2	3.87c	1.63	8.48	10.05	1.76	31.25%	1.24
T3/4	3.97c	1.62	8.78	25.50	3.25	35.35%	1.41
N Stage							
N0	3.55c	1.59	5.79	8.32	1.00	27.80%	1.05
N1–2	3.92c	1.65	8.35	12.78	2.20	33.06%	1.31
Number of affected lymph nodes							
0 Lymph nodes	3.55c	1.59	5.79	8.32	1.00	27.80%	1.05
1–3 Lymph nodes	4.04c	1.74	9.61	12.17	2.00	32.51%	1.34
> 3 Lymph nodes	3.78c	1.55	6.87	13.48	2.44	33.65%	1.28
Grading							
G1/G2	3.35c	*1.39*	7.27	5.77	1.55	24.25%	0.84
G2–3	3.43c	*1.50*	5.01	6.59	1.00	29.02%	1.02
G3	3.99c	*1.76*	7.91	14.02	1.83	32.38%	1.35
Histology							
Lobular	*3.13c*	1.43	3.56	4.24	0.55	26.48%	0.81
Ductal	*3.97c*	1.72	7.59	12.68	1.59	32.21%	1.34
Others	*3.94c*	1.62	10.73	13.48	3.05	29.35%	1.25
Menopausal status							
Pre-menopausal	4.11c	1.63	*10.97*	11.93	2.34	35.59%	*1.42*
Post-menopausal	3.57c	1.61	*5.49*	9.96	1.24	28.21%	*1.07*
ER Status							
ER–ve	3.65c	1.58	5.97	9.51	1.47	29.78%	1.16
ER+ve	3.72c	1.62	7.36	10.43	1.48	30.23%	1.16
PR Status							
PR–ve	3.87c	1.64	8.13	12.94	1.96	29.99%	1.26
PR+ve	3.59c	1.59	6.07	8.29	1.16	30.13%	1.10
ER/PR Status							
ER+ve/PR+ve	3.73c	1.66	7.12	10.18	1.33	30.48%	1.18
ER+ve/PR–ve	3.71c	1.56	7.79	10.86	1.72	29.78%	1.12
ER–ve/PR+ve	3.29c	1.46	3.84	4.29	0.79	29.39%	0.91
ER–ve/PR–ve	4.12c	1.75	8.66	16.11	2.32	30.39%	1.46

Abbreviations: DNA-AV = DNA Average value, 2c DI = 2c Deviation index, 5c EE = 5c Exceeding events, 9c EE = 9c Exceeding events, CV = Coefficient of variation, DNA-DM = DNA Degree of malignancy, ER status = Estrogen receptor status, PR-Status = Progesterone receptor status
(Statistically significant results are printed in italics.)

group estrogen-receptor-negative/progesterone-receptor-positive (ER–ve/PR+ve), the lowest average values of all DNA parameters were observed.

Table 2.28 shows significant difference of average values in a comparison of the DNA parameter average values in the various classes of the conventional prognostic factors ($p \leq 0{,}05$).

Table 2.29 shows a summary of all DNA parameter average values.

In addition, average values for age, size of tumour, estrogen and progesterone-receptors were produced in order to check these factors for significant differences in the various classes of the DNA parameters.

With regard to age, significant reductions of the average values with a corresponding increase of the DNA parameters 2c deviation index, 9c exceeding events and the coefficient of variation could be proven – in other words, an increase in DNA values in the direction of younger patients.

The comparison of the average values for tumour size showed such significant differences in the various classes of 5c exceeding events and the coefficient of variation that an association can be seen between increasing DNA values and an increase in the size of the tumour.

The investigation of the average values of the estrogen-receptors revealed significant differences in the three classes of the 2c deviation index. The lowest estrogen values were to be found in the class <1 and ≥5 2c deviation index.

With regard to the progesterone-receptors, numerous differences in average values could be detected. Whilst the PR average value increased slightly from 154 fmol/mg in the DNA average value range <2.5c to 165 fmol/mg in the range 2.5–3.99c, it fell sharply to an average of 60 fmol/mg in all tumours with an average DNA value ≥ 4c ($p = 0.01$). When the DNA index was subdivided into diploid, hyperdiploid, tetraploid and hypertetraploid categories, significantly higher average progesterone-receptor values were observed in the diploid and tetraploid group (196 and 204 fmol/mg) than in the hyperdiploid and hypertetraploid index ranges (89 and 41 fmol/mg) ($p = 0.003$, figure 2.41). Similarly, a decrease of the average progesterone-receptor value was observed in the 2c deviation index range ≥5, in the groups of 5c and 9c exceeding events and in the degree of malignancy.

Table 2.30 shows a summary of the average values of the conventional prognostic factors age, size of tumour, estrogen- and progesterone-receptor status in comparison to various classes of DNA imaging data.

Discussion

The quantitative determination of the DNA content of human tumours by means of flow or image cytometry has attracted increased interest in recent years. Since the chromosomal aneuploidy is regarded as a sign of neoplasia and aggressive tumour behaviour [9, 10], the DNA ploidies were examined with a view to the validity of the diagnosis or the malignancy grading of tumours.

Thus, a number of solid carcinomas e.g. mammary cancer, bladder carcinoma and stomach carcinoma were examined to determine their DNA content [11–13].

Some authors suggest that diploid mammary carcinoma demonstrates a better prognosis compared with aneuploid tumours with regard to the relapse-free interval and the total survival period [14–16]. In contrast with this view, other investigators observed no significant correla-

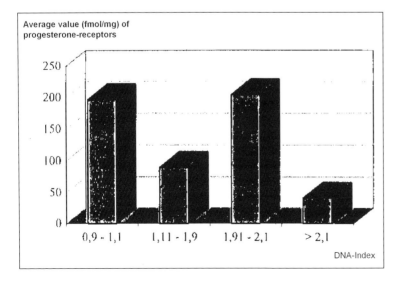

Figure 2.41: Average values (fmol/mg) of progesterone receptors of diploid, hyperdiploid, tetraploid and hypertetraploid mammary carcinomas.

Table 2.30, explanation see page 139

Prognostic factors ▶ DNA-Parameters ▼	Age (years)	p	Size of tumour (cm)	p	ER (fmol/mg)	p	PR (fmol/mg)	p
DNA Average value								
< 2.5 c	61.2		1.83		64.64		154.19	
2.5–3.99 c	58.8		2.18		85.87		165.69	
≥ 4 c	56.8		2.30		44.09		60.17	*0.01*
DNA Index								
0.9–1.1	56.5		2.39		61.67		196.80	
1.11–1.9	60.6		2.58		67.36		89.79	
1.91–2.1	56.6		2.58		107.41		204.56	
> 2.1	57.2		2.36		28.43		41.48	*0.003*
2c Deviation index								
< 1	63.2		1.89		59.13		154.54	
1–4.99	56.4		2.09		101.25		159.94	
≥ 5	56.4	*0.04*	2.35		45.49	*0.05*	70.75	*0.04*
5c Exceeding events								
0–2	60.5		1.93		68.21		188.35	
≥ 3	57.3		2.28	*0.05*	59.75		72.70	*0.0005*
9c Exceeding events								
0	61.3		2.02		68.51		159.69	
1–2	53.9		2.29		69.04		75.01	
≥ 3	54.7	*0.03*	2.36		38.13		32.39	*0.006*
Coefficient of variation								
< 20%	66.5		1.66		83.37		153.08	
20–39.99%	57.5		2.30		53.11		131.51	
≥ 40%	54.6	*0.006*	1.95	*0.007*	79.44		52.00	
DNA Degree of malignancy								
< 1	61.3		2.00		57.93		161.87	
1–2	57.1		2.20		79.47		110.21	
> 2	55.6		2.36		32.91		22.21	*0.02*
DNA Diagnosis								
diploid	57.8		1.95		57.69		172.28	
aneuploid	58.9		2.19		64.81		104.21	

(Statistically significant results are printed in italics. $p \leq 0.05$)

tion between the ploidy of the tumours and survival time [17, 18]. Some investigators reported a tendency for aneuploid tumours to recur faster, although they demonstrated no significant influence on the survival period after recurrence [19]. Hitchcock (1989) was of the opinion that differences in the ploidial pattern between the primary tumour and the metastases was responsible for this phenomenon [20].

Most cytometric studies carried out during recent years have restricted themselves to the evaluation of a small number of cytometric DNA parameters, such as the modal stem line ploidy and the DNA index, which is dependent upon this factor. With regard to analysis of DNA imaging the introduction of the 2c deviation index and the DNA malignancy grade by Böcking represented a considerable enlargement of the spectrum of objective, reproducible parameters [21]. These two parameters provide additional information in addition to the ploidy of the stem line, since they take into account the scattering of values around the diploid 2c value and permit a classification of the malignancy of tumours. The basis for this DNA malignancy grading lies in the observation that the modal chromosomal aneuploidy and the variation of the DNA values of many tumours can be correlated with the patient's prognosis [22].

Since the DNA parameters under investigation are obtained by image cytometry and therefore represent objective algorithmic histogram data, it was decided during the course of this investigation not to make use of the frequently employed histogram classification devised by Auer [11]. This discontinuous classification is a subjective method of interpretation which is subject to large variations within the individual data and between the various data. For this reason it is not recommended for an objective interpretation of DNA measurements (IAC/ASC Task Force on Standardization of Quantitative Methods for Diagnostic Pathology, Chicago, 1990).

The essential problem of the classical histological or cytological grading also lies in its unsatisfactory reproducibility both within the individual data and between the various data [6, 7]. Nonetheless, the prognostic significance of traditional tumour grading methods remains indisputable. Correlations were demonstrated with the survival period both in univariant and multivariant Cox analyses [8].

In view of the problems described above it seems desirable to seek objective, reproducible grading methods which possess a prognostic validity and offer the opportunity of classifying breast cancers according to new criteria.

The DNA average value represents the average DNA content of the measured tumour cells of a carcinoma preparation. In the investigation this figure produced values between 2.05c and 9.34c, with an average value of 3.71c. Taking into account the fact that euploid reference cells contain an average DNA content of 2c, the mere observation of the average figures obtained in the investigation permits the recognition of a significant divergence towards strongly aneuploid values.

Taking the DNA index as the quotient from the DNA content of the measured tumour cells and that of the diploid reference cell population permits the classic division into a diploid and an aneuploid group. In accordance with this subdivision, 24.8% of the carcinomas could be ascribed to the diploid index category. The classification of the aneuploid group into hyperdiploid, tetraploid and hypertetraploid takes into account the varying degrees and potential causes of the aneuploidy and has already been used in other cytometric studies [23].

The differentiated classification permits a quantification of the aneuploidy and gives an indication of potential differences in the subgroups with regard to prognosis. Thus, frequent reference has been made to the improved prognosis of tetraploid tumours compared with other aneuploid lesions, since tetraploidy frequently represents no more than the polyploidisation of a stem line which was originally diploid. The formation of hyperdiploid tumours could be based on the non-disjunction of certain chromosomes [10].

The 2c deviation index describes the variability of the DNA content of the cell nuclei around the normal 2c value and reflects the genetic instability of the carcinoma cells [21]. The large range of the indices between 0.1 and 71.2 with an average of 6.89 and a clustering in the range ≥ 5 is indicative of the considerable lack of homogeneity and variability not only within the group as a whole but also in the sub-group of aneuploid carcinomas.

As long ago as 1990, the IAC/ASC Task Force on Standardization of Quantitative Methods for Diagnostic Pathology named the 2c deviation index as an important prognostic criterion beside the root line ploidy with regard to objective and continuous interpretation of histograms.

In 1984, Böcking introduced the DNA degree of malignancy [21]. This is calculated by means of a logarithmic function of the 2c deviation index. Low values (< 1) are associated with a low risk with regard to the progress of the illness; values ≥ 1 are correspondingly associated with a high risk. Taking into account Böcking's remarks on the classification of DNA malignancy in tumours, a potentially increased risk with regard to the future course of the illness can be assumed for a relatively large percentage of patients (57%). In a prospective image cytometric study of 72 invasive breast cancers, Longin (1992) attributed a degree of malignancy >1 to only 36% of the tumours [24].

As a parameter for the interpretation of individual cells, the 5c exceeding events serves primarily for the dignity diagnosis or the early diagnosis of malignancy. For this purpose, evidence of at least three cells with a DNA content > 5c is required in order to diagnose aneuploidy. By analogy, tissues in which polyploidy up to 8c is diagnosed must demonstrate in at least three cells a DNA content > 9c [25]. In the present study, only malignant breast carcinomas of confirmed histology were investigated, so that a validity diagnosis was superfluous. Nonetheless, considerable differences were observed amongst the 125 carcinomas with regard to the number of 5c and 9c exceeding events. Thus, in 35 cases (28%) there were no exceeding events; in 16 cases (12.8%) there were one or two and in 74 cases (59.2%) there were three or more 5c exceeding events. With regard to the 9c exceeding events, 77 carcinomas (61.6%) displayed none, 25 carcinomas (20%) showed one or two and 23 tumours (18.4%) three or more 9c exceeding events.

The differences in the occurrence of the 5c and 9c exceeding events permit a classification of the carcinomas into different groups as well as supplying information concerning the variation in DNA content of individual tumour cells. In 1992, Kindermann et al. investigated various photocytometric criteria in 115 breast cancers with regard to their prognostic value [26]. They singled out DNA single-cell cytometry as the best parameter for the calculation of the risk of an early relapse. Similarly, a further image cytometric study of breast and stomach cancers demonstrated that only the 5c exceeding rate (percentage of cells above 5c) was of prognostic relevance [12]. In another study of 409 breast-cancer patients, Fallenius applied amongst other criteria the percentage of cells in excess of 5c in order to distinguish between low-grade and highly malignant tumours [15]. He found a very significant correlation between the percentage of cells above 5c and the survival rate of the patients.

Although in literature few statistics are quoted with regard to the varying coefficients of variation in the measured tumour preparations, frequent reference is made to the fact that the large scatter in some histograms should be interpreted as aneuploid peaks and the cause of large coefficients of variation [27]. This statement is further supported by our observations that large increases in the coefficients of variation demonstrate a highly significant correlation with large 2c deviation indices. A study which compared image and flow cytometry found in the case of near diploid-aneuploid peaks larger coefficients of variation than in diploid breast carcinomas [28]. In 1990, Crissmann and his team observed rising average values for the coefficient of variation in an investigation of 25 atypical hyperplasias and 35 intraductal carcinomas of the breast [29]. This figure rose from 5.5% in the diploid reference cell population through 9% for the atypical hyperplasias to 11% for the intraductal carcinomas. Both results indicate a correlation between the height of the coefficient of variation and the malignancy and ploidy of the tissue under examination.

The high percentage of diploid mammary carcinomas described in literature could not be confirmed in this study. Examples of high diploidy rates in malignant breast tumours as measured by flow cytometry range from 35% [30], 45% [18] to 64% [31]. The diploidy rate found in the present investigation was 24.8% [32–34], a figure which is considerably lower than that obtained in other studies.

When flow cytometry is used, no morphological classification or search for possible malignant cells can take place prior to measurement, in order that as far as possible surrounding blood and connective tissue cells as well as normal epithelia can be incorporated into the measurement [35]. Consequently, too many diploid cells are included in the measurement with the result that a number of essentially aneuploid tumours will be allocated a diploid DNA profile. The visualisation and morphological identification of a small number of aneuploid cells within diploid populations acquires particular significance in the analysis of pre-malignant lesions and micro-invasive tumours [27]. In this case, individual early changes can be detected with the help of single-cell interpretation. Flow cytometry cannot take these rare events into account.

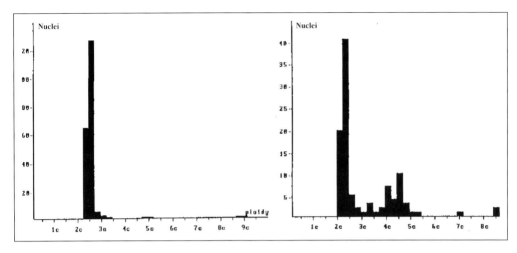

Figure 2.42: DNA Image cytograms. Left: Hyperdiploid mammary carcinoma showing little proliferation. Right: Hyperdiploid mammary carcinoma showing high proliferation.

Since image cytometry requires fewer cells for the measurement, it permits the analysis of smaller samples such as needle biopsies and impression preparations. This is particularly interesting with regard to the increasing number of small, unpalpable lesions. Furthermore, a re-examination of the measurement results and renewed measurement of the slide preparations is possible at any time if the measured images are saved in the computer beforehand. It follows that good reproducibility is therefore achieved.

If the stem line is separated from a duplication population, the use of image cell analysis also permits an opinion to be given with regard to the proportion of proliferating cells (figure 2.42).

Comparative investigations between proliferating cells (S-G2/M-Phase) using flow and image analysis show relatively close correlations [36] (figure 2.43).

The disadvantages of DNA image analysis lie in the small number of measured cells, which leads to a poorer histogram resolution and statistically less significant measurement results [23].

A significant relationship to the various T stages could only be demonstrated by a comparison of the average values of the 5c exceeding events. The lack of further correlation between DNA parameters and T stage is an important result because the size of the tumour is established as one of the most important prognostic factors. Most cytometry studies report a positive correlation between the T stage and ploidy. Thus, Beerman (1990) found after classifying the DNA indices of 690 breast cancer preparations an increased incidence of aneuploidy in tumour stage T2 to T4 [35]. Similarly, a DNA image analysis of 72 invasive breast tumours showed a positive correlation between the size of the tumour and the DNA degree of malignancy [24]. A study of 464 breast tumours demonstrated an increase in the average tumour size from 1,8 cm in the case of the Auer histogram type 1 [11] (diploid) to 2.2 cm in the aneuploid histogram types 3 and 4 [37]. In the present investigation, diploid and aneuploid tumours do not vary significantly as regards size. Thus, the diploid tumours had an average size of 1.95 cm compared with 2.19 cm in the case of the aneuploid growths. However, this result did not demonstrate any statistical significance.

In a flow-cytometry study of 56 cases of ductal carcinoma in situ, Killeen and Namiki (1991) report a lack of correlation between stem line ploidy and tumour size [38]. Mittra and McRae (1991) delivered a statistical summary of published results to provide a correlation between prognostic factors in breast cancer [39]. The authors distinguish between clinical-anatomical factors such as tumour size and the

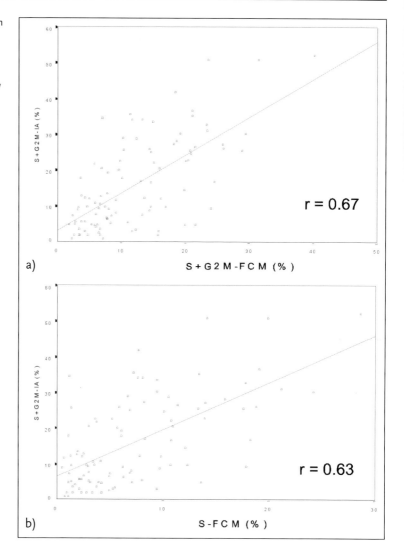

Figure 2.43: a) Correlation of proliferation phases S/G2/M (above); b) Correlation between S/G2/M (Image cytometry) and S-phase (Flow cytometry; bottom). [58]

status of the axillary lymph nodes and biological-prognostic factors, such as grading, hormone-receptor status and DNA ploidy (DNA index). Hereby, they found in only four out of a total of twenty papers a correlation between DNA index and tumour size. However, they discovered a relationship between the various biological prognostic factors themselves, whilst demonstrating a lack of correlation between biological and clinical-anatomical parameters. Breast cancer is probably determined by the individual biological aggressivity and metastasic potential on the one hand and the age of the tumour on the other.

With regard to the correlation between lymph node status and ploidy, literature to date reports various results. Whilst some authors report a positive correlation between ploidy and N stage as well as the number of affected lymph nodes [40, 41, 17], other investigators found no correlation between these two prognostic factors [35, 42, 43, 37]. The association of lymph node metastases with higher DNA malignancy grades and 5c and 9c exceeding events leads to the conclusion that major deviations from these cytometric parameters also represent an unfavourable factor with regard to prognosis. An interesting observation is that, at the time of investigation, only one of the tetraploid carcinomas had produced lymph node metastases. This correlation between tetraploidy and stage N0 is further evidence of the frequently described better prognosis of tetraploid tumours [10].

The lobular type of carcinoma correlated with lower DNA values, whilst the ductal type tended towards higher values. In contrast to the ductal carcinomas with an average DNA malignancy grading of 1.34, lobular tumours demonstrated an average malignancy grade of only 0.81. This value corresponds with a prognostic assessment as "low risk" tumours [22] since they lie in the DNA malignancy grade < 1.

Olszewski (1981) made similar observations in a flow cytometric study of 92 malignant breast tumours [44]. In addition he found a correlation between a lower ploidy and histological sub-types which demonstrate a better prognosis, such as colloid, tubular and ductal G1 carcinomas. Raju (1993) and Moran (1984) made comparable observations [45, 46]. A few less common special types of tumour – tubular, mucinous and cribriform carcinomas – demonstrate a much better prognosis, whilst lobular and medullary cancers occupy an intermediate position between the previously listed and ductal carcinomas as regards prognosis [47].

There is a good deal of literature describing the correlation between histological grading and the DNA content of the tumour [28, 41, 48]. Only a minority of authors saw no relationship between the two biological tumour parameters [49]. The literature study of Mittra and McRae (1991) discovered a correlation between DNA index and breast cancer grading in 16 out of 17 published studies [39]. Most investigators report an association between poor carcinoma differentiation and an aneuploid DNA content. Thus, Owainiti (1987) found diploidy in 78% of well differentiated breast cancers, compared with 74% aneuploidy in poorly differentiated tumours [19]. Moran (1984) and Sharma (1991) make similar observations. In the present study, a clear link was established between poorly differentiated carcinomas and divergent or higher DNA values [46]. This result supports the theory that poorly differentiated tumours are the biological or phenotyicpal result of aneuploidy. The clinical consequences are a shorter survival period and a polycentricity of the tumour [47, 48].

Although only some of the DNA parameters displayed a correlation with the menopausal status or the age of the patient at diagnosis (2c deviation index, coefficient of variation, DNA malignancy grade, 9c exceeding events), nonetheless there seems to be an association between relative youth and/or pre-menopausal status and higher DNA values. Other studies tend to report controversial results in this respect. Most studies differentiate only in general terms between euploid and aneuploid tumours. An investigation by Azavedo (1990) reported, as in the present study, a reduction of the average age by 10 years from 66 years in the case of diploid tumours to 56 years for aneuploid cancers [51]. A study of 464 patients calculated an average age of 62 years for histogram types 1 and 2 according to Auer, as opposed to an average age of 58–59 years for histogram types 3 and 4. Following Auer's interpretation this would reveal a correlation between aneuploidy (type 3 and 4) and relatively young age [37]. Coulsen (1984) published similar results [14]. Hedley (1987) found the opposite to be the case [41], as did Toikkanen (1990) [18]. Keyhani-Rofagha (1990) and Moran (1984) saw no link between these parameters [52, 46].

The significance of the present results lies firstly in the fact that a rough differentiation was arrived at between diploid and aneuploid tumours, and secondly in the fact that it takes into account parameters which have hitherto seldom been investigated, such as the 2c deviation index, the DNA degree of malignancy and the exceeding events. This is of particular importance in that a greater divergence of these parameters demonstrated a significant correlation with relatively young age and/or pre-menopausal status. These results agree with the opinion that pre-menopausal status is regarded as a high-risk factor when applied as a prognostic criterion [53, 54].

The estrogen-receptor status (ER) showed in the present investigation almost no correlation with the DNA parameters. It was merely observed that there was a reduction of the ER average value in the group of patients with a 2c deviation index ≥5 when compared with the group with a 2c deviation index < 5.

With regard to the progesterone-receptor status (PR), there was a significant clustering of PR negative values in the hyperdiploid and hypertetraploid DNA index range. The average progesterone-receptor values varied significantly in the various classes of DNA paramters; a reduction in the average value was observed in the DNA classes which are considered to be prognostically unfavourable.

The relationship between hormone receptor status and DNA content of the breast cancers is regarded as being a very important one because the estrogen-receptor status in particular is considered to be an important prognostic factor with regard to survival time and response to therapy [55].

In comparison with our observations, most investigators arrived at a different result. They saw a significant clustering of estrogen-positive values in the case of diploid tumours and a lack of hormone receptors in aneuploid tumours [35, 56, 57]. Whilst a majority of the investigations studied only the stem line ploidy or the DNA index, Longin (1992) demonstrated in a prospective image cytometry study a significant correlation between DNA degree of malignancy and hormone receptor status [24].

Analogous to our results, some investigators were unable to discover a relationship between estrogen-receptor status and ploidy [19, 52, 58]. In agreement with our results, Lee (1991) found a significant association between aneuploidy and progesterone-receptor negativity [28].

The distribution of the progesterone-receptor average values into the four different DNA index groups adopted in this paper emphasises once more the special position of tetraploid carcinomas within the aneuploid group. This sub-group even demonstrated a higher average progesterone-receptor value than diploid carcinomas. Bearing in mind the potentially favourable effect of high positive receptor values this could result in a better prognosis in future for tetraploid carcinomas. As early as 1964, Atkin reported on the improved prognosis for tetraploid carcinomas of the cervix compared with diploid tumours [59].

In the hypertetraploid index group, the average value of the progesterone-receptor was only half that found in the hyperdiploid group. This leads indirectly to the worst prognosis in the case of hypertetraploid carcinomas, because these were associated with particularly low progesterone-receptor values. Beerman (1990) also reported the least favourable prognosis for patients with hypertetraploid tumours within a pre-menopausal group [35].

There is still a lack of agreement as to whether DNA parameters should be used as prognostic factors in the assessment of breast cancers. In this study, it was possible to show significant links between DNA parameters and important prognostic factors such as lymph node status, histological typing and histological grading. Other factors, such as T stage and estrogen-receptor status, showed themselves to be on the whole independent of the ploidy of the tumour preparations. Interesting perspectives were discovered regarding the indices which to date have been relatively little investigated, such as the 2c deviation index, 5c exceeding events and DNA degree of malignancy, whilst simply classifying the tumours as diploid or aneuploid produced no statistically significant results. This observation underlines the fact that the large class of aneuploid breast cancers cannot be treated as a single group when it comes to prognosis. The sub-classification of the DNA index into four sub-groups as undertaken in the present study takes into account the different areas of aneuploidy; the results regarding the frequency of positive or negative progesterone-receptors and average progesterone value confirm the correctness of this sub-classification. It will be the object of future studies to examine, after lengthy periods of continued observation, the clinical relevance of image cytometric DNA parameters with regard to recurrence-free survival and total survival in single-variant and multi-variant analyses.

References: Page 206

2.3.6
The Influence of New Molecular Biological Parameters on Prognosis and Assessment in Primary Breast Cancers – Attempt at a Molecular Biological Classification

U. Vogt, C. M. Schlotter, U. Bosse

The discovery of specific changes in malignant tumours has given an important new impetus to oncological studies. New information regarding the function of oncogenes and oncoproteins has made a significant contribution to the understanding of the basis for malignant growth in the spheres of both cell biology and molecular biology. Based on this information, new approaches to the diagnosis, prognosis and therapy of malignant disease have been developed. In our study we should like to compare critically the value of new molecular biological parameters and their methods of determination with the results of other studies and to present a distinct new classification of breast cancer.

Patient Group

165 primary breast cancers were the subject of our study. According to the staging results, 86% of the patients were T1 or T2 (T1 → 71%; T2 → 15%), 6% of the cases presented with T3 or T4. There was no staging result in 8% of the cases. The grading indicated that 54% of the cases were G3 (which was taken to include G2–G3). 41% of the patients were G1 or G2. There was no grading in 5% of the cases. 121 patients were post-menopausal, 38 were pre-menopausal and 6 were peri-menopausal. The median of their age lay at 60 years (33–98 years). The following graph (fig. 2.44) shows the histological spread.

The following prognostic and predictory parameters were determined (table 2.31).

The following graph shows the distribution of the hormone receptors and of pS2 throughout the patient group (fig. 2.45).

Oncogenes

In 1983 the first report was published describing an amplification of the c-myc oncogenes in a human tumour [1]. Also in 1983, a study by Escot and others demonstrated the value of the c-myc amplification in breast cancer [2]. One-third of the tumours investigated demonstrated amplification of the c-myc gene. In subsequent clinical studies these results were substantiated. A relationship was demonstrated between the c-myc amplification and the progress of the disease and the survival rate in both nodally negative and nodally positive breast cancers. In the mid-1990s, studies by Berns and Klijn showed that c-myc amplified breast cancers responded less well to chemotherapy [3, 4]. The expression product of the c-myc oncogene is over-expressed in tumours with amplification. It represents a phosphoprotein found in the nucleus and is necessary for cell proliferation. If

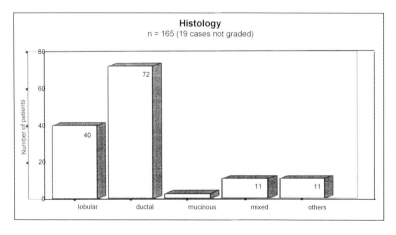

Figure 2.44: Histological Typing

Table 2.31: Determination of prognostic and predictive parameters

Parameter	Method of determination	Limit
Estrogen receptor	Biochemical (EIA)	20 fmol/mg
Progesterone receptor	Biochemical (EIA)	20 fmol/mg
pS2	Biochemical (EIA)	20 ng/mg
erb B-1	Double differential PCR (ddPCR)	> 0,4 <1,6
erb B-2	ddPCR	> 2.0
c-myc	ddPCR	> 3.0

Proliferation/DNA-Index flow cytometry			Proliferation/DNA-Index image analysis		
Equipment	Proliferation	DNA-Index	Equipment	Proliferation	DNA-Index
FacScan (BD) and CCA (Partec)	Proliferation S-Phase + G2/M-Phase > 12 % or S-Phase > 7%	Diploid 0.95–1.2 (incl. near diploid) Aneuploid > 1.2 < 1.95 Tetraploid 1.95–2.1 Hypertetraploid > 2.1 Hypoploid < 0.95	CYDOK (Hilgers)	S/G2/M-Phase > 18 %	Diploid 0.95–1.2 (incl. near diploid) Aneuploid > 1.2 < 1.9 Tetraploid 1.9–2.1 Hypertetraploid > 2.1 Hypoploid < 0.95

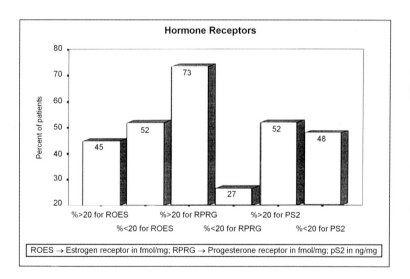

Figure 2.45, explanation see page 147

the myc protein is absent, the cell is removed from the cell division cycle. Through the function of the myc protein there is a relationship to a further oncogene for breast cancer, namely erb B-2. The expression product of the erb B-2 gene represents a membranous protein related to the epidermal growth factor (EGF-R). In a line of tumour cells, a negative regulation of the erb B-2 through the myc protein was observed. Denis Slalom reported in 1987 a pilot study in which he established a negative correlation between the grade of amplification of the erb B-2 gene and the disease-free interval and the survival time of nodally positive breast-cancer patients after operative therapy [5]. In 1989 he followed this study with a second, more extensive investigation. In it he demonstrates in 526 breast cancer cases the significance of the erb B-2 amplification and over-expression for the prognosis of nodally positive breast cancer [6]. There is considerable controversy in reports of the clinical relevance of erb B-2 for nodally negative breast cancer [7, 8, 9, 10].

The results of the international (Ludwig) breast-cancer study group [10] with 1506 patients demonstrate a negative predictive value of the erb B-2 expression in cancer tissue with regard to its response to polychemotherapy in both nodally positive and nodally negative breast cancer. The studies of Paik [11] showed that sub-groups with a high risk could be identified by means of the erb B-2 amplification or over-expression in patient groups with otherwise favourable prognostic factors. Paik found that patients with tumours with Grade 1 malignancy and an erb B-2 over-expression experienced a shortened interval without disease.

In Allred's study [12], in the group of nodally negative patients with T 1/2, few of the estrogen-receptor positive tumours demonstrated an erb B-2 amplification, and yet these patients too demonstrated a very short interval without recurrence of the disease. The work of Muss et al. [13] in 1994 demonstrated that the erb B-2 has not only a prognostic but also a predictive value. The EGF receptor (erb B-1) has a similar prognostic and predictive relevance to erb B-2.

As Wright (1992) [14] showed, erb B-1 over-expressed breast cancers respond less well to anti-hormone therapy. Klijn came to the same conclusions in 1993 [4].

Brand and others showed in 1995 [15] that a loss of the section of the erb B-1 gene is linked to a shorter disease-free interval. They also found that breast cancer patients with a ratio of erb B-1/erb B-2 less than 0.15 had a significantly shorter interval without recurrence of the disease. This also applied to nodally negative patients. The method of oncogene detection chosen by us is the double differential PCR, ddPCR [16, 17, 18].

The polymerase chain reaction (PCR) was developed by B. Mullis and H. A. Ehrlich in the mid-1980s [19]. It is a method for the propagation of DNA in vitro. It was not until 1988 that PCR became useful for medical diagnostics, with the discovery and isolation of thermally stable polymerase from the bacterium thermus aquaticus, the so-called taq-polymerase, which permitted an automatisation of the PCR. The principle of PCR is simple. The DNA with the desired target sequence is separated into complementary single strands by means of thermal denaturation. These strands are then copied by the Taq polymerase, and the DNA strands, thus retained, are used again as matrices. The DNA target sequence is thus propagated exponentially in this manner. The starting and finishing points of the DNA to be amplified are determined by means of chemically synthetic oligo-nucleotides (primers).

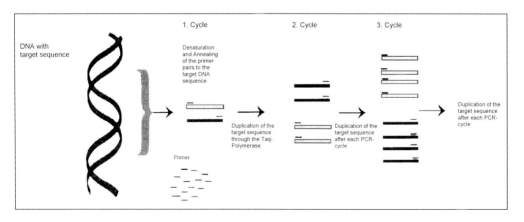

Figure 2.46: Sequence of a PCR Reaction

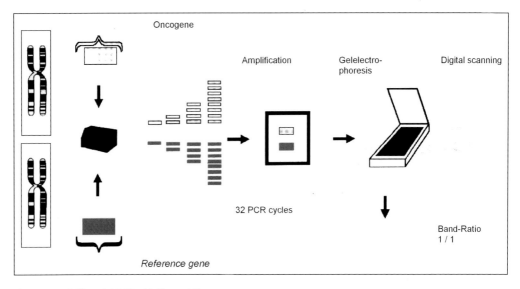

Figure 2.47: Differential PCR with Normal Tissues

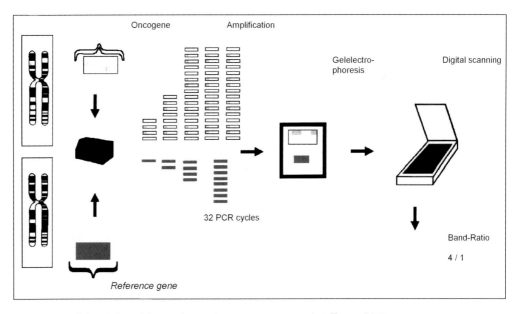

Figure 2.48: Detection of Amplification from Breast Cancer Tissues with Differential PCR

These are complementary to each of the DNA target strands in question and home in on their target sequence, like a probe, after each thermal denaturation. The Taq polymerase recognises the marked region after each target sequence has been thus marked, and replicates it [20]. The diagram demonstrates the various stages in the PCR reaction. Common replication produces two PCR products after a corresponding number of reaction cycles. These are separated with the help of gelelectrophoresis, and after they have been made visible their density is measured. The resulting ranges of values are finally differentiated from each

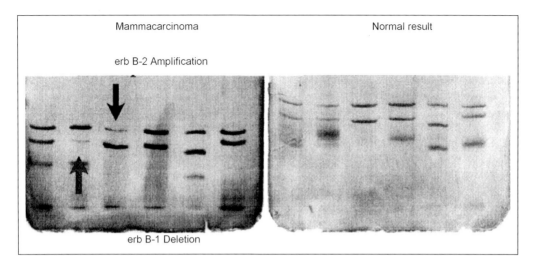

Figure 2.49

other, which explains the special name given to this type of PCR (fig. 2.46).

In a healthy or unchanged tissue sample the difference in value between the two PCR products is 1, as can be seen in figure 2.47.

If an amplification is present, as is the case in tumour samples, the difference between the two values will be greater than 1, whereby the deletion of an oncogene will lead to a difference in value of less than 1 (figure 2.48, figure 2.49). With the assistance of the quantitative differential PCR, amplifications or deletions of oncogenes in tumour samples can quickly be determined.

Theoretically, one cell from the tumour sample provides sufficient material for the investigation. In practical terms, specimens of 1 mg or more are adequate. This means that tumours smaller than 10 mm can also be examined for genetic aberrations by this method. The disadvantage of ddPCR compared with other methods (immunohistochemistry) lies in the use of native or cryo-prepared material. To date, samples which have been fixed with paraffin cannot be amplified reliably for reproduction. There follows another practical specimen from a patient following ddPCR and visualisation.

Results

In this section, the frequency of occurrence of events in percentages of the number of cases, or in the number of patients affected, are recorded. The reason for this is that the patient group was such that, of the 165 primary breast cancers, in some cases very small groups were formed in which a percentage evaluation would lead to a false positive or negative interpretation. Furthermore, image and flow cytometry were used in an attempt to divide the subjects into genetic classes. In doing so, one aim was a comparison between image and flow cytometry and their correlation with other prognostic factors; another was an attempt at the classification of breast cancers by means of a subdivision into genetic classes. The investigation was based on works by Schenk (1994), Sinn (1997) and Dawson (1990) [19,20,21]. The following genetic classes were formed and the distribution compared with other prognostic factors investigated:

- Diploid breast cancer with high and low proliferation
- Aneuploid breast cancer with high and low proliferation
- Tetraploid breast cancer with high and low proliferation
- Hypertetraploid breast cancer with high and low proliferation

For the definition of the individual classes see the table above. No classification of the hypoploid breast cancers was undertaken since the group included only two cases of this type. The old histological classification, together with all the prognostic factors under investigation, was correlated with the new genetic classification. All results are presented in tabular or graphic form (fig. 2.50–2.58).

References: Page 209

Summary of results for the hormone receptor status (HR)

The hormone receptor status is defined as positive when all three parameters (estrogen receptor, progesterone receptor and pS2) lie above their cut-off value (compare the table above). All patients were defined as having a negative hormone receptor status if at least one parameter was negative. In the case of a negative status, no further subdivision was made to indicate patients with two or three negative parameters since too few cases were involved (fig. 2.59–2.66).

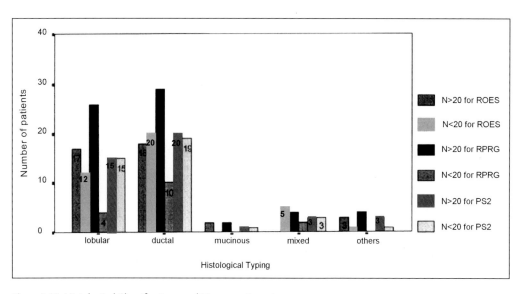

Figure 2.50: Histological Classifications and Hormone Receptors

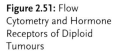

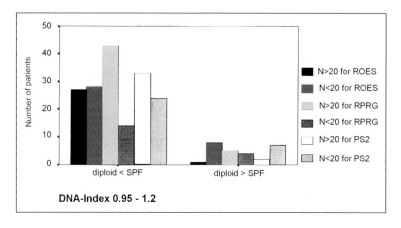

Figure 2.51: Flow Cytometry and Hormone Receptors of Diploid Tumours

Oncogene aberration and ploidy/proliferation. The following oncogenes were subjected to analysis: c-myc, erb B-1, erb B-2 and the factor erb B-1/erb B-2. The cut-off values of the oncogenes have been taken from the publication by Brandt and others [17]. The same primers and PCR conditions were chosen as in the publication. All results are shown as bar charts (fig. 2.67–2.72).

References: Page 209

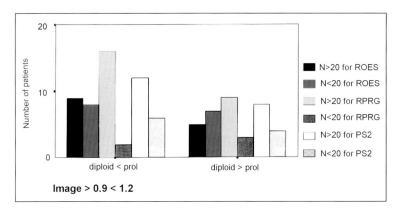

Figure 2.52: Image Analysis and Hormone Receptors of Diploid Tumours

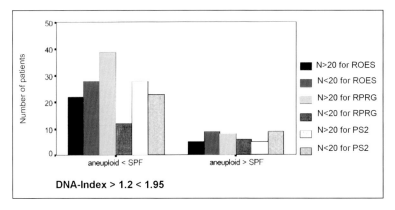

Figure 2.53: Flow Cytometry and Hormone Receptors of Aneuploid Tumours

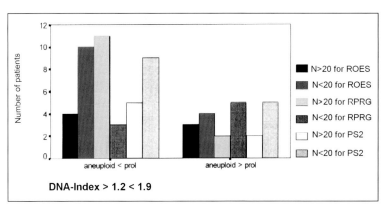

Figure 2.54: Image Analysis and Hormone Receptors of Aneuploid Tumours

Figure 2.55: Flow Cytometry and Hormone Receptors of Tetraploid Tumours

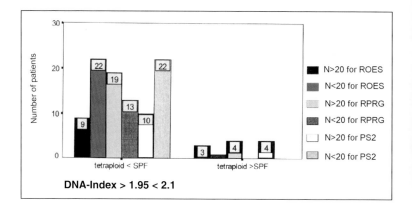

Figure 2.56: Image Analysis and Hormone Receptors of Tetraploid Tumours

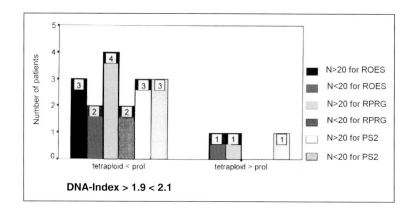

Figure 2.57: Flow Cytometry and Hormone Receptors of Hypertetraploid Tumours

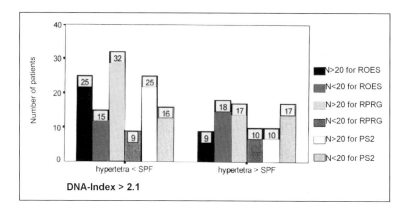

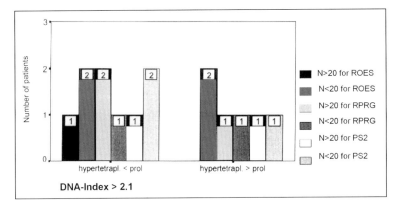

Figure 2.58: Image Analysis and Hormone Receptors of Hypertetraploid Tumours

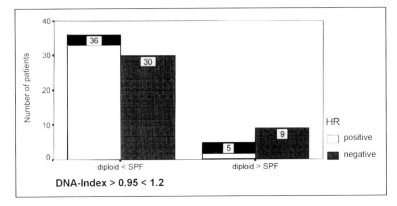

Figure 2.59: Flow Cytometry and HRS of Diploid Tumours

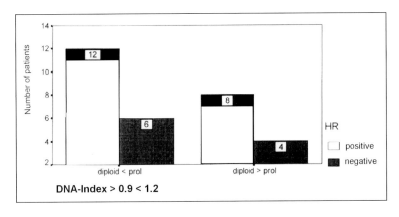

Figure 2.60: Image Analysis and HRS of Diploid Tumours

Figure 2.61: Flow Cytometry and HRS of Aneuploid Tumours

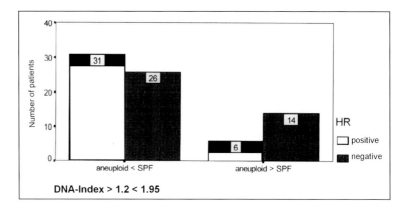

Figure 2.62: Image Analysis and HRS of Aneuploid Tumours

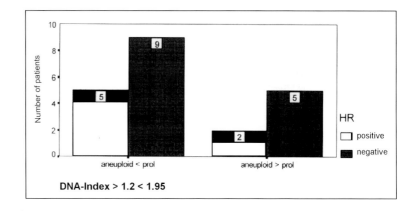

Figure 2.63: Flow Cytometry and HRS of Tetraploid Tumours

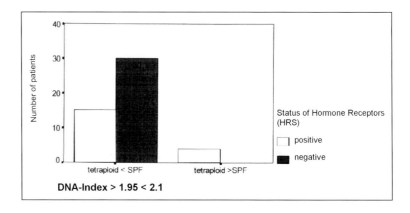

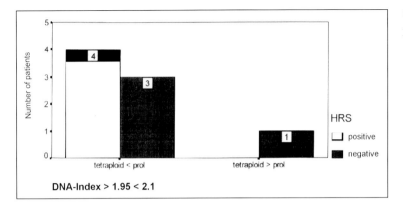

Figure 2.64: Image Analysis and HRS of Tetraploid Tumours

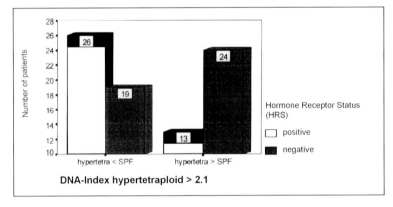

Figure 2.65: Flow Cytometry and HRS of Hypertetraploid Tumours

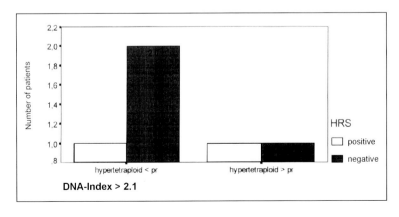

Figure 2.66: Image Analysis and HRS of Hypertetraploid Tumours

Figure 2.67: Flow Cytometry and Oncogenes of Diploid Tumours

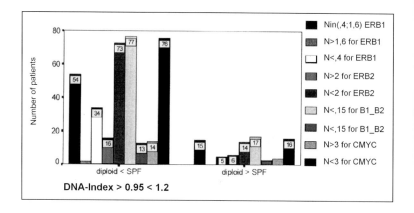

Figure 2.68: Image Analysis and Oncogenes of Diploid Tumours

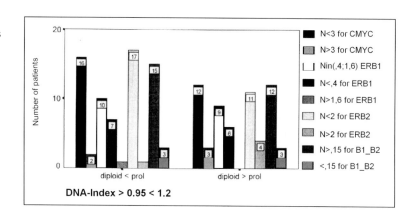

Figure 2.69: Flow Cytometry and Oncogenes of Aneuploid Tumours

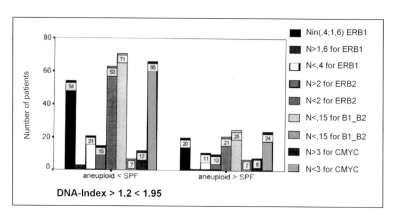

Quality Assurance Recommendations for an Objective Diagnosis 159

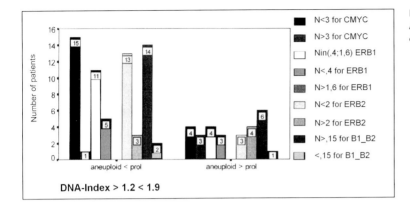

Figure 2.70: Image Analysis and Oncogenes of Aneuploid Tumours

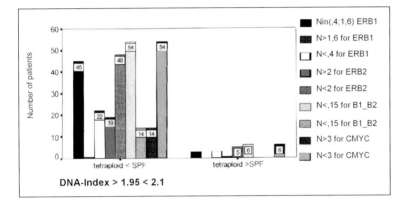

Figure 2.71: Flow Cytometry and Oncogenes of Tetraploid Tumours

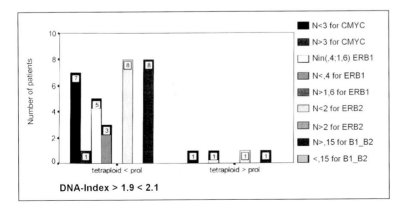

Figure 2.72: Image Analysis and Oncogenes of Tetraploid Tumours

Appendices

Appendices 2.1.1

Appendix 1

National Coordinating Group for Breast Screening Pathology

Chairman:
- Professor J. P. Sloane, Department of Pathology, University of Liverpool, Royal Liverpool University Hospital, Liverpool L69 3BX
- Dr T. J. Anderson, Department of Pathology, University Medical School, Teviot Place, Edinburgh EH8 9AG
- Dr L. Bobrow, Department of Histopathology, Addenbrooke's Hospital, Cambridge CB2 2QQ
- Dr C. L. Brown, Institute of Pathology, The London Hospital Medical College, Turner Street, London EI 1 BB
- Professor R. L. Carter, Department of Histopathology, Royal Surrey County Hospital, Egerton Road, Guildford, Surrey GU2 5XX
- Dr C. E. Connolly, Department of Pathology, Clinical Sciences Institute, University College Hospital, Costello Road, Galway, Republic of Ireland
- Dr J. Coyne, Department of Histopathology, University Hospital of South Manchester, West Didsbury, Manchester M20 8LR
- Dr N. S. Dallimore, Department of Histopathology, Llandough Hospital, Penarth, South Glamorgan CF6 IXX
- Dr J. D. Davies, Breast Pathology Unit, University of Bristol, Southmead Hospital, Bristol BSIO 5NB
- Dr P. M. Dennis, Department of Histopathology, Peterborough District Hospital, Thorpe Road, Peterborough, Cambridgeshire PE3 6DA
- Professor P. Dervan, Pathology Department, Mater Misericordiae Hospital, Eccles Street, Dublin 7, Republic of Ireland
- Dr I. O. Ellis, Department of Histopathology, City Hospital, Hucknall Road, Nottingham NG5 1 PB
- Professor C. W. Elston, Department of Histopathology, City Hospital, Hucknall Road, Nottingham NG5 1 PB
- Dr S. Humphreys, Department of Histopathology, King's College Hospital, Denmark Hill, London SE5 9RS
- Dr J. Lowe, Department of Histopathology, Bradford Royal Infirmary, Duckworth Lane, Bradford, West Yorks BD9 6RJ
- Professor R. E. Mansel, Department of Surgery, University of Wales College of Medicine, Heath, Cardiff CF4 4XW
- Dr J. McCartney, Department of Histopathology, Walsgrave Hospital, Cufford Bridge Road, Walsgrave, Coventry CV2 2DX
- Professor J. O. D. McGee, Nuffield Department of Pathology and Bacteriology, John Radcliffe Hospital, Oxford 0X3 9DU
- Dr M. Michell, Department of Radiology, King's College Hospital, Denmark Hill, London SE5 9RS
- Dr S. Moss, Cancer Screening Evaluation Unit, The Institute of Cancer Research, Block D, Cotswold Road, Sutton, Surrey SM2 5NG
- Miss C. Munt, Cancer Screening Evaluation Unit, The Institute of Cancer Research, Block D, Cotswold Road, Sutton, Surrey SM2 5NG
- Mrs J. Patrick, NHS Breast Screening Programme, The Manor House, 260 Ecclesall Road South, Sheffield S 1 1 9PS
- Dr D. J. Scott, Department of Histopathology, Newcastle General Hospital, Westgate Road, Newcastle upon Tyne NE4 6BE

- Dr S. M. Shousha, Department of Histopathology, Charing Cross Hospital, Fulham Palace Road, London W6 8RF
- Dr J. M. Sloan, Department of Histopathology, Royal Victoria Hospital, Belfast, Northern Ireland BT 1 2 6BA
- Dr C. Swinson, Department of Health, Weilington House, 135–155 Waterloo Road, London SEI 8UG
- Dr J. Theaker, Department of Histopathology, Southampton General Hospital, Tremona Road, Southampton, Hampshire SO9 4XY
- Dr P. A. Trott, Department of Cytopathology, Royal Marsden Hospital, Fulham Road, London SW3 6JJ
- Professor J. C. E. Underwood, Department of Pathology, University of Sheffield Medical School, Beech Hill Road, Sheffield S 10 2RX
- Dr R. A. Walker, University of Leicester, Department of Pathology, School of Medicine, Robert Kilpatrick Building, Leicester Royal Infirmary, PO Box 65, Leicester LE2 7LX
- Dr C. A. Wells, Department of Histopathology, St. Bartholomew's Hospital Medical School, West Smithfield, London EC 1 A 7BE
- Dr H. D. Zakhour, Department of Histopathology, Arrowe Park Hospital, Arrowe Park Road, Upton, Wirral, Merseyside L49 5PE

Writing group

- Dr T. J. Anderson
- Professor R. W. Blamey
- Dr J. Coyne
- Dr J. D. Davies
- Dr I. O. Ellis
- Professor C. W. Elston
- Dr S. Humphreys
- Dr J. Lowe
- Dr J. Nottingham
- Professor J. P. Sloane (chairman)
- Dr C. A. Wells

Appendix 2

Reporting Forms

NHSBSP Histopathology Reporting Form:

NATIONAL HEALTH SERVICE BREAST SCREENING PROGRAMME

HISTOPATHOLOGY

Surname .... Forenames .... Date of Birth ....
Screening No. .... Hospital No. .... Report No. ....
PATHOLOGIST .... Date of reporting .... Report No. ....

Histological calcification   ☐ Absent   ☐ Benign   ☐ Malignant   ☐ Both

Specimen radiograph seen?   ☐ Yes ☐ No   Mammographic abnormality present in specimen? ☐ Yes ☐ No ☐ Unsure

Specimen Type   ☐ Localisation biopsy   ☐ Open biopsy   ☐ Segmental excision   ☐ Mastectomy   ☐ Wide bore needle core

Specimen Weight .... g

Benign lesions present   ☐ Yes   ☐ No   Malignant lesions present   ☐ Yes   ☐ No

---

BENIGN LESIONS

☐ Complex sclerosing lesion/radial scar   ☐ Multiple papilloma
☐ Periductal mastitis/duct ectasia   ☐ Solitary papilloma
☐ Fibroadenoma   ☐ Sclerosing adenosis
☐ Fibrocystic change   ☐ Solitary cyst
☐ Other (please specify) ....

EPITHELIAL PROLIFERATION

☐ Not present   ☐ Present with atypia (ductal)
☐ Present without atypia   ☐ Present with atypia (lobular)

MALIGNANT LESIONS

NON-INVASIVE

☐ Not present
☐ Ductal, high grade   ☐ Ductal, other
☐ Lobular   ☐ Paget's   SIZE (Ductal only) .... mm
MICROINVASION (< 1mm)   ☐ Not present   ☐ Present   ☐ Possible

INVASIVE

☐ Not present   ☐ Mucinous carcinoma
☐ "Ductal"/no specific type (NST)   ☐ Tubular carcinoma
☐ Lobular carcinoma   ☐ Mixed (Please tick component types present)
☐ Medullary carcinoma   ☐ Not assessable
Other primary carcinoma (please specify) ....
Other malignant tumour (please specify) ....
MAXIMUM DIAMETER OF INVASIVE TUMOUR .... mm
WHOLE SIZE OF TUMOUR (to include DCIS extending >1mm beyond invasive area) .... mm
AXILLARY NODES PRESENT   ☐ Yes   ☐ No   Number positive .... Total number ....
OTHER NODES PRESENT   ☐ Yes   ☐ No   Number positive .... Total number ....
                                            Site of other nodes ....
EXICISION MARGINS   ☐ Reaches margin   ☐ Uncertain   Does not reach margin (nearest .... mm)

GRADE   ☐ I   ☐ II   ☐ III   ☐ Not assessable
DISEASE EXTENT   ☐ Localised   ☐ Multiple   ☐ Not assessable
VASCULAR INVASION   ☐ Present   ☐ Not seen
(blood or lymphatic)

COMMENTS/ADDITIONAL INFORMATION

HISTOLOGICAL DIAGNOSIS   ☐ NORMAL   ☐ BENIGN   ☐ MALIGNANT

NHSBSP Wide Bore Needle Biopsy Form:

BREAST SCREENING CYTOPATHOLOGY

Surname .... Forenames .... Date of Birth ....
Screening No. .... Hospital No. .... Centre .... Report No. ....

Side	☐ Right	☐ Left		Number of cores ....
Calcification present on specimen X-ray?	☐ Yes	☐ No	☐ Radiograph not seen	
Histological calcification	☐ Absent	☐ Benign	☐ Malignant	☐ Both
Localisation techique	☐ Palpation	☐ X-ray guided	☐ Ultrasound guided	☐ Stereotaxis

Opinion
 ☐ B1. Unsatisfactory/Normal tissue only
 ☐ B2. Benign
 ☐ B3. Benign but of uncertain malignant potential
 ☐ B4. Suspicious of malignancy
 ☐ 5. Malignant　　　　　　　　　　　　　a. ☐ In-situ
 　　　　　　　　　　　　　　　　　　　　b. ☐ Invasive

PATHOLOGIST .... Operator taking biopsy .... Date ....
Comment ....

NHSBSP Cytology Reporting Form:

BREAST SCREENING CYTOPATHOLOGY

Surname .... Forenames .... Date of Birth ....
Screening No. .... Hospital No. .... Centre .... Report No. ....

Side	☐ Right	☐ Left		
Specimen Type	☐ FNA (Solid lesion)	☐ FNA (Cyst)	☐ Nipple discharge	☐ Nipple or skin scrapings
Localisation techique	☐ Palpation	☐ X-ray guided	☐ Ultrasound guided	☐ Stereotaxis

Opinion
 ☐ 1. Unsatisfactory　　　　　　　　Comment
 ☐ 2. Benign
 ☐ 3. Atypia probably benign
 ☐ 4. Suspicious of malignancy
 ☐ 5. Malignant
 　　　　　　　　　　　☐ Case for review?

PATHOLOGIST .... NAME OF ASPIRATOR .... DATE ....

Appendices

Histology EQA reporting form

NHSBSP HISTOPATHOLOGY EQA SCHEME

Slide no./yr. [ ] / [ ]

Mark for review (CSEU use only) [ ]

Participant's name [   ] Participant's code no. [   ]

Please SHADE the circles (using BLACK INK) to indicate lesions present. Any text should be written WITHIN boxes.

BENIGN LESIONS

- ○ Fibroadenoma
- ○ Solitary papilloma
- ○ Multiple papilloma
- ○ Complex sclerosing lesion/radial scar
- ○ Fibrocystic change
- ○ Solitary cyst
- ○ Periductal mastitis/duct ectasia
- ○ Sclerosing adenosis

○ Other (please specify) [   ]

CSEU use only [   ]

Epithelial proliferation

- ○ Not present
- ○ Present without atypia
- ○ Present with atypia ('ductal')
- ○ Present with atypia ('lobular')
- ○ Present with atypia ('ductal' & 'lobular')

MALIGNANT LESIONS

Non-invasive

- ○ Not present
- ○ Lobular
- ○ Paget's

CSEU use only [   ]

- ○ Ductal — Growth pattern (please specify) [   ]

  Nuclear grade   ○ High   ○ Intermediate   ○ Low

  Maximum diameter (ductal insitu only) [ ] mm (please round up/down to the nearest mm)

Microinvasion (<=1mm)   ○ Not present   ○ Possible   ○ Present

Invasive

- ○ Not present
- ○ Ductal/no specific type (NST)
- ○ Lobular carcinoma
- ○ Medullary carcinoma
- ○ Tubular carcinoma
- ○ Mucinous carcinoma
- ○ Mixed (please shade circles for component types present)
- ○ Not assessable

CSEU use only [   ]

○ Other primary carcinoma (please specify) [   ]

○ Other malignant tumour (please specify) [   ]

Maximum diameter (invasive component) [ ] mm (please round up/down to the nearest mm)

Whole size of invasive tumour (to include DCIS extending >1mm beyond invasive area) [ ] mm

Grade   ○ I   ○ II   ○ III   ○ Not assessable

Vascular invasion (blood or lymphatic)   ○ Present   ○ Not present

OVERALL DIAGNOSIS
(If more than one category is present, please indicate the MOST SIGNIFICANT only)

- ○ BENIGN
- ○ ATYPICAL HYPERPLASIA
- ○ INSITU or MICROINVASIVE CARCINOMA
- ○ INVASIVE CARCINOMA

Appendix 3

Specimen Service Level Agreement for a Regional Coordinator in Breast Screening Pathology

Agreement Objective. To provide a regional coordinator in the quality assurance aspects of breast screening pathology for the Regional Quality Assurance Programme for Breast Screening. Agreements should normally be for a minimum period of three years.

Definition of the Service to be Provided
- The postholder will develop and manage quality assurance initiatives in pathology in the breast screening programme.
- They will be a member of the multidisciplinary quality assurance team and will be involved in assessing performance of all the breast screening centres in the region, which includes monitoring and evaluating results and reporting findings and implications to the regional quality assurance manager. They will also be involved in making formal quality assurance visits with other members of the regional team.
- They will ensure that the NHSBSP guidelines for pathologists are communicated and understood and will monitor their implementation.
- The postholder will represent the region on the National Coordinating Group for Breast Screening Pathology.
- The postholder will coordinate the national EQA scheme within the region but will have no role in identifying substandard performance. They will hold meetings (at least twice yearly) to discuss the circulated slides and accompanying analyses and ideally circulate and discuss additional cases for discussion.
- They will assist screening units and the regional cancer registry in maintaining a complete, accurate and timely record of all pathologically confirmed breast cancers detected by the screening programme.
- They will provide advice for health authorities on matters of breast care quality assurance.
- The postholder will manage, initiate, lead and develop all other regional quality assurance initiatives of the screening programme relevant to pathology for the whole region.
- The coordinator should facilitate applied and fundamental research within their region as appropriate. They should also ensure that the necessary specialised diagnostic techniques (e.g. hormone receptor determinations) are available to regional pathologists where required.

Outcome. Accurate and standardised pathology data from the whole of the region from the breast screening programme.

Standards. The postholder will follow the guidelines for breast pathology services agreed by the Royal College of Pathologists and the NHSBSP National Coordinating Group for Breast Screening Pathology and set out in this document.

Administrative and Technical Support. The administrative and technical support necessary for the post will be provided by the breast screening Programme and should include a secretary (0.3 WTE) and laboratory technician (0.1 WTE).

Location of Post. It is expected that the postholder will be undertaking the histological and/or cytological reporting of biopsies and aspirates from screened women from an assessment centre in the region and be based in a department undertaking such work.

Variation/Exceptional Circumstances. It may be necessary from time to time for either party to seek to vary or cancel one or more of the provisions of the agreement. In such instances, notice should be given in writing of any proposed variations to the other party. Such variations will only occur by agreement. If agreement cannot be reached, the following procedures should be followed.

Resolution of Disputes. Any dispute between the parties concerning or arising out of this agreement or its construction, or effect, or concerning the rights, duties or liabilities of either of the parties, shall be referred to arbitration in accordance with this clause. Any dispute should be referred in the first instance to the lead health authority and the national coordination team then, if not resolved, to the regional director of public health.

Term of Agreement. This agreement would be subject to annual review. It is envisaged that the funding will be available at least for a further seven years to allow the breast screening programme to be evaluated according to the national recommendations.

Financial Allocation. The Regional Quality Assurance Programme will pay n[1] of a WTE of an NHS consultant post to the employer.

Appendix 4

External Quality Assessment Scheme in Breast Histology

Introduction

The EQA scheme in breast histology is of the "consensus" variety, there being no prejudgment about the correct diagnosis which is generally accepted to be that made by the majority of participants unless there is clear evidence to the contrary. This contrasts with the so-called "proficiency testing" schemes where the correct diagnoses are determined in advance by the organisers who thus function similarly to examiners conducting an examination. Although the breast histology scheme is able to identify substandard performance, it also has significant educational value by allowing participants regularly to compare and discuss their diagnoses with other participants. Furthermore, not every case needs to be suitable for assessing performance and some rare and difficult lesions can be included. Unsuitable cases are simply identified by an inadequate level of agreement by the participants. Another advantage is that it allows valid studies of diagnostic consistency to be made as cases are selected in a random manner within diagnostic categories. Consistency studies undertaken during the first three years of the scheme have been published [6].

Operation of the Scheme. Three sets of 12 slides are sent to each of 17 regional coordinators every six months. The coordinators represent the 14 old English health regions and the three Celtic nations. They distribute the slides to as many consultant pathologists as possible within their regions over a period of about four months. Cases are randomly selected but specific diagnostic categories may be chosen. Occasionally cases are selected because they are thought to be particularly difficult or interesting examples but are generally not included in the assessment of participants' performance.

Participants report the sections using the EQA reporting form shown in Appendix 2 which is a modified version of the standard reporting form in which data are excluded which cannot be supplied by examining histological sections alone. The completed forms are sent to the Cancer Screening Evaluation Unit where the responses are analysed.

Apart from investigating the consistency with which major diagnoses are made, the scheme can also be used to determine the level of agreement in reporting prognostic features such as tumour size, grade and type [6].

Determination of Substandard Performance. This is determined from four major diagnostic categories: benign (including radial scar), atypical hyperplasia, in situ carcinoma (including microinvasive carcinoma) and invasive carcinoma. Only cases where there is a majority diagnosis of at least 80% in any of these groups are included in the assessment. If the participant's diagnosis accords with the majority opinion, a score of 3 is given. A score of 2 is awarded if the diagnosis deviates by one group, 1 if it deviates by two groups and 0 if it deviates by three groups. Thus, for a majority diagnosis of inva-

---

[1] Figure to be agreed between commissioner and host hospital and should be at least 0.3 WTE and in some centres 0.5 WTE where the coordinator is playing a more extensive role in implementing and developing the pathology QA Programme.

sive carcinoma, scores of 3, 2, 1 and 0 would be awarded for diagnoses of invasive carcinoma, in situ carcinoma, atypical hyperplasia and benign respectively. Each participant's scores are then added together. A participant is deemed to be a "persistent substandard performer" if his/her total score for a circulation falls below the fifth percentile of the whole group and remains below this level for a further circulation. In every round, each participant is informed of their score and whether it is above or below the fifth percentile.

Although trainees may participate in the scheme, their scores are not included in this assessment process. Only those participants (generally consultants) who take ultimate responsibility for their diagnoses in their normal working practice will be assessed.

Release of Results. The general analyses of consistency of diagnosis and reporting prognostic features on individual cases are sent to all participants who are thus able to see the spread of opinions on each case and how theirs' relate to those of the majority. There is evidence that this process improves diagnostic consistency. A secretary in the Cancer Screening Evaluation Unit links participants' codes to their names and addresses so that the scheme organiser and other members of the Cancer Screening Evaluation Unit are unaware of individual participants' opinions.

Definition of Participation. It is unreasonable to expect all participants to take part in each circulation and participation is thus defined as taking part in two out of every three circulations. Given the large size of the scheme and the occasional logistical difficulties of reaching all participants this definition may rarely have to be relaxed. A certificate of participation is issued where required to those who fulfil this criterion. Given that all those taking part in the scheme will regularly be reporting breast specimens, and cases are included for scoring only where the majority opinion is made by 80% of participants, it is not acceptable for participants to omit any cases.

Action to be Taken on Identifying a Substandard Performer. At the time of writing the action to be taken on identifying a substandard performer is being considered by the Royal College of Pathologists, the National Quality Assurance Advisory Panel and the Joint Working Group. It should be stressed that external quality assessment schemes are a convenient but artificial mechanism for auditing the performance of histopathologists. There are several reasons why the standard achieved in a scheme may not reflect performance in daily diagnostic practice. Knowing that no clinical action will follow the reporting of the EQA slides, some participants devote little effort to them, whereas others may spend a disproportionately long time for fear of being deemed substandard. Only one slide per case is circulated in the EQA scheme and no clinical data are provided. There are no opportunities to undertake further investigations or express uncertainty.

The EQA scheme must therefore be seen as a screening procedure designed to identify a small number of pathologists who **may** be performing inadequately in their clinical practice. The first step must therefore be to determine if this is indeed the case and, if it is, then the second must be to determine the cause of the problem in order that appropriate remedial action may be taken. This description is accurate at the time of writing. The operation of the scheme is under continual review and may change in the light of experience and future developments.

Appendices 2.1.2

Appendices of the National Health Service Breast Screening Programme (NHSBSP), UK[2]

Dr T. J. Anderson (Chairman), Dr J. Coyne, Dr J. C. Davies, Dr I. O. Ellis, Professor C. W. Horne, Dr J. M. Theaker, Professor J. C. E. Underwood

Introduction

The following appendices have been prepared to address new developments in histological examination that are not accepted as standard practice, but could become so. Consequently, they constitute brief reviews on selected topics rather than guidance, although a few recommendations are made. Some have lengthly reference lists to assist interested readers in drawing their own conclusions. Appendices 2, 4 and 5 have immediate relevance in the screening context, whilst the other two are not satisfactorily established with regard to definition (intraductal component) or methology (steroid receptor) to find general application.

Appendix 1: Steroid Receptor Determination in Breast Lesions

The steroid receptor status of breast carcinomas should be determined in those cases in which it will influence clinical management.

For many year, steroid receptor assays of breast lesions have been performed by homogenising fresh tissue samples and adding low concentrations of radioactively-labelled steriod: the unbound or loosley bound steriod is then removed by a variety of techniques (e. g. dextran-coated charcoal) and the amount of specifically receptor-bound steriod determined.

---

[2] Publication: National Coordinating Group for Breast Screening Pathology (1997): Pathology Reporting in Breast Cancer Screening. NHSBSP Publication* No. 3, 2nd Edition, 65 pages. (ISBN 1871 997 22 4) Copyright © 1997 by NHSBSP
* NHSBSP Publications, National Breast Screening Programme, The Manor House, 260 Ecclesall Road South, Sheffield S11 9PS, UK
Reprint by permission

Tumours with a receptor concentration greater than 10 fmoles/mg protein are regarded as positive.

Using monoclonal antibodies or polyclonal antisera, it is now possible to detect and localise steroid receptors in cytological or histological preparations [1]. Most of these reagents work reliably only with cryostat sections or cytological preparations. However, these immunohistochemical methods have various advantages over biochemical assays:

- Positive cells are directly visualised so that any tumour cell heterogeneity can be detected.
- The presence of viable tumour tissue in the assessed sample is confirmed.
- Any stromal contribution can be discounted.
- Receptors already occupied by the relatively high levels of sex steroids in premenopausal women can still be detected.
- They can be applied to cytological material.

The preparations are assessed by estimating the proportion of stained cells and the staining intensity. The results show good correlation with biochemical assays and are predictive of responses to endocrine therapy [2].

The lesions detected by mammographic screening are frequently so small that samples for any biochemical receptor assay are either inadequate or their acquisition compromises the subsequent histological diagnosis. Frozen section examination of small breast lesions discovered by mammography should not generally be performed. The immunohistochemical methods can, however, be adapted to reveal ER and PR in routinely prepared paraffin sections of formalin-fixed tissues [3].

Immunostaining for ER and PR in fine needle aspirates is especially valuable when non-surgical treatment is contemplated, such as in very frail or otherwise debilitated patients.

Standardisation of methodology, with inter-laboratory and intra-laboratory quality assurance, is necessary for routine clinical applications. This standardisation applies not only to tissue fixation and processing but also to immunohistochemical techniques and evaluation of staining, both semi-quantitative and qualitative. Quality assurance equivalent to that operating for the biochemical evaluation is obligatory.

References page 209

Appendix 2: Marking the Margins of Breast Biopsies

Major emphasis is often given to histological determination of margin "clearance" of lesions but it should be recognized that all methods have limited sensitivity and specificity [1]. Major problems include sampling errors and the apparently discontinuous nature of several varieties of breast cancer. Furthermore, it should be recognized that various factors may make assessment superfluous, e. g. metastases already known, mammographic evidence of partial excision, extensive vascular invasion in the histological sections. A combination of radiological, surgical and pathological information is likely to prove most effective.

There are many ways to mark the planes of surgical excision of biopsies. No single method is ideal, each having advantages and disadvantages. Practical advice and comments are contained in reviews listed at the end of this appendix [2, 3, 4]. These should be consulted to determine the method most appropriate to local circumstances. Some biopsies are submitted fresh, others in the fixed state, The requirement from fresh tissues of material for biochemical analysis may be adversely affected by the marking paints.

India ink is widely used but is slow to dry and thus has the tendency to penetrate the planes of the tissue close to the site of its application. In consequence, some regard it as an unreliable marker of the external plane of surgical excision. Nevertheless, preliminary drying of the specimen or coating with alcohol can obviate this problem. Non-aqueous solvents like acetone [5, 6] and ethanol have been tried and allow the ink to dry more quickly. The specimen should not, of course, be sliced until the ink is dry.

Another recommended method is to coat the specimen with warm gelatin [7]. Instead of relying upon the evaporation of a solvent, the use of a gelatin depends on the setting of the gel. This is facilitated by preliminary chilling of the tissue. Fixation of the coated specimen apparently increases polymerisation in the gel, thus rendering it still more durable. The well-known typists' aid "Tippex" has also been tried [8] but, unfortunately, is densely radio-opaque on account of its titanium content. The dye Alcian blue [9] and inorganic pigments are fast drying and the latter can be used for differential colour marking [10]. Commercially available pigment markers have been recommended [2] which also have the advantage of being able to identify different planes for clearance.

The evaluation of surgical margins of biopsies is to be encouraged given the provisos stated above. Except in cases where the margin passes directly through a focus of cancer, the findings should, however, be interpreted with circumspection. The histopathology report should comment on the closest margin giving distance in mm, and specifying whether any involvement is by invasive or non-invasive cancer. The information should be related to orientation markers if given.

References page 209

Appendix 3: Extensive Intraduct Carcinoma

With the increasing use of conservation surgery for breast cancer, the identification of histological features associated with an increased risk of local recurrence is clearly important. A feature identified in many studies is the extent of the ductal carcinoma in situ in a local excision specimen [1–12]. The Boston group defines extensive intraduct carcinoma (EIC) as that comprising more than 25 % of the main invasive tumour mass **and** extending beyond it into surrounding breast tissue or a tumour which shows foci of invasion but is predominantly of intraduct type [10]. A recent EORTC consensus meeting concluded that "the principle risk factor for local relapse after breast conserving treatment is large residual burden, and the main source of this burden is an extensive in situ component which is found adjacent to 10–15 % of all invasive breast carcinomas" [13]. Data from one large group shows a local recurrence rate of 34% at 5 years and 40% at 10 years for tumours with an EIC, compared to 2 and 3% respectively for those without [14]. However, another study reported locally recurrent carcinoma after a maximum of 7 years (mean 3.7) at a rate of 13% with EIC and 3.7% without [15]. A significant proportion of such cases relapse as invasive carcinoma. These findings suggest that part of the routine histological assessment of breast tumours should include information about the nature of the intraduct component.

DCIS commonly extends beyond the confines of microcalcification apparent radiologically and of abnormal breast tissue palpable at surgery [15]. It is thus of little surprise that studies of re-excision specimens following an initial limited local excision show a high incidence of residual DCIS when this was an important component of the original specimen. Most local recurrences, therefore, probably relate to incomplete primary excision rather than the development of a new primary tumour. The identification of tumours with an EIC may therefore be an indication for more extensive local surgery.

It is recommended that pathologists take blocks from macroscopically normal tissue between an excised tumour and excision margins in all three planes of section. This allows for specific comment on the extent DCIS within a specimen, and its relationship with excision margins. Slice specimen radiology is a useful supplement to this assessment.

References page 210

Appendix 4: Histological Examination of Lymph Nodes for Cancer Metastasis

Lymph node staging provides powerful prognostic information in primary breast cancer, which can be used to determine the appropriateness of therapy and the extent of surgery [1]. It is axiomatic that the proportion of cancers with negative nodes is increased by mammographic screening. The detection of metastases in regional lymph nodes depends on surgical technique (which differs throughout the UK) and the thoroughness of pathological examination. Standardisation of lymph node processing does not exist between, and perhaps within, U.K. laboratories, and this factor may affect the quality of information recorded on the screening programme pathology database. Attention has recently focused on the deficiencies of routine histological assessment in detecting small deposits of tumour.

This appendix is not concerned with techniques to improve the **yield** of lymph nodes in tissues submitted from surgery but with factors which influence the likelihood of identifying cancer metastasis within lymph nodes. Lists reports from various groups that have employed serial sectioning or immunohistochemistry to increase the proportion of cases classified as lymph nodes "positive". Distinctions may need to be drawn between "gross, microscopic and single cell" metastasis, since clinical relevance may differ. For example, there is evidence that survival is not adversely affected by deposits of 1 mm or less [2, 3]. Further studies are thus required to define and evaluate the relevance of "occult" lymph node metastasis. Mathematical considerations of probability can be applied to the sampling process [4].

Immunohistological examination has cost benefits over serial sectioning but its use is still not clearly established in cases negative by conventional methods (Table A.1).

Furthermore, it should be remembered that other factors such as peritumoural lymphatic/vascular invasion detected on H&E sections may prove equally informative in prognostication of "node negative" cases (see Appendix 5).

References page 211

Appendix 5: Evaluating Lymphatic and Blood Vessel Invasion

A majority of reports has found that lymphatic and/or blood vessel invasion is an adverse prognostic feature in women with and without axillary lymph node involvement [1–7]. Some studies have combined lymphatic and blood vessel invasion as peritumoural "vascular invasion" [1, 3] while others have investigated them separately [4, 5, 6]. In one of the latter studies, the prognostic significance was found to apply to

Table A.1: Detection of Lymph Node Metastases by Serial Sectioning and Immunohistology

Pathological techniques	No. cases	% increased detection	Surgical techniques	Survival effect	Reference
SS	83/921	9	All	Yes	[5]
SS	7/50	14	AX cl	–	[6]
SS	19/78	24	–	No	[7]
IH	21/150	14	AX cl	Yes	[8]
IH	7/45	15	All	Yes	[9]
IH	8/40	20	AX cl	Yes	[10]
IH	9/98	9	BX	No	[11]
IH	37/91 (lobular)	41	AX cl	No	[12]

both lymphatic and blood vessel involvement individually [5]. In a further investigation by Weigand et al., an assessment was made of the importance of blood vessel invasion alone [7]. The findings of these studies are summarized in Table A.2 together with two further investigations in which lymphatic invasion was found not to be a useful prognostic indicator [8, 9].

Lymphatic and blood vessel invasion by cancer is said to have prognostic significance similar to that axillary lymph node involvement [4]. Although lymphatic invasion correlates with the presence of lymph node metastases [10], the adverse prognostic effects are considered to be independent of occult axillary node involvement [11]. In addition, a significant association has been reported between peritumoural vascular invasion and the presence of micrometastases in the bone marrow [12]. There is a 20–30% recurrence rate in patients with lymph node negative breast cancer and it is among these Stage I cases that lymphatic invasion has been found to be the most significant predictor of recurrence [4]. However, a wide range in the incidence of vascular invasion in breast cancer has been noted which appears to be related to significant interobserver variation in the recognition of blood and lymphatic spaces [13].

Several factors contribute to this interobserver variation but useful morphologic criteria for the correct identification of invasion of small vessels have been delineated [14]. Immunohistochemistry has been used in several studies to improve the identification of vascular spaces [5, 15–19]. Staining with antibodies against Factor VIII rag, blood group isoantigens A, B and H and Ulex Europaeus I Agglutinin appear to be most effective in localising small lymphatic and blood vessels [15,16]. These methods probably give only small increases in the number of cases detected as many can be discerned with H&E alone [4, 16]. Disadvantages include the staining of other cells such as myoepithelial and tumour cells [15]; false positives and false negatives have been reported [18]. In a recent study, both topographic as well as morphologic criteria were used to improve identification of lymphatic vascular spaces and an 82% interobserver reproducibility rate was achieved [20].

Further work is clearly required in this area but present evidence suggests that adequate sampling and careful examination of routine H&E preparation is a reliable and cost effective method of detecting vascular invasion (Table A.2).

References page 211

EUROPEAN BREAST SCREENING

HISTOPATHOLOGY

Surname .... Forenames .... Date of birth ....
Screening no .... Hospital No .... Side: ☐ RIGHT   ☐ LEFT
PATHOLOGIST .... Date of reporting .... Report No ....
Histological calcification   ☐ Absent ☐ Benign ☐ Malignant   ☐ Both
Specimen radiograph seen?   ☐ Yes   ☐ No   Mammographic abnormality present in specimen   ☐ Yes   ☐ No   ☐ Both
Specimen type   ☐ Localisation biopsy   ☐ Open biopsy   ☐ Segmental excision   ☐ Mastectomy   ☐ Wide bore needle core

Specimen Weight ....g   Size ....mm x ....mm x ....mm

BENIGN LESION PRESENT
☐ Complex sclerosing lesion/radial scar   ☐ Multiple papilloma
☐ Periductal mastitis/duct ectasia   ☐ Solitary papilloma
☐ Fibroadenoma   ☐ Sclerosing adenosis
☐ Fibrocystic change   ☐ Solitary cyst
☐ Other (please specify)

EPITHELIAL PROLIFERATION
☐ Not present   ☐ Present with atypia (ductal)
☐ Present without atypia   ☐ Present with atypia (lobular)

Malignant lesions non-invasive
☐ Not present
☐ Ductal, high grade   ☐ Ductal, other
Growth pattern(s) ....   Cell type/pattern..
☐ Lobular   ☐ Paget´s   SIZE (Ductal only) ....

MICROINVASION   ☐ Not present   ☐ Present   ☐ Possible
INVASIVE
☐ Not present   ☐ Mucinous carcinoma
☐ Ductal/no specific type (NST)   ☐ Tubular carcinoma
☐ Lobular carcinoma   ☐ Mixed (please tick component types present)
☐ Medullary carcinoma   ☐ Not assessable

☐ Other primary carcinoma (please specify) ....
☐ Other malignant tumour (please specify) ....

MAXIMUM DIAMETER OF INVASIVE TUMOUR ....mm
WHOLE SIZE OF TUMOUR (to include DCIS extending > 1 mm beyond invasive area) ....mm

AXILLARY NODES PRESENT   ☐ Yes   ☐ No   Number positive ....Total number..............
OTHER NODES PRESENT   ☐ Yes   ☐ No   Number positive ....Total number..............
                                   Site of other nodes ....
EXCISION MARGINS   ☐ Reaches margin   ☐ Uncertain   ☐ Does not reach margin (nearest ....mm)
GRADE   ☐ I   ☐ II   ☐ III   ☐ Not assessable
DISEASE EXTENT   ☐ Localised   ☐ Multiple   ☐ Not assessable
VASCULAR INVASION (blood or lymphatic)   ☐ Present   ☐ Not seen
COMMENTS/ADDITIONAL INFORMATION

HISTOLOGICAL DIAGNOSIS   ☐ NORMAL   ☐ BENIGN   ☐ MALIGNANT

Table A.2

Author	Study	Vessel Type	Method	Conclusion
Bettelheim et al. [1]	232 Stage I, II, III breast cancers. Local excision and mastectomy	VI	H&E immuno-histochemistry	Decreased DFS with VI
Davis et al. [2]	1510 axillary VI node positive cancers. Mastectomy		H&E	Decreased DFS with VI
Pinder et al. [3]	1704 Stage I breast cancers. Local excision and mastectomy	VI	H&E	Decreased DFS and survival with VI. Independent prognostic indicator on multivariate analysis
Roses et al. [4]	122 Stage I breast cancers. Mastectomy	LVI BVI	H&E	Decreased DFS with LVI. BVI not statistically significant as prognostic indicator
Lee et al. [5]	220 node negative breast cancers. Mastectomy	LVI	H&E immuno-histochemistry	Decreased DFS with both LVI and BVI independently
Rosen et al. [6]	382 Stage I breast cancer BVI	LVI	H&E. Elastic tissue stains	Decreased DFS with LVI. BVI not statistically significant as prognostic indicator
Weigand et al. [7]	175 Stage I–IV cancers	BVI	Elastic tissue stains	Decreased DFS with BVI
Sears et al. [8]	275 node negative breast cancers. Mastectomy	LVI BVI	H&E	LVI not an indicator of poor prognosis
Dawson et al. [9]	93 Stage I, II & III breast cancers. Radical mastectomy	LVI BVI	H&E and elastic stain	LVI not an indicator of poor prognosis

LVI = lymphatic vessel invasion
BVI = blood vessel invasion
VI = vascular invasion (both lymphatic vessels and blood vessels)
DFS = disease free survival

Appendices 2.1.3

Appendix 1: Breast Cancer Check List

Name: _____ SP No.: _____

Breast	(1) Left	(2) Right	
Specimen	(1) Excisional (for palpable mass)	(2) Mammographic localization	
	(3) Incisional (includes core needle and FNA)		
	(4) Re-excisional	(5) Mastectomy	(6) Chest wall

Specimen size

Tumor size(s)

Tumor type
    (1) DCIS   (5) Mixed NOS/ILC   (9) Papillary
    (2) LCIS   (6) Tubular   (10) Cribiform
    (3) Infiltrating ductal (NOS)   (7) Mucinous   (11) Other (specify)
    (4) Infiltrating lobular   (8) Medullary

Grade of invasive   (1) I   (2) II   (3) III

Gross margin   (1) Free (specify distance)   (2) Involved

Margins invasive (specify type of margin evaluation)
    (1) Free (specify distance)   (2) Focal   (3) >Focal   (4) Unevaluable

Margins DCIS (specify type of margin evaluation)
    (1) Free (specify distance)   (2) Focal   (3) >Focal   (4) Unevaluable

DCIS nuclear morphology
    (1) High grade   (2) Intermediate grade   (3) Low grade

DCIS patterns
    (1) Large areas of central necrosis (comedo)
    (2) Small areas of central necrosis
    (3) Cribriform   (4) Solid   (5) Micropapillary   (6) Papillary
    (specify all that apply)

Calcification *in situ*
    (1) Absent   (2) Prominent in DCIS   (3) Focal in DCIS
    (4) in LCIS   (5) Prominent in benign breast tissue
    (6) Focal in benign breast tissue

Peritumoral lymphatic invasion
    (1) Absent   (2) Present   (3) Dermal

Peritumoral vascular invasion
    (1) Absent   (2) Present

Extent DCIS within invasive tumor
    (1) Absent   (2) Slight   (3) Moderate-marked
    (4) Tumor primarily DCIS with focal invasion

Extent DCIS adjacent to invasive tumor
    (1) Absent   (2) Slight   (3) Moderate-marked

EIC status   (1) EIC negative   (2) EIC positive   (3) EIC indeterminate

NOTE: If a tumor is primarily DCIS with focal invasion or has a moderate or marked amount of DCIS within the infiltrating tumor and any in the adjacent tissue, it is EIC positive.

Appendix (continues)

Appendix 1: Breast Cancer Check List *(continued)*

Skin	(1) Not sampled	(2) Free	(3) Invasive	(4) Dermal lymphatic		____
Nipple	(1) Not sampled	(2) Free	(3) Invasive	(4) Dermal lymphatic		
	(5) DCIS	(6) Paget's				____
Muscle	(1) Not sampled	(2) Free	(3) Involved			____

Mastectomy
  Tumor location
        (1) Central   (2) UOQ   (3) UIQ   (4) LOQ   (5) LIQ   ____
  Multiple areas involved
        (1) Central   (3) UOQ   (3) UIQ   (4) LOQ   (5) LIQ
        (6) Only 1 area involved   ____

Lymph nodes (no. of involved nodes in relation to total no. examined)
  Total
  Level I
  Level II
  Level III
  Other (specify)   ____

Extranodal extension
        (1) Absent   (2) Present   ____

Metastatic cancer in   ____

Nature of nontumorous breast tissue (describe)   ____

Comments:

Ancillary studies (results and methodology used)

Appendix 2

Membership of E. C. Working Group

- Chairman: Prof J. P. Sloane, University of Liverpool, United Kingdom.
- Dr I. Amendoeira, Institute of Molecular Pathology and Immunology of the University of Porto, Porto, Portugal.
- Dr N. Apostolikas, Hellenic Anticancer Institute, Athens, Greece.
- Professor J. P. Bellocq, Hôpital de Hautepierre, Strasbourg, France.
- Dr S. Bianchi, Italian Breast Screening Programme and Istituto di Anatomia e Istologia Patologica, Firenze, Italy.
- Professor W. Böcker, Gerhard-Domagk-Institut für Pathologie, Münster, Germany.
- Professor G. Bussolati, Istituto di Anatomia e Istologia Patologica, Torino, Italy.
- Dr C. E. Connolly, Associate Professor of Pathology, University College Hospital, Galway, Ireland.
- Dr C. De Miguel, Hospital Virgen del Camino, Pamplona, Spain.
- Professor P. Dervan, The Eccles Breast Screening Project, Mater Hospital and University College, Dublin, Ireland.
- Dr R. Drijkoningen, Pathologische Ontleedkunde 1, Leuven, Belgium.
- Dr C. W. Elston, City Hospital, Nottingham, United Kingdom.
- Dr D. Faverly, Projet Bruxellois de Däpistage du Cancer du Sein and C. M. P. Laboratory, Bruxelles, Belgium.
- Dr A. Gad, Falun Hospital, Falun, Sweden.
- Dr R. Holland, National Expert and Training Centre for Breast Cancer Screening, Nijmegen, The Netherlands.
- Dr J. Jacquemier, Institut Paoli Calmette and Breast Histological Registry, Marseille, France.
- Dr M. Lacerda, Centro de Oncologia de Coimbra, Coimbra, Portugal.
- Dr A. Lindgren, University Hospital, Uppsala, Sweden.

- Dr J. Martinez-Peñuela, Hospital de Navarra, Pamplona, Spain.
- Dr J. L. Peterse, The Netherlands Cancer Institute, Amsterdam, The Netherlands.
- Dr F. Rank, Bispebjerg Hospital and Danish Cancer Society, Copenhagen, Denmark.
- Dr V. Tsakraklides, Hygeia Hospital, Athens, Greece.
- Dr C. de Wolf, European Commission, Luxembourg.
- Dr B. Zafrani, Institut Curie, Paris, France.

Membership of National Coordinating Group for Pathology in Breast Screening

- Chairman: Prof. J. P. Sloane, University of Liverpool, Department of Pathology, Duncan Building, Royal Liverpool University Hospital, Liverpool L69 3BX.
- Dr T. J. Anderson, Department of Pathology, University Medical School, Teviot Place, Edinburgh EH8 9AG
- Prof. R. W. Blamey, City Hospital, Hucknall Road, Nottingham NG5 1PB
- Dr C. L. Brown, Institute of Pathology, The London Hospital Medical College, Turner Street, London E1 1BB
- Dr J. Coyne, Department of Histopathology, University Hospital of South Manchester, West Didsbury, Manchester M20 8LR
- Dr N. S. Dallimore, Department of Histopathology, Llandough Hospital, Penarth, S. Glam CF6 1XX
- Dr D. R. Davies, Department of Cellular Pathology, Level 1, The John Radcliffe Hospital, Headley Way, Headington Oxford OX3 9DU
- Dr J. D. Davies, Breast Pathology Unit, S. W. Regional Health Authority, Southmead Hospital, Bristol BS10 5NB
- Dr P. M. Dennis, Department of Histopathology, Peterborough District Hospital, Thorpe Road, Peterborough, Cambs PE3 6DA
- Dr I. O. Ellis, Department of Histopathology, City Hospital, Hucknall Road, Nottingham NG5 1PB
- Dr C. W. Elston, Department of Histopathology, City Hospital, Hucknall Road, Nottingham NG5 1PB
- Dr S. Humphreys, Department of Histopathology, King's College Hospital, Denmark Hill, London SE5 9RS
- Dr D. Lawrence, Department of Histopathology, Luton and Dunstable Hospital, Lewsey Road, Luton, Beds LU4 0DZ
- Dr J. Lowe, Department of Histopathology, Bradford Royal Infirmary, Duckworth Lane, Bradford, West Yorks BD9 6RJ
- Prof. J.O'D. McGee, Nuffield Department of Pathology & Bacteriology, John Radcliffe Hospital, Oxford OX3 9DU
- Dr M. Michell, Department Radiology, King's College Hospital, Denmark Hill, London SE5 9RS
- Dr R. R. Millis, ICRF Clinical Oncology Unit, Guy's Hospital, London SE1 9RT
- Dr J. Nottingham, Department of Histopathology, George Eliot Hospital, College Road, Nuneaton CV10 7BL
- Mrs J. Patnick, NHS Breast Screening Programme, Fulwood House, Old Fulwood Road, Sheffield S10 3TH
- Dr N. Ryley, Department of Histopathology, Royal Surrey County Hospital, Egerton Road, Park Barn, Guikdford, Surey GU2 5XX
- Dr D. J. Scott, Department of Histopathology, Newcastle General Hospital, Westgate Road, Newcastle upon Tyne NE4 6BE
- Dr J. M. Sloan, Department of Histopathology, Royal Victoria Hospital, Belfast, N. Ireland BT12 6BA
- Dr J. Theaker, Department of Histopathology, Southampton General Hospital, Tremona Road, Southampton, Hants SO9 4XY
- Dr P. A. Trott, Department of Cytopathology, Royal Marsden Hospital, Fulham Road, London SW3 6JJ
- Dr C. A. Wells, Department of Histopathology, St. Bartholomew's Hospital Medical School, West Smithfield, London ED1A 7BE
- Dr H. D. Zakhour, Department of Histopathology, Arrowe Park Hospital Road, Upton, Wirral, Merseyside L49 5PE

Membership of Writing Committee

- Dr J. P. Sloane
- Dr T. J. Anderson
- Dr J. D. Davies
- Dr I. O. Ellis
- Dr C. W. Elston
- Dr R. R. Millis
- Dr C. A. Wells

Appendices 2.1.5

Acknowledgement

The conference gratefully acknowledges The Breast Health Institute, Philadelphia, PA; The Fashion Group International, Philadelphia, PA; and the Jefferson Medical College and Thomas Jefferson University Hospital, Philadelphia, PA for their sponsorship and additional grant support from the following companies:

- Biopsys Medical, Inc., Irvine, CA
- Oxford Health Plans, Philadelphia, PA
- Zeneca, Wimington, DE

Conference Chairman:

Gordon F. Schwartz, M. D., M. B. A., Jefferson Medical College, Philadelphia, PA

Conference Cochairman:

Michael D. Lagios, M. D., St Mary's Medical Center, San Francisco, CA

Pathologists:

- Darryl Carter, M. D., Yale University School of Medicine, New Haven, CT
- James Connolly, M. D., Beth Israel Deaconess Medical Center, Boston, MA
- Ian O. Ellis, M. D., City Hospital NHS Trust, Nottingham, United Kingdom
- Vincenzo Eusebio, M. B., Universita di Bologna, Bologna, Italy
- Gerald C. Finkel, M. D., Thomas Jefferson University Hospital, Philadelphia, PA
- Fred Gorstein, M. D., Thomas Jefferson University Hospital, Philadelphia, PA
- Roland Holland, M. D., University Hospital Nijmegen, Nijmegen, The Netherlands
- Robert V. P. Hutter, M. D., Saint Barnabas Medical Center, Livingston, NJ
- Michael D. Lagios, M. D., St Mary's Medical Center, San Francisco, CA
- Shahla Masood, M. D., University of Florida Health Science Center, Jacksonville, FL
- Rosemary R. Millis, M. D., Guy's Hospital, London, United Kingdom
- Frances P. O'Malley, M. B., FRCPC, London Health Science Centre, London, Ontario, Canada
- Juan Palazzo, M. D., Thomas Jefferson University Hospital, Philadelphia, PA
- Arthur S. Patchefsky, M. D., Fox Chase Cancer Center, Philadelphia, PA
- Juan Rosai, M. D., Memorial Sloan-Kettering Cancer Center, New York, NY
- Stuart J. Schnitt, M. D., Beth Israel Deaconess Medical Center, Boston, MA
- Roland Schwarting, M. D., Thomas Jefferson University Hospital, Philadelphia, PA
- John P. Sloane, M. D., Royal Liverpool University Hospital, Liverpool, United Kingdom
- Fattaneh A. Tavassoli, M. D., Armed Forces Institute of Pathology, Washington, DC

Mammographer

- Stephen A. Feig, M. D., Thomas Jefferson University Hospital, Philadelphia, PA
- Daniel B. Kopans, Massachusetts General Hospital, Boston, MA

Radiation Oncologist

Beryl McCormick, Memorial Sloan-Kettering Cancer Center, New York, NY

Surgeons

- Edward M. Copeland, III, University of Florida College of Medicine, Gainesville, FL
- Armando, E. Guiliano, John Wayne Cancer Institute, Santa Monica, CA
- Gordon R. Schwartz, M. D., M. B. A., Jefferson Medical College, Philadelphia, PA

- Melvin J. Silverstein, The Breast Center, Van Nuys, CA
- Joop A. van Dongen, The Netherlands Cancer Institute, Amsterdam, The Netherlands

Biostatistician

Carol Bodian, The Mount Sinai Medical Center, New York, NY

Appendices 2.2.3

Appendix 1: Aspiration Procedure

- 1. Locate the lesion (fig. A.1).
- 2. Clean the skin.
- 3. Local anaesthetic may be used but may make the lesion difficult to feel. Inject the skin and immediate subcutaneous tissue only. Avoid injecting the lesion.
- 4. Place syringe and needle into holder if used.
- 5. Fix the lesion between the index finger and the thumb.
- 6. Choosing the shortest direction introduce the needle through the skin and subcutaneous tissue into lesion. Enter lesion with needle point.
- 7. Aspirate by exerting gentle negative pressure through the syringe and moving the needle tip gently by short back and forth movements within the lesion.
  Aspirate using negative pressure and short back and forth movements rotating the needle to cut with the bevel.
- 8. Maintain negative pressure and withdraw the needle point just out of the lesion. Re-insert at a slightly different angle and repeat above procedure. Repeat at least twice at different angles without withdrawing needle from skin.
- 9. Release negative pressure from syringe before withdrawing the needle.
- 10. Then withdraw the needle from the skin.

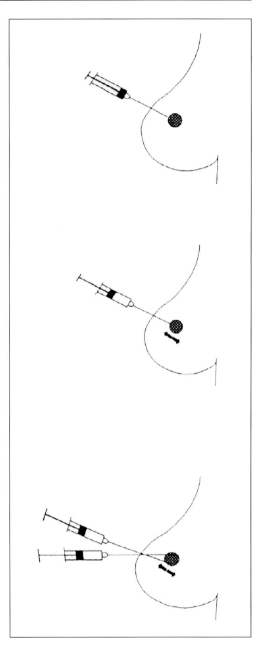

Figure A.1: Aspiration Procedure

Appendix 2: Spreading the slides

A number of methods can be used to spread the slides obtained by placing a drop of aspirated material from the needle on a glass slide. Many of these are variations on a theme but the essential problem is to get a thin layer of material on the slide to allow rapid drying for air-dried fixation without appreciable squash artefacts due to excess pressure (fig. A.2).

Spreading with a slide.

Three basic methods all producing similar effects can be used (1, 2, or 3).

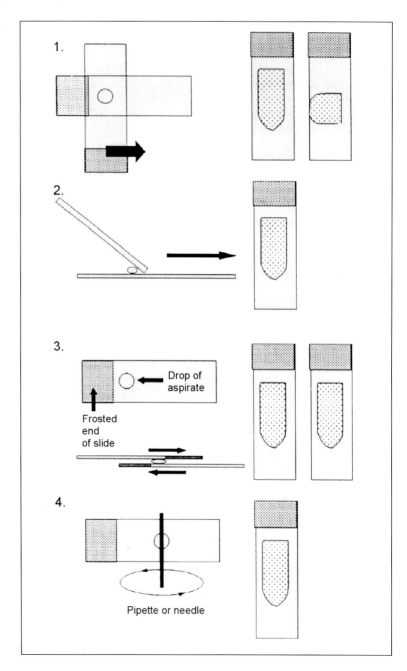

Figure A.2: Spreading the slides

Alternatively the slide may be spread using a pipette or a needle (4).

Whichever method is used it is imperative that no excess downward pressure or surface squash or distort the cells as this may render the slides uninterpretable.

All pathologists have received slides from clinicians where the aspirate has been well taken but has been ruined by poor spreading technique. It is sometimes difficult to remedy this but multidisciplinary discussion and making aspirators aware of the problems, especially visually and microscopically often helps to alleviate the problem.

Appendix 3: Fixation Methods

Wet fixed smears

These smears must be fixed **immediately** after spreading and before they have a chance to dry, by dropping into a pot of fixative or flooding the slide with a drop of fixative if no container is available. Spray fixation can be used (fig. A.3).

Air dried smears

After spreading, the slide should be dried rapidly by waving in the air or by using a fan. (Some units use a hair drier but this should be done only on a cold setting as warm air will "cook" the cells and lead to artefacts.) (fig. A.3)

Transport medium

In some units transport medium is used for specimens which means that optimum preparations can be made in the laboratory after cytocentrifugation. This method is best used where clinicians are not used to making cytological smears and do not follow proper fixation techniques. It can be superior to delayed fixation of wet preparations where air-drying can make interpretation difficult (fig. A.3).

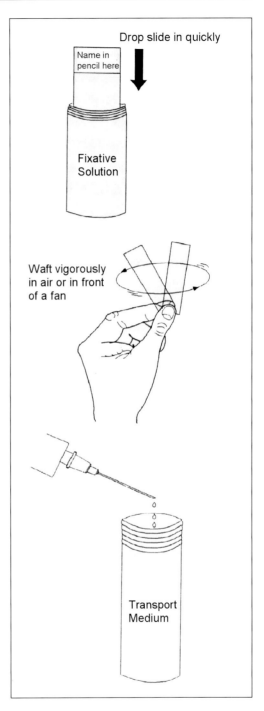

Figure A.3: Fixation Methods

Appendix 4: How the national screening system treats the information

The National Computer System, designed in Oxford, and used in most regions for the recording of breast screening, stores fine needle aspiration results as a diagnostic set (FINE) which is part of the assessment module. While specimen type and cytological diagnosis are obviously recorded along with the comment field, other information is also recorded on the radiological side. Thus the method of localisation of the lesion, whether by clinical, ultrasound, perforated plate or stereotaxis, is recorded and the radiation dosage (number of exposures, films, kV and Mas) is similarly recorded. The system records not only a cytological opinion (C 1, C2 etc.) but also an overall opinion after full assessment which is entered after a multidisciplinary decision is taken. This opinion then forms the basis for an action which may range from routine recall (RR) to surgical treatment (ST) depending on the outcome of assessment. The date of the aspiration and report, the pathologist, aspirator and the specimen number are also recorded.

The cytological opinion forms part of a field in the software which is called "episode endpoint". In this, cytology is not treated the same as in the program itself, being separated from assessment. Examples of the coding of this field would be S+, Aabn, C-, H- where a lesion was thought positive on screening films (S), was thought benign in nature after assessment (A), was thought overall to be benign after cytology (NB this does not necessarily mean that cytology was benign) (C) and was histologically benign (H), or S+, A+, C+, H+ for a malignancy identified as such by screening (S), assessment (A), cytology (C) (NB this does not mean that cytology was necessarily malignant) and histology (H). This field can be downloaded in a batch along with patient identifiers and other fields as a "file of episodes" from the software onto a PC for further analysis and further releases intend to explain this facility.

In the newest version of the software (2.3) it is possible to download a "file of assessment details" which contains all the fields present on the cytology form.

Because of a problem on conversion of the database from version 2.0 to version 2.1 where the assessment and cytology record structure were changed a number of cytology results which were originally "benign" on the system were recorded as "suspicious probably benign (C3)". This error occurred at a date of conversion in each unit which generally varies from August 1990 to December 1990, although some units may be even later than this. Records entered before that date may be subject to this error and data obtained from the computer before 1991 may contain a high number of suspicious results due to this date conversion.

It is recommended therefore that data downloaded or patient episodes reviewed from the national system pertaining to results entered before 1991 be treated with caution. Also some of these records may be lacking certain data items which were not part of the previous software.

It is not possible to run a general correction for these results as the dates at which the conversion was done varies from unit to unit but it is possible to run an FNAC program which will list all FNAC performed with their dates to allow correction of these. If this is required then information may be obtained from the Oxford Level Two Support Team in your region. This error does not apply to other systems but information on those may be obtained from regional computer management teams.

Appendix 5: Further rules used in deriving the statistics from the computer system

- Cases with both a non-invasive cancer and an invasive cancer in the pathology database should count as invasive unless they are opposite sides where they would be counted twice (once in each).
- In cases with a malignant diagnosis the malignant findings override benign findings unless they are opposite sides.
- Cytology cases with open episodes are listed at the bottom of the report.
- Cases with two or more FNA records for the same side are listed at the bottom of the report with the corresponding C score and worst histological diagnosis for each record.

- The table should be capable of being produced for all cases, for all cases performed by any one aspirator, for all cases reported by any one pathologist, and for cases by any one localisation method (palpable, ultrasound, X-ray guided perforated plate) or stereotaxis).
- The table should be producible for any data range, the date taken being the date of aspiration or, if that is not available, the date of reporting and for any location.
- Ideally the table should be producible for any one of the radiological appearances by method of localisation also. (The radiological appearances being: Stellate opacity, rounded opacity, microcalcification, or asymmetrical density.)
- It should be possible to list the screening numbers of clients involved in any of the cells on request.
- A list of cases in cell no. **26** is essential with the title:
  - **Cases with C4 cytology not biopsied but with closed episodes**
  - All cases in box **25** are regarded as malignant
  - All cases in box **27** are regarded as benign

Appendix 6

Membership of working party
Editorial group:
- Dr C. A. Wells – Consultant Pathologist, St Bartholomew's Hospital, West Smithfield, London EC1A 7BE
- Dr I. O. Ellis – Consultant Pathologist, City Hospital, Hucknall Road, Nottingham NG5 1PB
- Dr H. D. Zakhour – Consultant Pathologist, Arrowe Park Hospital, Upton, Wirral, Merseyside L49 5PE
- Dr R. Wilson – Consultant Radiologist, Helen Garrod Breast Screening Unit, City Hospital, Hucknall Road, Nottingham NG5 1PB

Members of the cytology sub-group of the National Co-ordinating Committee for Breast Cancer Screening Pathology

- Dr C. L. Brown (Chairman) – The Royal London Hospital, Whitechapel, London
- Dr Grace McKee – The Royal Surrey County Hospital, Guildford, Surrey
- Dr Peter Trott – The Royal Marsden Hospital, Fulham Road, London
- Dr C. A. Wells – Consultant Pathologist, St Bartholomew's Hospital, London
- Dr I. O. Ellis – Consultant Pathologist, City Hospital, Hucknall Road, Nottingham NG5 1PB
- Dr H. Zakhour – Consultant Pathologist, Arrowe Park Hospital, Merseyside
- Dr Ruth Ellman – Breast Cancer Screening Evaluation Unit, Cotswold Road, Belmont, Sutton, Surrey

The authors also wish to thank the numerous people who sent in comments on these guidelines from the UK, Europe and the United States. These comments have been invaluable in preparing this manuscript. Dr Wells would also like to acknowledge the late Dr Vincenzo Crucioli whose teaching and views have been extensively incorporated into this document and without which this task would have been infinitely more difficult.

Appendices 2.2.4

List of Subcommittee Members

- Andrea Abati, M. D. (Conference Coordinator, Chairman Editorial/Publication Subcommittee)
- John Abele, M. D. (Indications Subcommittee, Fine Needle Aspiration Technique Subcommittee)
- Sarah S. Bacus, Ph. D. (Ancillary Studies Subcommittee)
- Carlos Bedrossian, M. D. (Editorial/Publication Subcommittee)
- Donald Beerline, M. D. (Post-FNA Recommendations Subcommittee)
- Marluce Bibbo, M. D., Sc. D. (Editorial/Publication Subcommittee)

- Blake Cady, M. D. (Post-FNA Recommendations Subcommittee)
- Jamie Covell, C. T., ASCP (Post-FNA Recommendations Subcommittee)
- Diane Davey, M. D. (Indications Subcommittee)
- Andrea Dawson, M. D. (Terminology Committee)
- Bruno Fornage, M. D. (Indications Subcommittee)
- Roger Foster, M. D. (Conference Moderator)
- William Frable, M. D. (Chairman, Indications Subcommittee, Co-Chairman, Training and Credentialing Subcommittee)
- Mindy Goldfischer, M. D. (Indications Subcommittee)
- Heinz Grohs, M. D. (Indications Subcommittee, Fine Needle Aspiration Technique Subcommittee)
- Michael Henry, M. D. (Terminology Subcommittee)
- Yasmine Hijazi, M. D. (Ancillary Studies Subcommittee)
- William Hindle, M. D. (Indications Subcommittee)
- Lydia Howell, M. D. (Fine Needle Aspiration Technique Subcommittee)
- David Kaminsky, M. D. (Ancillary Studies Subcommittee)
- Ruth Katz, M. D. (Chairman, Ancillary Studies Subcommittee)
- Tilde Kline, M. D. (Fine Needle Aspiration Technique Subcommittee, Training and Credentialing Subcommittee)
- Leopold G. Koss, M. D. (Ancillary Studies Subcommittee)
- Donald R. Lannin, M. D. (Post-FNA Recommendations Subcommittee)
- Lester Layfield, M. D. (Chairman, Post-FNA Recommendations Subcommittee)
- Gladwyn Leiman, M. D. (Terminology Subcommittee)
- Melinda Lewis, M. D. (Indications Subcommittee)
- Karin Lindholm, M. D. (Terminology Subcommittee)
- Britt-Marie Ljung, M. D. (Chairman, Fine Needle Aspiration Technique Subcommittee, Co-Chairman, Training and Credentialing Subcommittee)
- Shahla Masood, M. D. (Co-Chairman, Terminology Subcommittee, Editorial/Publication Subcommittee)
- Jane Miyazaki, C. T. (Terminology Subcommittee)
- Gillian Newstead, M. D. (Indications Subcommittee)
- Joyce O'Shaughnessy, M. D. (Ancillary Studies Subcommittee)
- David Page, M. D. (Terminology Subcommittee)
- Celeste Powers, M. D., Ph. D. (Indications Subcommittee)
- Susan Rollins, M. D. (Fine Needle Aspiration Technique Subcommittee, Ancillary Studies Subcommittee)
- Dorothy Rosenthal, M. D. (Ancillary Studies Subcommittee)
- Miguel A. Sanchez, M. D. (Vice-Chairman, Indications Subcommittee)
- Waldemar Schmidt, M. D. (Editorial/Publication Subcommittee)
- Mary Sidawy, M. D. (Terminology Subcommittee)
- Jan Silverman, M. D. (Indications Subcommittee)
- Nour Sneige, M. D. (Co-Chairman, Terminology Subcommittee)
- Rosalyn E. Stahl, M. D. (Indications Subcommittee)
- Michael Stanley, M. D. (Steering Committee Chairman, Terminology Subcommittee)
- Patricia Thomas, M. D. (Fine Needle Aspiration Technique Subcommittee)
- Madeline Vazquez, M. D. (Post-FNA Recommendations Subcommittee)
- Jerry Waisman, M. D. (Conference Moderator, Terminology Subcommittee)
- Sandra Wolman, M. D. (Ancillary Studies Subcommittee)
- Caryn Wunderlich, M. D. (Fine Needle Aspiration Technique Subcommittee)
- Barbara Yawn, M. D. (Indications Subcommittee, Training and Credentialing Subcommittee)

Appendices 2.2.5

Standards of Practice Task Force Members

- Kenneth C. Suen, M. D. (chair)
- Fadi W. Abdul-Karim, M. D.
- David B. Kaminsky, M. D.
- Lester J. Layfield, M. D.
- Theodore R. Miller, M. D.
- Susan E. Spires, M. D.
- Donald E. Stanley, D. O.

Consultant Members

- Carlos W. M. Bedrossian, M. D.
- Michael B. Cohen, M. D.
- William J. Frable, M. D.
- Tilde S. Kline, M. D.
- Virginia A. LiVolsi, M. D.
- G.-Khanh Nguyen, M. D.
- Celeste N. Powers, M. D.
- Jan F. Silverman, M. D.
- Michael W. Stanley, M. D.
- Thomas A. Thomson, M. D.

- Department of Pathology, Vancouver Hospital and Health Sciences Centre, Vancouver, British Columbia, Canada
- Institute of Pathology, Case Western Reserve University, Cleveland, Ohio
- Department of Pathology, Eisenhower Medical Center, Rancho Mirage, California
- Department of Pathology, Duke University Medical Center, Durham, North Carolina
- Department of Pathology. University of California San Francisco Medical Center, San Francisco, California
- Department of Pathology, Saint Joseph Hospital Lexington, Kentucky
- Department of Pathology, Rutland Regional Medical Center, Rutland, Vermont
- Department of Pathology, Wayne State University, Detroit, Michigan
- Department of Pathology, University of Iowa Hospitals and Clinics, Iowa City, Iowa
- Department of Pathology, Medical College of Virginia Hospital, Richmond, Virginia
- Department of Pathology, Lankenau Hospital, Wynnewood, Pennsylvania
- Department of Pathology, University of Pennsylvania, Philadelphia, Pennsylvania
- Department of Pathology, University of Alberta Hospitals, Edmonton, Alberta, Canada
- Department of Pathology, State University of New York, Syracuse, New York
- Department of Pathology, Last Carolina University School of Medicine, Greenville. North Carolina
- Department of Pathology, University of Arkansas for Medical Sciences, Little Rock, Arkansas
- Department of Pathology, British Columbia Cancer Agency, Vancouver, British Columbia, Canada

Correspondence to: Dr Kenneth Suen, Department of Pathology, Vancouver Hospital, 855 West 12th Ave., Vancouver, British Columbia, V5Z 1 M9, Canada.

References

References 1.1.1

- 1 Degrell I. (1976): *Atlas of Disease of the Mammary Gland*. S. Karger, Basel.

References 1.2.1

- 1 Burke H. B., Henson D. E. (1993): Criteria for prognostic factors and for an enhanced prognostic systems. *Cancer* **72**: 3131–3135.
- 2 Burke H. B., Hutter R. V. P., Henson D. E. (1995): *Breast carcinoma, Prognostic Factors in Cancer*. Springer Verlag.
- 3 CEC (Commission of the European Communities) (1993): European guidelines for quality assurance in mammography screening. *Report EUR* 14821.
- 4 Page D. L., Anderson T. J. (1987): *Diagnostic Histopathology of the breast*. Churchill Livingstone.
- 5 Ellis I. O., Galea M., Broughton N., Locker A., Blamey R. W., Elston C. W. (1992): Pathological prognostic factors in breast cancer. II. Histological type. Relationship with survival in a large study with long-term follow-up. *Histopathology* **20**: 479–489.
- 6 Ellis I. O., Elston C. W. (1995): Tumours of the breast. In: Fletcher C. (editor): *Diagnostic Histopathology of tumours*. Churchill Livingstone.
- 7 Bässler R. (1978): *Pathologie der Brustdrüse*. Springer Verlag.
- 8 Rosen P. P., Oberman H. A. (1993): Tumours of the mammary gland. *Atlas of tumour pathology*. Armed Forces Institute of Pathology.

References 1.2.2

- 1 Page D. L., Dupont W. D., Rogers L. W., Landenberger M. (1982): Intraductal carcinoma of the breast: follow-up after biopsy only. *Cancer* **49**: 751–758.
- 2 Page D. L., Dupont W. D., Rogers S. W., Rados M. S. (1985): Atypical hyperplastic lesions of the female breast. A long-term follow-up study. *Cancer* **55**: 2698–2708.
- 3 Page D. L., Anderson T. J., Rogers L. W. (1988): Epithelial hyperplasia. In: Page D. L., Anderson T. J. (editors): *Diagnostic Histopathology of the Breast*. Churchill Livingstone, Edinburgh, 120–156.
- 4 Page D. L., Rogers L. W. (1992): Combined histologic and cytologic criteria for the diagnosis of mammary atypical ductal hyperplasia. *Hum. Pathol.* **23**: 1095–1097
- 5 Page D. L., Kidd T. E., Dupont W. D., Simpson J. F., Rogers L. W. (1991): Lobular neoplasia of the breast: Higher risk for subsequent invasive cancer predicted by more extensive disease. *Hum. Pathol.* **222**: 1232–1239.
- 6 Tavassoli F. A., Norris H. J. (1990): A comparison of the results of long-term follow-up for atypical intraductal hyperplasia and intraductal hyperplasia of the breast. *Cancer* **65**: 518–529.
- 7 McDivitt R. W., Stevens J. A., Lee N. C., Wingo P. A., Rubin G. L., Gersell D., Cancer and Steroid Hormone Study Group (1992): Histologic types of benign breast disease and the risk for breast cancer. *Cancer* **69**: 1408–1414.
- 8 Dupont W. D., Parl F. F., Hartmann W. H., Brinton L. A., Winfield A. C., Worrell J. A., Schuyler P. A., Plummer W. D. (1993): Breast cancer risk associated with proliferative breast disease and atypical hyperplasia. *Cancer* **71**: 1258–1265.
- 9 O'Malley F. P., Page D. L., Nelson E. H., Dupont W. D. (1994): Ductal carcinoma in situ of the breast with apocrine cytology: de-

finition of a borderline category. *Hum. Pathol.* **25**: 164–168.

- 10 Guerry P., Erlandson R. A., Rosen P. P. (1988): Cystic hypersecretory hyperplasia and cystic hypersecretory duct carcinoma of the breast: Pathology, therapy, and follow-up of 39 patients. *Cancer* **61**: 1611–1620.

References 2.1.1

- 1 Galea M. H. et al. (1992): The Nottingham Prognostic Index. *Breast Cancer Research and Treatment* **22**: 187–191.
- 2 Moss S. M. et al. (1995): Results from the NHS Breast Screening Programme 1990–1993. *Journal of Medical Screening* **2**: 186–190.
- 3 National Health Service Breast Screening Programme (1995): Pathology Reporting in Breast Cancer Screening. 2nd ed. *NHSBSP Publication No 3*, ISBN 1871997 22 4.
- 4 National Health Service Breast Screening Programme (1993): Guidelines for Cytology Procedures and Reporting in Breast Cancer Screening. *NHSBSP Publication No 22*, ISBN 1871997 26 7.
- 5 Medical Devices Directorate (1991): Guidance Notes on Specimen Radiography Cabinets. MDD/91/13.
- 6 Sloane J. P. and members of the UK Coordinating Group for Breast Screening Pathology (1994): Consistency of Histopathological Reporting of Breast Lesions Detected by Screening. Findings of the UK National External Quality Assessment (EQA) Scheme. *European Journal of Cancer* **30A**: 1414–1419.
- 7 Kocjan G. (1991): Evaluation of the cost effectiveness of establishing a fine needle aspiration cytology clinic in a hospital out-patient department. *Cytopathology* **2/1**: 13–18.
- 8 Brown L. A., Coghill S. B. (1992): Cost effectiveness of a fine needle aspiration clinic. *Cytopathology* **3**: 275–280.
- 9 Expert Advisory Group on Cancer to the Chief Medical Officers of England and Wales (1995): A Policy Framework for Commissioning Cancer Services. HMSO.
- 10 Richards M. A. et al. (1994): Provision of Breast Services in the UK. – The Advantages of Specialist Breast Unit. *British Breast Group*.
- 11 National Health Service Breast Screening Programme. Quality (1995): Assurance in the NHS Breast Screening Programme. (Internal guidance).
- 12 Wells C. A. (1995): Quality Assurance in Breast Cancer Screening Cytology: A Review of the Literature and a Report on The UK National Cytology Scheme. *European Journal of Cancer* **31A**: 273–280.
- 13 Royal College of Pathologists (1992): Medical and Scientific Staffing of National Health Service Pathology Departments.
- 14 NHS Executive EL(96)66 (1996): Improving Outcomes in Breast Cancer: *Guidance for Purchasers*. Leeds, Department of Health.

References 2.1.2

- 1 Andersen J., Poulsen H. S. (1989): Immunohistochemical oestrogen receptor determination in paraffinembedded tissue: prediction of response to hormonal treatment in advanced breast cancer. *Cancer* **64**: 1901–1908.
- 2 Snead D. R. J., Bell J. A., Dixon A. R., Nicholson R. I., Eiston C. W., Blamey R. W., Ellis I. O. (1993): Methodology of immunohistological detection of oestrogen receptor in human breast carcinoma in formalin-fixed, paraffin-embedded tissue: a comparison with frozen section methodology. *Histopathology* **23**: 233–238.
- 3 Anderson T. J. (1989): Breast cancer screening: principles and practicalities for histopathologists. Churchill Livingstone, *Recent Advances in Histopathology* **14**: 43–61.
- 4 Armstrong J. S., Davies J. D. (1991): Laboratory handling of impalpable breast lesions: A review. *J. Clin. Pathol.* **44**: 89–93.
- 5 Department of Health Medical Devices Directorate (1991): Evaluation of specimen radiography cabinets: reports and guidance notes. *Blue book* (MDD/91/13) London: Department of Health: 1–33, 1–13.
- 6 Schnitt S. J., Wang H. H. (1989): Histologic sampling of grossly benign breast biopsies: how much is enough? *Am. J. Surg. Pathol.* **13**: 505–512.

- 7 Gad A. (1993): Pathology in breast cancer screening: A 15-year experience from a Swedish programme. In: Gad A., Rosselli del Turco M. (editors): *Breast Cancer Screening in Europe.* Springer-Verlag, 87–101.
- 8 Frappart L., Boudeulle M., Boumendil J. et al. (1984): Structure and composition of microcalcifications in benign and malignant lesions of the breast. *Human. Pathol.* **15**: 880–889.
- 9 Nielsen B. B. (1987): Adenosis tumour of the breast – a clinicopathological investigation of 27 cases. *Histopathology* **11**: 1259–1275.
- 10 Simpson J. F., Page D. L., Dupont W. D. (1990): Apocrine adenosis: a mimic of mammary carcinoma. *Surg. Pathol.* **3**: 289–299.
- 11 Page D. L., Rogers L. W. (1992): Combined histologic and cytologic criteria for the diagnosis of mammary atypical ductal hyperplasia. *Human. Pathol.* **23**, 1095–1097.
- 12 Böcker W., Bier B., Freytag G., Brömmelkamp B., Jarasch E.-D., Edel G., Dockhorn-Dworniczak B., Schmid K. W. (1992): An immunohistochemical study of the breast using antibodies to basal and luminal keratins, alpha-smooth muscle actin, vimentin, collagen IV and laminin. Part 1: normal breast and benign proliferative lesions. Virchows Archiv A. *Pathol. Anat.* **421**: 315–322.
- 13 Lagios M. D. (1990): Duct carcinoma in situ. *Surg. Clin. N. Am.* **70**: 853–871.
- 14 Bellamy C. O. C., McDonald C., Salter D. M., Chetty U., Anderson T. J. (1993): Noninvasive ductal carcinoma of the breast: the relevance of histologic categorization. *Human. Pathol.* **24**: 16–23.
- 15 Holland R., Peterse J. L., Millis R. R., Eusebi V., Faverly D., van de Vijver M. J., Zafrani B. (1994): Ductal carcinoma in situ: a proposal for a new classification. *Semin. Diagn. Pathol.* **11**: 167–180.
- 16 Page D. L., Anderson T. J. (1987): *Diagnostic Histopathology of the Breast.* Churchill Livingstone, Edinburgh, London, Melbourne, New York, 193–268.
- 17 Ellis I. O., Galea M., Broughton N., Locker A., Blamey R. W., Elston C. W. (1992): Pathological prognostic factors in breast cancer. 11. Histological type. Relationship with survival in a large study with long term follow-up. *Histopathology* **20**: 479–489.
- 18 Martinez V., Azzopardi J. G. (1979): Invasive lobular carcinoma of the breast: incidence and variants. *Histopathology* **3**: 467–488.
- 19 Fechner R. E. (1975): Histologic variants of infiltrating lobular carcinoma of the breast. *Human. Pathol.* **6**: 373–378.
- 20 Fisher E. R., Gregorio R. M., Redmond C., Fisher B. (1977): Tubulolobular invasive breast cancer: a variant of lobular invasive cancer. *Human. Pathol.* **8**: 679–683.
- 21 Fisher E. R., Gregorio R. M., Fisher B., Redmond C., Vellios F., Sommers S. C., co-operating investigators (1975): The pathology of invasive breast cancer: a syllabus derived from findings of the National Surgical Adjuvant Breast Project (Protocol No 4). *Cancer* **36**: 1–84.
- 22 Ridolfi R. L., Rosen P. P., Port A., Kinne D., Mike V. (1977): Medullary carcinoma of the breast: a clinicopathologic study with 10-year follow-up. *Cancer* **40**: 1365–1385.
- 23 Parl F. F., Richardson L. D. (1983): The histological and biological spectrum of tubular carcinoma of the breast. *Human. Pathol.* **14**: 694–698.
- 24 Elston C. W., Ellis I. O. (1991): Pathological prognostic factors in breast cancer. 1. The value of histological grade in breast cancer: experience from a large study with long term follow up. *Histopathology* **19**: 403–410.

References 2.1.3

- 1 Elston C. W., Ellis I. O. (1991): Pathological prognostic factors in breast cancer. I. The value of histological grade in breast cancer: Experience from a large study with long-term follow-up. *Histopathology* **19**: 403–410.
- 2 Schnitt S. J., Connolly J. L. (1992): Processing and evaluation of breast excision specimens: A clinically oriented approach. *Am. J. Clin. Pathol.* **98**: 125–137.
- 3 Association of Directors of Anatomic and Surgical Pathology (1993): Immediate man-

agement of mammographically detected breast lesions. *Am. J. Surg. Pathol.* **17**: 850–851.
- 4 Association of Directors of Anatomic and Surgical Pathology (1993): Immediate management of mammographically detected breast lesions. *American College of Surgeons Bulletin* **78**: 16–17.
- 5 Association of Directors of Anatomic and Surgical Pathology (1993): Immediate management of mammographically detected breast lesions. *Hum. Pathol.* **24**: 689–690.
- 6 Association of Directors of Anatomic and Surgical Pathology (1993): Immediate management of mammographically detected breast lesions. *Am. J. Clin. Pathol.* **100**: 92–93.
- 7 Bellamy C. O. C., McDonald C., Salter D. M. et al. (1994): Non-invasive ductal carcinoma of breast: The relevance of histological categorization. *Hum. Pathol.* **24**: 16–23.
- 8 Holland R., Peterse J. L., Millis R. R., Eusebi V., Faverly D., van de Vijver M. J. and Zafrani B. (1994): Ductal Carcinoma In Situ: A Proposal for a New Classification. *Seminars in Diagnostic Pathology* **11/3**: 167–180.

References 2.2.2

- 1 Schöndorf H. (1977): *Die Aspirationszytologie der Brustdrüse*. F. K. Schattauer Verlag, Stuttgart, New York.
- 2 Kreuzer G., Boquoi E. (1981): *Zytologie der weiblichen Brustdrüse*, Grundriß und Atlas. Georg Thieme Verlag, Stuttgart, New York.
- 3 Mouriquand J., Mermet M. A., Brocard M. C., Collomb N., Payan R., Panh H. (1986): Interet de l'examen cytologique systematique des secretions mammaires: 60 cancers diagnostiques sur 2120 ecoulements examines. *Rev. Fr. Gynecol. Obstet.* **81**: 41–45.
- 4 Wunderlich M. (1990): Diagnostische Leistungsfähigkeit und Ergebnisse der Exfoliativzytologie bei sezernierender Mamma. *GBK Mitteilungsdienst* **18**: 6–10.
- 5 Wells C. A., Ellis I.O., Zakhour H. D., Wilson A. R. (1994): Guidelines for cytology procedures and reporting on fine needle aspirates of the breast. *Cytopathology* **5**: 316–334.
- 6 Sneige N. (1996): A comparison of fine needle aspiration, core biopsy and needle localization biopsy techniques in mammographically detectable nonpalpable breast lesions. *Pathology Case Reviews* **1**: 6–11.
- 7 Papanicolaou G. N., Holmquist D. G., Bader G. M., Falk E. A. (1958): Exfoliative cytology of the human mammary gland and its value in the diagnosis of cancer and other diseases of the breast. *Cancer* **11**: 377–409.

References 2.2.3

- 1 The Royal College of Pathologists Working Group. February (1990): Guidelines for pathologists. *NHSBSP Screening Publications* (ISBN 1871997 65 8).
- 2 The Royal College of Pathologists Working Group. February (1990): Pathology reporting in breast cancer screening. *NHSBSP Screening Publications* (ISBN 1871997 70 4) (also published in abridged form with photographs in *J. Clin. Pathol.* 1991, 44, 710–725).
- 3 Warren R. and members of the Epping breast screening service (1991): Team learning and breast cancer screening. *Lancet* **338/24**: 514.
- 4 The Royal College of Radiologists (1990): Quality assurance guidelines for radiologists. *NHSBSP Screening Publications* (ISBN 1 872 263 208).
- 5 Lamb J., Anderson T. J., Dixon M. J., Levack RA. (1987): Role of fine needle aspiration cytology in breast cancer screening. *Clin. Pathol.* **40**: 705–709.
- 6 Zajdela A., Chossein N. A., Pillerton J. P. (1975): The value of aspiration cytology in the diagnosis of breast cancer. *Cancer* **35**: 499–506.
- 7 Azavedo E., Svane G., Auer G. (1989): Stereotactic fine-needle biopsy in 2594 mammographically detected non-palpable lesions. *Lancet* **1/8646**: 1033–1036.
- 8 Stewart F. W. (1933): The diagnosis of tumours by aspiration. *Am. J. Pathol.* **9**: 801–812.
- 9 Zajdela A., Zillhardt P., Voillemot N. (1987): Cytological diagnosis by fine needle

sampling without aspiration. *Cancer* **59**: 1201–1205.
- 10 Jackson V. P. (1990): Mammographically guided fine-needle aspiration cytology of non-palpable breast lesions. *Current Opinion in Radiology* **2**: 741–745.
- 11 Lofgren M., Andersson I., Lindholm K. (1990): Stereotactic X-ray guided fine needle aspiration biopsy of non-palpable breast lesions: comparison with the coordinate grid localisation technique. In: Brunner S. and Langfield B. (eds.): *Recent Results in Cancer Research* **119**: 100–104.
- 12 Catania S., Boccato P., Bono A., De Pietro S. D., Pilotti S., Ravetto C. (1989): Pneumothorax: A rare complication of fine needle aspiration of the breast. *Acta Cytol.* **33**: 140.
- 13 Peterse J. L., Koolman-Schellekens M. A., van-de-Peppel-van-de-Ham T., van-Heerde P. (1989): Atypia in fine needle aspiration cytology of the breast: a histologic follow-up study of 301 cases. *Semin. Diagn. Pathol.* **6/2**: 126–34.
- 14 Simpson J. F., Page D. L., Dupont W. D. (1990): Apocrine adenosis – a mimic of mammary carcinoma. *Surgical Pathology* **3**: 289–299.
- 15 Oertel Y. Butterworth: *Fine needle aspiration cytology of the breast.*
- 16 Salhany K. E.; Page D. L. (1989): Fine needle aspiration of mammary lobular carcinoma in situ and atypical lobular hyperplasia. *Am. Clin. Pathol.* **92&1**: 22–26.
- 17 Wells C. A., Wells C. W., Yeomans P., Vina M., Jordan S., d'Ardenne A. J. (1990): Spherical connective tissue inclusions in epithelial hyperplasia of the breast ("collagenous spherulosis"). *Clin. Pathol.* **43**: 905–908.
- 18 Tyler X., Coghill S. B. (1991): Fine needle aspiration cytology of collagenous spherulosis of the breast. *Cytopathology* **2**: 159–162.
- 19 *Cytopathology* 1990, 1, 311–316: A microglandular adenosis-like lesion simulating tubular adenocarcinoma of the breast. A case report with cytological and histological appearances.
- 20 Lamb J., Anderson T. J. (1989): Influence of cancer histology on the success of fine needle aspiration of the breast. *J Clin. Pathol.* **42/7**: 733–735.
- 21 Bondeson L., Lindholm K (1990): Aspiration cytology of tubular breast carcinoma. *Acta Cytol.* **34/1**: 15–20.
- 22 Sneige-N., Zachariah S., Fanning T. V., Dekmezian R. H., Ordonez N. G. (1989): Fine needle aspiration cytology of metastatic neoplasms in the breast. *Am. J. Clin. Pathol.* **92/1**: 27–35.
- 23 Weintraub J., Weintraub D., Redard M., Vassilakos P. (1987): Evaluation of oestrogen receptors by immunocytochemistry on fine needle aspiration biopsy specimens from breast tumours. *Cancer* **60**: 1163–1172.
- 24 Redard M., Vassilakos P., Weintraub J. (1989): A simple method for oestrogen receptor antigen preservation in cytologic specimens containing breast carcinoma cells. *Diagnostic Cytopathology* **5**: 188–193.
- 25 Cytological grading of breast carcinoma – a feasible proposition? Hunt C. M., Ellis I. O., Elston C. W., Locker A., Pearson D., Blamey R. W. (1990): *Cytopathology* **1**: 287–295.
- 26 Thomas J. S. J., Mallon E. A., George W. D. (1989): Semi-quantitative analyses of fine needle aspirates from benign and malignant breast lesions. *J. Clin. Pathol.* **42**: 28–34.
- 27 Mapstone N. P., Zakhour H. D. (1990): Morphometric analysis of fine needle aspirates from breast lesions. *Cytopathology* **1**: 349–355.
- 28 Barrows G. H., Anderson T. J., Lamb J. L., Dixon J. M. (1986): Fine needle aspiration of breast cancer – Relationship of clinical factors to cytology results in 689 primary malignancies. *Cancer* **58**: 1493–1498.
- 29 Elston C. W. (1991): Training for breast screening pathology. *The Bulletin of the Royal College of Pathologists*, 76.
- 30 Karainsky D. B. (1984): Aspiration biopsy in the context of the new Medicare riscal policy. *Acta Cytologica* **28**: 333–337.
- 31 Kocjan G. (1991): Evaluation of the cost-effectiveness of establishing a fine needle aspiration cytology clinic in a hospital out patient department. *Cytopathology* **2**: 13–18.

- 32 McKee G., Thomas B., Cooke J. (1991): Stereotactic cytology – Results of the first 250 cases. Abstract presented at 3rd annual B. S. C. C. meeting – Sheffield.
- 33 Brown L. A., Coghill S. B., Powis S. A. J. (1991): Audit of diagnostic accuracy of FNA cytology specimens taken by the histopathologist in a symptomatic breast clinic. *Cytopathology* **2**: 1–7.
- 34 Powles T. J., Trott P. A., Cherryman G., Clarke S., Ashley S., Coombes R. C., Jones A. L., Sinnett H. D., Nash A. G. (1991): Fine needle aspiration cytodiagnosis as a prerequisite for primary medical treatment of breast cancer. *Cytopathology* **2**: 7–13.
- 35 Lofgren M., Andersson I., Lindhold K. (1990): Stereotactic fine-needle aspiration for cytologic diagnosis of non-palpable breast lesions. *Am. J. of Radiol.* **154**: 1191–1195.
- 36 Bibbo M., Scheiber M., Cajulis R., Keebler C. M., Wied G. L., Dowlatshahi K. (1988): Stereotaxic fine needle aspiration cytology of clinically occult malignant and pre-malignant breast lesions. *Acta Cytologica* **32/2**: 193–201.
- 37 Dent D. M., Kirkpatrick A. E., McGoogan E., Chetty U., Anderson T. J. (1989): Stereotaxic localisation and aspiration cytology of impalpable breast lesions. *Clin. Radiol.* **40/4**: 380–382.
- 38 Masood S., Frykberg E. R., McLellan G. L., Scalapino M. C., Mitchum D. G., Bullard J. B. (1990): Prospective evaluation of radiologically directed fine-needle aspiration biopsy of non-palpable breast lesions. *Cancer* **66**: 1480–1487.

References 2.2.5

- 1 Saleh H. A., Khatib G. (1996): Positive economic and diagnostic accuracy impacts of on-site evaluation of fine needle aspiration biopsies by pathologists. *Acta Cytol.* **40**: 1227–1230.
- 2 Brown L. A., Coghill S. B. (1992): Cost effectiveness of a fine needle aspiration clinic. *Cytopathology* **3**: 275–280.
- 3 Kaminsky D. B. (1984): Aspiration biopsy in the context of the new medicare fiscal policy. *Acta Cytol.* **28**: 333–336.
- 4 Sneige N., Staerkel G. A., Caraway N. P., Fanning T. V., Katz R. L. (1994): A plea for uniform terminology and reporting of breast fine needle aspirates. The M. D. Anderson Cancer Center's proposal. *Acta Cytol.* **38**: 971–972.
- 5 Wells C. A., Ellis I. O., Zakhour H. D., Wilson A. R. (1994): Guidelines for cytology procedures and reporting on fine needle aspirates of the breast. *Cytopathology* **5**: 316–334.
- 6 Suen K. C., Abdul-Karim F. W., Kaminsky D. B., et al. (1996): Guidelines of the Papanicolaou Society of Cytopathology for the examination of fine needle aspiration specimens from thyroid nodules. *Mod. Pathol.* **9**: 710–715 and *Diagn. Cytopathol.* **15**: 84–89 (simultaneous publication).
- 7 The National Committee for Clinical Laboratory Standards (1996): Fine needle aspiration biopsy (FNAB) techniques; approved guideline. *NCCLS document GP20–A*.
- 8 Abati A., Abele J., Bacus S. S., Bedrossian C., Beerline D., et al. (1996): The uniform approach to breast fine needle aspiration biopsy: a synopsis. *Acta Cytol.* **40**: 1120–1126.
- 9 Frable W. J. (1983): Fine needle aspiration biopsy. A review. *Hum. Pathol.* **14**: 9–28.
- 10 DeMay R. M. (1996): The art and science of cytopathology. Volume 11: *aspiration cytology*. Chicago: ASCP Press: 464–474.
- 11 Stanley M. W. (1992): Inappropriate referrals for fine needle aspiration: the need for expert clinical skills in the cytopathologist who sees patients. *Acta Cytol.* **36**: 615.
- 12 Stanley M. W., Abele J., Kline T. S., Silverman J. F., Skoog L. (1995): What constitutes adequate sampling of palpable breast lesions that appear benign by clinical and mammographic criteria? *Diagn. Cytopathol.* **13**: 473–485.
- 13 Silverman J. F., Lannin D. R., O'Brien K., Norris H. T. (1987): The triage role of fine needle aspiration biopsy of palpable breast masses. *Acta Cytol.* **31**: 731–736.
- 14 Layfield L. J., Chrischilles E. A., Cohen M. B., Bottle K. (1993): The palpable breast nodule. A cost effectiveness analysis of

alternate diagnostic approaches. *Cancer* **72**: 1642–1651.
- 15 Geier G. R., Strecker J. R. (1981): Aspiration cytology and E2 content in ovarian tumors. *Acta Cytol.* **25**: 400–406.
- 16 Suen K. C. (1990): *Atlas and text of aspiration cytology*. Baltimore: Williams & Wilkins: 254–263.
- 17 Greenebaum E. (1996): Aspirating non-neoplastic ovarian cysts. Rationale, technique, and controversy. *Lab. Med.* **27**: 462–467.
- 18 Greenebaum E. (1996): Aspirating malignant ovarian cysts. *Lab. Med.* **27**: 607–611.
- 19 Trimbos J. B., Hacker N. E. (1993): The case against aspirating ovarian cysts. *Cancer* **72**: 838–831.
- 20 Hajdu S. I., Melamed M. R. (1984): Limitations of needle aspiration cytology in the diagnosis of primary neoplasms. *Acta Cytol.* **28**: 337–345.
- 21 Highman W. J., Oliver R. T. (1987): Diagnosis of metastases from testicular germ cell tumors using fine needle aspiration cytology. *J. Clin. Pathol.* **40**: 1324–1333.
- 22 Jadusingh I. H. (1996): Fine needle aspiration biopsy of superficial sites in patients with hemostatic defects. *Acta Cytol.* **40**: 472–474.
- 23 Engzell U., Franzen S., Zajicek J. (1971): Aspiration biopsy of tumors of the cytologic findings in 13 cases of carotid body tumor. *Acta Cytol.* **15**: 25–30.
- 24 Jamieson W. R. E., Suen K. C., Hicken P., Martin A. L. P., Burr L. H., Munro A. I. (1981): Reliability of percutaneous needle aspiration biopsy for diagnosis of bronchogenic carcinoma. *Cancer Detect. Prev.* **4**: 331–336.
- 25 Lalli A. F., McCormack L. J., Zelch M., Reich N. E., Belovich D. (1978): Aspiration of chest lesions. *Radiology* **127**: 35–40.
- 26 Westcott J. L. (1980): Direct percutaneous needle aspiration of localized pulmonary lesions. *Radiology* **137**: 31–35.
- 27 Sinner W. N. (1976): Complications of percutaneous transthoracic needle aspiration biopsy. *Acta Radiol. Diagn.* **17**: 813–828.
- 28 Livraghi T., Damascelli B., Lombardi C., Spagnoli I. (1983): Risk in fine-needle abdominal biopsy. *J. Clin. Ultrasound* **11**: 77–81.
- 29 Fornari F., Civardi G., Cavanna L., et al. (1989): Complications of ultrasonally guided, fine-needle abdominal biopsy. *Scand. J. Gastroenterol.* **24**: 949–955.
- 30 Smith E. H. (1984): The hazards of fine-needle aspiration biopsy. *Ultrasound Med. Biol.* **10**: 629–634.
- 31 Smith E. H. (1991): Complications of percutaneous abdominal fine-needle biopsy: review. *Radiology* **178**: 253–258.
- 32 Glasgow B. J., Brown H. H., Zargoza A. M., Foos R. Y. (1988): Quantitation of tumor seeding from fine needle aspiration of ocular melanomas. *Am. J. Ophthalmol.* **105**: 538–546.
- 33 Glaser K. S., Weger A. R., Schmid K. W., Bodner E. (1989): Is fine needle aspiration of tumors harmless? *Lancet* **1**: 620.
- 34 Hales M. S., Hsu F. S. F. (1990): Needle tract implantation of papillary carcinoma of the thyroid following aspiration biopsy. *Acta Cytol.* **34**: 801–804.
- 35 Von Schreeb T., Arner O., Skovsted G., Wikstad N. (1967): Renal adenocarcinoma. Is there a risk of spreading cells in diagnostic puncture? *Scand. J. Nephrol.* **1**: 270–276.
- 36 Sinner W. N. (1973): Transthoracic needle biopsy of small peripheral malignant lung lesions. *Invest. Radiol.* **8**: 305–314.
- 37 Kini S. R. (1996): Postfine-needle biopsy infarction of thyroid neoplasms. *Diagn. Cytopathol.* **15**: 211–220.
- 38 LiVolsi V. A., Merino M. J. (1994): Worrisome histologic alterations following fine needle aspiration of thyroid. *Pathol. Ann.* **29**: 99–120.
- 39 Layfield L. J., Lones M. A. (1991): Necrosis in thyroid nodules after fine needle aspiration biopsy. Report of two cases. *Acta Cytol.* **35**: 427–430.
- 40 Davies J. D., Webb A. J. (1982): Segmental lymph node infarction after fine needle aspiration. *J. Clin. Pathol.* **35**: 855–857.
- 41 Grohs H. K. (1988): The interventional cytopathologist. A new clinician/pathologist hybrid. *Am. J. Clin. Pathol.* **90**: 351–354.
- 42 Frable W. J. (1993): Aspiration cytology. In: Keebler C. M., Somrak T. M., eds.:

Manual of cytotechnology. 7th ed. Chicago: ASCP: 239–251.
- 43 Japko L. (1986): Aspiration biopsy: the pathologist as hands-on consultant. *Diagn. Cytopathol.* **2**: 233–235.
- 44 Davey D. D., Talkington S., Kannan V., Masood S., Davila R., Cohen M. B. (1996): Cytopathology and the pathology resident. A survey of residency program directors. *Arch. Pathol. Lab. Med.* **120**: 101–104.
- 45 Cohen M. B., Perez-Reyes N., Stoloff A. C. (1995): The status of residency training in cytopathology. *Diagn. Cytopathol.* **12**: 186–187.
- 46 Hoda R. S. (1995): Steps for residency training in cytology. *Diagn. Cytopathol.* **13**: 277.
- 47 Cohen M. (1987): Influence of training and experience in fine-needle aspiration biopsy of breast. *Arch. Pathol. Lab. Med.* **111**: 518–520.
- 48 Lee K. R. (1987): Fine needle aspiration biopsy of breast: importance of aspirator. *Acta Cytol.* **31**: 281–284.
- 49 Suen K. C., Wood W. S., Syed A. A., Quenville N. F., Clement P. B. (1978): Role of imprint cytology in intraoperative diagnosis. *J. Clin. Pathol.* **31**: 328–337.
- 50 Blaustein P. A., Silverberg S. G. (1977): Rapid cytologic examination of surgical specimens. *Pathol. Annu.* **12**: 251–278.
- 51 Fitzpatrick B. T., Bibbo M. (1996): Superficial fine needle aspiration by clinicians: a survey of utilization. *Acta Cytol.* **40**: 1092.
- 52 Stanley M. M., Lowhagen T. (1993): *Fine needle aspiration of palpable masses.* Boston: Butterworth-Heinemann: 1–65.
- 53 Schultenover S. J., Ramzy I., Page C. P., LeFebre S. M., Cruz A. B. Jr. (1984): Needle aspiration biopsy: role and limitations in surgical decision making. *Am. J. Clin. Pathol.* **82**: 405–410.
- 54 Abele J. S., Miller T. R. (1993): Implementation of an outpatient needle aspiration biopsy service and clinic: a personal perspective. *Cytopathol. Annu.*: 43–71.
- 55 Hall T. L., Layfield L. J., Philippe A., Rosenthal D. L. (1989): Sources of diagnostic error in fine needle aspiration of the thyroid. *Cancer* **63**: 18–25.
- 56 Stanley M. W. (1990): Who should perform fine-needle aspiration biopsy? *Diagn. Cytopathol.* **6**: 215–217.
- 57 Coghill S. B., Brown L. A. (1995): Editorial: why pathologists should take needle aspiration specimens. *Cytopathology* **6**: 1–4.
- 58 Dixon J. M., Lamb J., Anderson T. J. (1983): Fine needle aspiration of the breast: importance of the operator. *Lancet* **2**: 564.
- 59 Carson H. J., Saint Martin G. A., Castelli M. J., Gattuso P. (1995): Unsatisfactory aspirates from fine-needle aspiration biopsies: a review. *Diagn. Cytopathol.* **12**: 280–284.
- 60 Kline T. S. (1988): *Handbook of fine needle aspiration biopsy cytology.* 2nd ed. New York: Churchill Livingstone: 9–16.
- 61 Ljung B. M. (1992): Techniques of aspiration and smear preparation. In: Koss L. G., Woyke S., Olszewski W., eds.: *Aspiration biopsy. Cytologic interpretation and histologic bases.* 2nd ed. New York: Igaku-Shoin: 12–38.
- 62 National Committee for Clinical Laboratory Standards. Protection of laboratory workers from infectious disease transmitted by blood, body fluids, and tissue; tentative guideline. *NCCLS document* M29-T, 1989.
- 63 Zajdela A., Zillhardt P., Voillemot N. (1987): Cytologic diagnosis by fine-needle sampling without aspiration. *Cancer* **59**: 1201–1205.
- 64 Akhtar M., Ali M. A., Huq M., Faulkner C. (1989): Fine-needle biopsy: comparison of cellular yield with and without aspiration. *Diagn. Cytopathol.* **5**: 162–165.
- 65 Santos J. E. C., Leiman G. (1988): Non-aspiration fine-needle cytology: application of a new technique to nodular thyroid disease. *Acta Cytol.* **32**: 353–356.
- 66 Cajulls R. S., Sneige N. (1993): Objective comparison of cellular yield in fine-needle biopsy of lymph nodes with and without aspiration. *Diagn. Cytopathol.* **9**: 43–45.
- 67 Fagelman D., Chess Q. (1990): *Non-aspiration fine needle cytology of the liver.* A new technique for obtaining diagnostic samples. AJR 155: 1217–1219.
- 68 Dey P., Shashirekha R. R. (1994): Fine needle sampling without suction in intraabdominal lesions. Comparison with fine needle aspiration. *Acta Cytol.* **38**: 495–496.

- 69 Chess Q. (1996): Intraabdominal lesions: fine needle sampling without suction vs. fine needle aspiration. *Acta Cytol.* **40**: 610.
- 70 Yang G. C. H., Alvarez I. I. (1995): Ultrafast Papanicolaou stain. An alternative preparation for fine needle aspiration cytology. *Acta Cytol.* **39**: 55–60.
- 71 McGoogan E., Reith A. (1996): Would monolayers provide more representative samples and improved preparations for cervical screening? Overview and evaluation of systems available. *Acta Cytol.* **49**: 107–119.
- 72 Papillo J. L., Lee K. R., Manna E. A. (1992): Clinical evaluation of the ThinPrep method for the preparation of nongynecologic material. *Acta Cytol.* **36**: 651–652.
- 73 Perez-Reyes N., Mulford D. K., Rutkowski M. A., Logan-Young W., Dawson A. E. (1994): Breast fine needle aspiration: a comparison of thin-layer and conventional preparation. *Am. J. Clin. Pathol.* **102**: 349–353.
- 74 Lee K. R., Papillo J., St. John T., Eyerer G. J. A. (1996): Evaluation of the ThinPrep processor for fine needle aspiration specimens. *Acta Cytol.* **40**: 895–899.
- 75 Yazdi H. M., Dardick I. (1992): *Guides to clinical aspiration biopsy*: diagnostic immunocytochemistry and electron microscopy. New York: IgakuShoin, 1992.
- 76 Fowler L. J., Valente P. T., Schantz H. D. (1996): Cell block techniques and immunocytochemistry. *Diagn. Cytopathol.* **14**: 281.
- 77 Moriarty A. T., Wiersema L., Snyder W., et al. (1993): Immunophenotyping of cytologic specimens by flow cytometry. *Diagn. Cytopathol.* **9**: 252–258.
- 78 Skoog L., Humla S., Isaksson S., Tani E. (1990): Immunocytochemical analysis of receptors for estrogen and progestrone in fine-needle aspirates from human breast carcinomas. *Diagn. Cytopathol.* **6**: 95–98.
- 79 Greiner T. C. (1992): Polymerase chain reaction: uses and potential applications in cytology. *Diagn. Cytopathol.* **8**: 61–65.
- 80 Abati A., Sanford J. S., Fetsch P., Marincola F. M., Wolman S. R. (1995): Fluorescence in situ hybridization (FISH): a user's guide to optimal preparation of cytologic specimens. *Diagn. Cytopathol.* **13**: 486–492.
- 81 Suen K. C. (1992): Seeing, not just looking (editorial). *Diagn. Cytopathol.* **7**: 335–336.
- 82 Kline T. S. (1995): Adequacy and aspirates from the breast – A philosophical approach. *Diagn. Cytopathol.* **13**: 470–472.
- 83 Hajdu S. I. (1995): Malpractice vs. Benepractice (letter to the editor). *Am. J. Surg. Pathol.* **19**: 481.
- 84 Moriarty A. T. (1995): Fine-needle biopsy of breast: when is enough, enough? *Diagn. Cytopathol.* **13**: 373–374.
- 85 Hermansen C., Poulsen H. S., Jensen J., et al. (1987): Diagnostic reliability of combined physical examination, mammography and fine needle punctate ("triple test") in breast tumors. *Cancer* **60**: 1866–1871.
- 86 Henry-Stanley M. J., Beneke J., Bardales R. H., Stanley M. W. (1995): Fine-needle aspiration of normal tissue from enlarged salivary glands: sialosis or missed target? *Diagn. Cytopathol.* **13**: 300–303.
- 87 Kline T. S., Bedrossian C. W. M. (1996): Editorial: communication and cytopathology. *Diagn. Cytopathol.* **14**: 7–10.
- 88 Skoumal S. M., Florell S. R., Bydalek M. K., Hunter W. J. III (1996): Malpractice protection. Communication of diagnostic uncertainty. *Diagn. Cytopathol.* **14**: 385–389.
- 89 Silverman J. F., Frable W. J. (1990): The use of the Diff-Quik stain in the immediate interpretation of fine-needle aspiration biopsies. *Diagn. Cytopathol.* **6**: 366–369.
- 90 Miller D. A., Carrasco C. H., Katz R. L., Cramer F. M., Wallace S., Charnsangavej C. (1986): Fine needle aspiration biopsy: the role of immediate cytologic assessment. *AJR* 147: 155–158.
- 91 Yang G. C. H., Liebeskind D., Messina A. (1996): On-site immediate diagnosis for fine needle aspiration biopsy: experience at an outpatient radiology clinic. *Acta Cytol.* **40**: 1099.
- 92 US Department of Helath and Human Services Services, Medicare, Medicaid and CLIA programs (1992): Clinical Laboratory Improvement Amendments of 1988 (CLIA '88) final rules. *Fed. Regist.* **57**: 7137–7186.
- 93 Quality improvement manual in anatomic pathology. 2nd ed. Northfield, Ill. *College of American Pathologists*, 1993.

- 94 Kline T. S., Nguyen G. K. (1996): *Critical issues in cytopathology*. New York: Igaku-Shoin: 42–61.
- 95 Inhorn S. I., Shalkham J. E., Mueller G. B. (1994): Quality assurance programs to meet CLIA requirements. *Diagn. Cytopathol.* 11: 195–200.
- 96 Lachowicz C. M., Kline T. S. (1996): Quality improvement principles in cytopathology. In: Kline T. S., Nguyen G. K., eds.: *Critical issues in cytopathology*. New York: Igaku-Shoin 42–61.

References 2.3.1

- 1 Ali I. U., Lidereau R., Theillet C., Callahan R. (1987): Reduction to homozygosity of genes on chromome 11 in human breast neoplasia. *Science* 238: 185–188.
- 2 American Society of Clinical Oncology (1996): Statement of the American Society of Clinical Oncology: Genetic testing for cancer susceptibility. *J. Clinical Oncology* 14: 1730–1736.
- 3 Andersen T. I., Gautsad A., Ottestad L., Farrants G. W., Nesland J. M., Tveit K. M., Børresen A.-L. (1992): Genetic alterations of the tumor suppressor gene regions 3p, 11p, 13q, 17p, and 17q in human breast carcinomas. *Genes Chrom. Cancer* 4: 113–121.
- 4 Andersen T. I., Holm R., Nesland J. M., Heimdal K. R., Ottestad L., Børresen A.-L. (1993): Prognostic significance of TP53 alterations in breast carcinoma. *Br. J. Cancer* 68: 540–548.
- 5 Baak J. P. A. (1990): Mitosis counting in tumors. *Hum. Pathol.* 21: 683–685.
- 6 Barker P. E. and Hsu T. C. (1978): Are double minutes chromosomes? *Exp. Cell Res.* 113: 456–458,
- 7 Bártek J., Bártková B., Vojtesek B., Stasková Z., Lukás J., Rejthar A., Kovarik J., Midgley C. A., Gannon J. V., Lane D. P. (1991): Aberrant expression of the p53 oncoprotein is a common feature of a wide spectrum in human malignancies. *Oncogene* 6: 1699–1703.
- 8 Beerman H., Kluin Ph. M., Hermans J., Van de Velde C. J. H., Cornelisse C. J. (1990): Prognostic significance of DNA-ploidy in a series of 690 primary breast cancer patients. *Int. J. Cancer* 45: 34–39.
- 9 Bertwistle D. and Ashworth A. (1998): Functions of the BRCA1 and BRCA2 genes. *Curr. Opin. Genet. Dev.* 8: 14–20.
- 10 Bhargava V., Thor A., Deng G., Ljung B.-M., Moore D. H., Waldman F., Benz C., Goodson W., Mayall B., Chew K., Smith H. S. (1994): The association of p53 immunopositivity with tumor proliferation and other prognostic indicators in breast cancer. *Modern Pathol.* 7: 361–368.
- 11 Børresen A.-L. (1992): Role of genetic factors in breast cancer susceptibility. *Acta Oncologica* 31: 151–155.
- 12 Buchhagen D. L., Qiu L., Etkind P. (1994): Homozygous deletion, rearrangement and hypermethylation implicate chromosome region 3p14.3–3p21.3 in sporadic breast-cancer development. *Int. J. Cancer* 57: 473–479.
- 13 Bullerdiek J., Leuschner E., Taquia E., Bonk U., Bartnitzke S. (1993): Trisomy 8 as a recurrent clonal abnormality in breast cancer? *Cancer Genet. Cytogenet.* 65: 64–67.
- 14 Callahan R., Cropp C., Sheng Z. M., Merlo G., Steeg P., Liscia D., Lidereau R. (1993): Definition of regions of the human genome affected by loss of heterozygosity in primary human breat tumors. *J. Cellular Biochemistry* 17G: 167–172.
- 15 Casey G., Plummer S., Hoeltge G., Scanlon D., Fasching C., Stanbridge E. J. (1993): Functional evidence for a breast cancer growth suppressor gene on chromome 17. *Human Molecular Genetics* 2: 1921–1927.
- 16 Cattoretti G., Becker M. H. G., Key G., et al. (1992): Monoclonal antibodies against recombinant parts of the Ki-67 antigen (MIB 1 and MIB 3) detect proliferating cells in microwave-processed formalin-fixed paraffin sections. *J. Pathol.* 168: 357–363.
- 17 Chen L.-C., Dollbaum C., Smith H. S. (1989): Loss of heterozygosity on chromome 1q in human breast cancer. *Proc. Natl. Acad. Sci. USA* 86: 7204–7207.
- 18 Chen L.-C., Matsumara K., Deng G., Kurisu W., Ljung B.-M., Lerman M. I., Waldman F. M., Smith H. S. (1994): Deletion of two separate regions on chromo-

some 3p in breast cancers. *Cancer Res.* **54**: 3021–3024.
- 19 Cleton-Jansen A.-M., Collins N., Lakhani S. R., Weissenbach J., Devilee P., Cornelisse C. J. (1995): Loss of heterozygosity in sporadic brest tumours ate the BRCA2 locus on chromosome 13q12–q13. *Br. J. Cancer* **72**: 1241–1244.
- 20 Collins, F. S. (1996): BRCA1 – Lots of mutations, lots of dilemmas. *New England J. Med.* **334**: 186–188.
- 21 Cornelisse C. J., Van de Velde C. H. J., Caspers R. J. C., Moolenaar A. J., Hermans J. (1987): DNA ploidy and survival in breast cancer patients. *Cytometry* **8**: 225–234.
- 22 Cox L. A., Chen G., Lee E. Y.-H. P. (1994): Tumor suppressor genes and their roles in breast cancer. *Breast Cancer Res. Treat.* **32**: 19–38.
- 23 Devilee P. and Cornelisse C. J. (1990): Genetics of human breast cancer. *Cancer Surveys* **9**: 605–630.
- 24 Dressler L. G., Seamer L. C., Owens M. A., Clark G. M., McGuire W. L. (1988): DNA flow cytometry and prognostic factors in 1331 frozen breast cancer specimens. *Cancer* **1988**: 420–427.
- 25 Easton D., Ford D., Peto J. (1993): Inherited susceptibility to breast cancer. *Cancer Surveys* **18**: 95–113.
- 26 Eeles R. A., Bartkova J., Lane D. P., Bartek J. (1993): The role of TP53 in breast cancer. *Cancer Surveys* **18**: 57–75.
- 27 Eisinger F., Jacquemier J., Charpin C., Stoppa-Lyonnet D., Bressac-de Paillerets B., Peyrat J. P., Longy M., Guinebretiere J. M., Sauvan R., Noguchi T., Birnbaum D., Sobol H. (1998): Mutations at BRCA1: the medullary breast carcinoma revisited. *Cancer Res.* **58**: 1588–1592.
- 28 Eisinger F., Stoppa-Lyonnet D., Longy M., Kerangueven F., Noguchi T., Bailly C., Vincent-Salomon A., Jacquemier J., Birnbaum D., Sobol H. (1996): Germ line mutation at BRCA1 affects the histoprognostic grade in hereditary breast cancer. *Cancer Res.* **56**: 471–474.
- 29 Elledge R. M. and Allred D. C. (1994): The p53 tumor suppressor gene in breast cancer. *Breast Cancer Res. Treat.* **32**: 39–47.
- 30 Elledge R. M., McGuire W. L., Osborne C. K. (1992): Prognostic factors in breast cancer. *Seminars in Oncology* **19**: 244–253.
- 31 Ewers S.-B., Attewell R., Baldetorp B., Borg A., Langström E., Kilander D. (1991): Prognostic potential of flow cytometric S-phase and ploidy prospectively determined in primary breast carcinomas. *Breast Cancer Res. Treat.* **20**: 93–108.
- 32 Finley C. A., Hinds, P. W., Levine, A. J. (1989): The p53 proto-oncogene can act as a supppressor of transformation. *Cell* **57**: 1083–1093.
- 33 Futreal P. A., Liu Q., Shattuck-Eidens D., Cochran C., Harshman K., Tavtigian S., Bennett L. M., Haugen-Strano A., Swensen J., Miki Y., Eddington K., McClure M., Frye C., Weaver-Feldhaus J., Ding W., Gholami Z., Söderkvist P., Terry L., Jhanwar S., Berchuck A., Iglehart J. D., Marks J., Ballinger D. G., Barrett J. C., Skolnick M. H., Kamb A., Wiseman R. (1994): BRCA1 mutations in primary breast and ovarian carcinomas. *Science* **266**: 120–122.
- 34 Futreal P. A., Söderkvist P., Marks J. R., Iglehart J. D., Cochran C., Barrett J. C., Wiseman R. W. (1992): Detection of frequent allelic loss on proximal chromosome 17q in sporadic breast carcinoma using microsatellite length polymorphisms. *Cancer Res.* **52**: 2624–2627.
- 35 Gasparini G., Boracchi P., Verderio P., Bevilacqua P. (1994): Cell kinetics in human breast cancer: comparison between the prognostic value of the cytofluorimetric S-phase fraction and that of the antibodies to Ki-67 and PCNA antigens detected by immunocytochemistry. *Int. J. Cancer* **57**: 822–829.
- 36 Gasparini G., Pozza F., Bevilacqua P., Meli S., Boracchi P., Reitano M., Santini G., Marubini E., Sainsbury J. R. C. (1992): Growth fraction (Ki-67 antibody) determination in stage-I–II breast carcinoma: histologic, clinical and prognostic correlations. *Breast* **1**: 92–99.
- 37 Gasparini G., Pozza F., Harris A. L. (1993): Evaluating the potential usefulness of new prognostic and predictive indicators in node-negative breast cancer patients. *J. Natl. Cancer Inst.* **85**: 1206–1219.

- 38 Gebhart E., Brüderlein S., Augustus M., Siebert E., Feldner J., Schmidt W. (1986): Cytogenetic studies on human breast carcinomas. *Breast Cancer Res. Treat.* **8**: 125–138.
- 39 Geleick D., Müller H., Matter A., Torhost J., Regenass U. (1990): Cytogenetics of breast cancer. *Cancer Genet. Cytogenet.* **46**: 217–229.
- 40 Ghali V. S., Liau S., Teplitz C., Prudente R. (1992): A comparative study of DNA ploidy in 115 fresh-frozen breast carcinomas by image analysis versus flow cytometry. *Cancer* **70**: 2668–2672.
- 41 Goodson W. H., Ljung B.-M., Moore D. H., Mayall B., Waldman F. M., Chew K., Benz C. C., Smith H. S. (1993): Tumor labeling indices of primary breast cancers and their regional lymph node metastases. *Cancer* **71**: 3914–3919.
- 42 Grade K., Jandrig B., Scherneck S. (1996): BRCA1 mutation update and analysis. *J. Cancer Res. Clin. Oncol.* **122**: 702–706.
- 43 Hainsworth P. J., Raphael K. L., Stillwell R. G., Bennett R. C., Garson O. M. (1991): Cytogenetic features of twenty-six primary breast cancers. *Cancer Genet. Cytogenet.* **52**: 205–218.
- 44 Hainsworth P. J., Raphael K. L., Stillwell R. G., Bennett R. C., Garson O. M. (1992): Rearrangement of chomosome 1p in breast cancer correlates with poor prognostic features. *Br. J. Cancer* **66**: 131–135.
- 45 Hall J. M., Lee M. K., Newman B., Morrow J. E., Anderson L. A., Huey B., King M. C. (1990): Linkage of early-onset familial breast cancer to chromosome 17q21. *Science* **250**: 1684–1689.
- 46 Hampton G. M., Mannermaa A., Winquist R., Alavaikko M., Blanco G., Taskinen P. J., Kiviniemi H., Newsham I., Cavenee W. K., Evans G. A. (1994): Loss of heterozygosity in sporadic human breast carcinomas: a common region between 11q22 and 11q23.3. *Cancer Res.* **54**: 4586–4589.
- 47 Hartwell L. (1994): Defects in a cell cycle checkpoint may be responsible for the genomic instability of cancer cells. *Cell* **71**: 543–546.
- 48 Hedley D. W., Clark G. M., Cornelisse C. J., Killander D., Kute T., Merkel D. (1993): DNA Cytometry Consensus Conference. Consensus review of the clinical utility of DNA cytometry in carcinoma of the breast. *Breast Cancer Res. Treat.* **28**: 55–59.
- 49 Hedley D. W., Rugg C. A., Gelber R. D. (1987): Association of DNA index and S-phase fraction with prognosis of node-positive early breast cancer. *Cancer Res.* **47**: 4729–4735.
- 50 Heim S. and Mitelman F. (1995): *Cancer cytogenetics.* Alan R. Liss, New York.
- Hill S. M., Rodgers C. S., Hultén M. A. (1987): Cytogenetics analysis in human breast carcinoma. II. Seven cases in the triploid/tetraploid range investigated using direct preparations. *Cancer Genet. Cytogenet.* **24**: 45–62.
- 51 Hollstein M., Sidransky D., Vogelstein B., Harris C. C. (1991): p53 mutations in human cancers. *Science* **253**: 49–53.
- 52 Jones-Cruciger Q. V., Pathak S., Cailleau R. (1976): Human breast carcinomas: marker chromosomes involving 1q in seven cases. *Cytogenet. Cell Genet.* **17**: 231–235.
- 53 Kallioniemi, O.-P., Blanco G., Alavaikko M., Hietanen T., Mattila J., Lauslahti K., Lehtinen M., Koivula T. (1988): Improving the prognostic value of DNA flow cytometry in breast cancer by combining DNA index and S-phase fraction. *Cancer* **62**: 2183–2190.
- 54 Keshgegian A. A. and Cnaan A. (1995): Proliferation markers in breast carcinoma. Mitotic figure count, S-phase fraction, proliferating cell nuclear antigen, Ki-67 and MIB-1. *Am. J. Clin. Pathol.* **104**: 42–49.
- 55 Key G., Becker M. H. G., Baron B., et al. (1993): New Ki-67-equivalent murine monoclonal antibodies (MIB 1–3) generating against bacterially expressed parts of the Ki-67 cDNA containing three 62 base pair repetitive elements encoding for the Ki-67 epitope. *Lab. Invest.* **68**: 629–636.
- 56 King M.-C. (1992): Breast cancer genes: how many, where and who are they? *Nature Genet.* **2**: 89–90.
- 57 Klijn J. G. M., Berns E. M. J. J., Foekens J. A. (1993): Prognostic factors and response to therapy in breast cancer. *Cancer Surveys* **18**: 165–197.
- 58 Koutselini H., Malliri A., Field J. K., Spandidos D. A. (1991): p53 expression in

cytologic specimens from benign and malignant breast lesions. *Anticancer Res.* **11**: 1415–1420.
- 59 Kreipe H., Alm P., Olsson H., Hauberg M., Fischer L., Parwaresch R. (1993): Prognostic significance of a formalin-resistant nuclear-proliferation antigen in mammary carcinomas as determined by the monoclonal antibody Ki-S1. *Am. J. Pathol.* **142**: 651–657.
- 60 Lane D. P. and Crawford L. V. (1979): T antigen is bound to a host protein in SV40-transformed cells. *Nature* **278**: 261–263.
- 61 Luzi P., Bruni A., Mangiavacchi P., Cevenini G., Marini D., Tosi P. (1994): Ploidy pattern and cell cycle in breast cancer as detected by image analysis and flow cytometry. *Cytometry* **18**: 79–87.
- 62 Lynch H. T., Lemon S. J., Durham C., Tinley S. T., Connolly C., Lynch J. F., Surdam J., Orinion E., Slominski-Caster S., Watson P., Lerman C., Tonin P., Lenoir G., Serova O., Narod S. (1997): A descriptive study of BRCA1 testing and reactions to disclosure of test results. *Cancer* **79**: 2219–2228.
- 63 Malkin D., Li F. P., Strong L. C., Fraumeni J. F., Nelson C. E., Kim D. H., Kassel J., Gryka M. A., Bischoff F. Z., Tainsky M. A., Friend S. H. (1990): Germ-line p53 mutations in a familial syndrome of breast cancer, sarcomas, and other neoplasms. *Science* **250**: 1233–1238.
- 64 Marcus J. N., Watson P., Page D. L., Narod S. A., Lenoir G. M., Tonin P., Linder-Stephenson L., Salerno G., Conway T. A., Lynch H. T. (1996): Hereditary breast cancer. Pathobiology, prognosis, and BRCA1 and BRCA2 gene linkage. *Cancer* **77**: 697–709.
- 65 Matsumara K., Kallioniemi A., Kallioniemi O., Chen L., Smith H. S., Pinkel D., Gray J., Waldman F. M. (1992): Deletion of chromosome 17p loci in breast cancer cells detected by fluorescence in situ hybridization. *Cancer Res.* **52**: 3474–3477.
- 66 McGuire W. L. and Clark G. M. (1992): Prognostic factors and treatment decisions in axillary-node-negative breast cancer. *New Engl. J. Med.* **326**: 1756–1761.
- 67 Meyer J. S. and Province M. A. (1994): S-phase fraction and nuclear size in long term prognosis of patients with breast cancer. *Cancer* **74**: 2287–2299.
- 68 Miki Y., Swensen J., Shattuck-Eidens D., Futreal P. A., Harshman K., Tavtigian S., Liu Q., Cochran C., Bennett L. M., Ding W., Bell R., Rodenthal J., Hussey C., Tran T., McClure M., Frye C., Hattier T., Phelps R., Strano-Haugen A., Katcher H., Yakumo K., Gholami Z., Shaffer D., Stone S., Bayer S., Wray C., Bogden R., Dayananth P., Ward J., Tonin P., Narod S., Bristow P. K., Norris F. H., Helvering L., Morrison P., Rosteck P., Lai M., Barrett C., Lewis C., Neuhausen S., Cannon-Albright L., Goldgar D., Wiseman R., Kamb A., Skolnick M. H. (1994): A strong candidate for the breast and ovarian susceptibility gene BRCA1. *Science* **266**: 66–71.
- 69 Mirecka J., Korabiowska M., Schauer A. (1993): Correlation between the occurrence of Ki-67 antigen and clinical parameters in human breast carcinoma. *Folia Histochemica et Cytobiologica* **31**: 83–86.
- 70 Negrini M., Sabbioni S., Haldar S., Possati L., Castagnoli A., Corallini A., Barbanti-Brodano G., Croce C. M. (1994): Tumor and growth suppression of breast cancer cells by chromosome 17-associated functions. *Cancer Res.* **54**: 1818–1824.
- 71 Noguchi M., Thomas M., Kitagawa H., Kinoshita K., Ohta N., Earashi M., Miyazaki I., Mizukami Y. (1993): The prognostic significance of proliferating cell nuclear antigen in breast cancer: correlation with DNA ploidy, c-erB-2 expression, histopathology, lymph node metastases and patient survival. *Int. J. Oncol.* **2**: 985–989.
- 72 Ogata K., Kurki P., Celis J. E., Nakamura T. E. M. (1987): Monoclonal antibodies to a nuclear protein (PCNA/Cyclin) associated with DNA replication. *Exp. Cell Res.* **168**: 475–486.
- 73 Osborne R. J., Merlo G. R., Mitsudomi T., Venesio T., Liscia D. S., Cappa A. P. M., Chiba I., Takahashi T., Nau M. M., Callahan R., Minna J. D. (1991): Mutations in the p53 gene in primary human breast cancers. *Cancer Res.* **51**: 6194–6198.

- 74 Pandis N., Heim S., Bardi G., Idvall I., Mandahl N., Mitelman F. (1993): Chromosome analysis in 20 breast carcinomas: cytogenetic multiclonality and karyotypic-pathologic correlations. *Genes Chrom. Cancer* **6**: 52–57.
- 75 Pandis N., Idvall I., Bardi G., Jin Y., Gorunova L., Mertens F., Olsson H., Ingvar C., Beroukas K., Mitelman F., Heim S. (1996): Correlation between karyotypic pattern and clinicopathologic features in 125 breast cancer cases. *Int. J. Cancer* **66**: 191–196.
- 76 Pandis N., Jin Y., Gorunova L., Petersson C., Bardi G., Idvall I., Johansson B., Ingvar C., Mandahl N., Mitelman F., Heim S. (1995): Chromosome analysis of 97 primary breast carcinomas: identification of eight karyotypic subgroups. *Genes Chrom. Cancer* **12**: 173–185.
- 77 Poller D. N., Hutchings C. E., Galea M., Bell J. A., Nicholson R. A., Elston C. W., Blamey R. W., Ellis I. O. (1992): p53 protein expression in human breast carcinoma: relationship to expression of epidermal growth factor receptor, c-erB-2 protein overexpression, and oestrogen receptor. *Br. J. Cancer* **66**: 583–588.
- 78 Rodgers C. S., Hill S. M., Hultén M. A. (1984): Cytogenetic analysis in human breast carcinoma. I. Nine cases in the near-diploid range investigated using direct preparations. *Cancer Genet. Cytogenet.* **13**: 95–116.
- 79 Rohen C., Meyer-Bolte K., Bonk U., Ebel T., Staats B., Leuschner E., Gohla G., Caselitz J., Bartnitzke S., Bullerdiek J. (1994): Trisomy 8 and 18 as frequent clonal and single-cell aberrations in 185 primary breast carcinomas. *Cancer Genet. Cytogenet.* **80**: 33–39.
- 80 Rudas M., Gnant M. F. X., Mittlböck M., Neumayer R., Kummer A., Jakesz R., Reiner G., Reiner A. (1994): Thymidine labeling index and Ki-67 growth fraction in breast cancer: comparison and correlation with prognosis. *Breast Cancer Res. Treat.* **32**: 165–175.
- 81 Runnebaum I. B., Nagarajan M., Bowman M., Soto D., Sukumar S. (1991): Mutataions in p53 as potential molecular markers for human breast cancer. *Proc. Natl. Acad. Science* **88**: 10657–10661.
- 82 Sahin A. A., Ro J., Ro J. Y., Blick M. B., El-Naggar A. K., Ordonez N. G., Fritsche H. A., Smith T. L., Hortobagyi G. N., Ayala A. G. (1991): Ki-67 immunostaining in node-negative stage-I/II breast carcinoma. *Cancer* **68**: 549–557.
- 83 Sarli G., Benazzi C., Preziosi R., Marcato P. S. (1995): Assessment of proliferative activity by Anti-PCNA monoclonal antibodies in formalin-fixed, paraffin-embedded samples and correlation with mitotic index. *Vet. Pathol.* **32**: 93–96.
- 84 Schubert E. L., Lee M. K., Mefford H. C., Argonza R. H., Morrow J. E., Hull J., Dann J. L., King M. E. (1997): BRCA2 in American families with four or more cases of breast or ovarian cancer: Recurrent and novel mutations, variable expression, penetrance, and the possibility of families whose cancer is not attributable to BRCA1 or BRCA2. *Am. J. Genet.* **60**: 1031–1040.
- 85 Serova O. M., Mazoyer S., Puget N., Dubois V., Tonin P., Shugart Y. Y., Goldgar D., Narod S. A., Lynch H. T., Lenoir G. M. (1997): Mutations in BRCA1 and BRCA2 in breast cancer families: are there more breast cancer-susceptibility genes? *Am. J. Genet.* **60**: 486–495.
- 86 Shattuck-Eidens D., McClure M., Simard J., Labrie F., Narod S., Couch F., Hoskins K., Weber B., Castilla L., Erdos M., Brody L., Friedman L., Ostermeyer E., Szabo C., King M.-C., Jhanwar S., Offit K., Norton L., Gilewski T., Lubin M., Osborne M., Black D., Boyd M., Steel M., Ingles S., Haile R., Lindblom A., Olsson H., Borg A., Bishop D. T., Solomon E., Radice P., Spatti G., Gayther S., Ponder B., Warren W., Stratton M., Liu Q., Fujimura F., Lewis C., Skolnick M., Goldgar D. E. (1995): A collaborative survey of 80 mutations in the BRCA1 breast and ovarian susceptibility gene – implications for presymptomatic testing and screening. *J. A. M. A.* **273**: 535–541.
- 87 Siddique H., Zou J. P., Rao V. N., Reddy E. S. (1998): The BRCA2 is a histone acetytransferase. *Oncogene* **16**: 2283–2285.
- 88 Sobczak K., Kozlowski P., Napierala M., Czarny J., Kapuscinska M., Losko M., Koziczak M., Jasinsk A., Powierska J.,

Braczkowski R., Breborowski L., Godlewski D., Mackiewicz A., Kryzyzosiak W. (1997): Novel BRCA1 mutations and more frequent intron-20 alteration found among 236 women from Western Poland. *Oncogene* **15**: 1773–1779.

- 89 Sommer S. S., Cunningham J., McGovern R. M., Saitoh S., Schroeder J. J., Wold L. E., Kovach J. S. (1992): Pattern of p53 gene mutataions in breast cancers of Women of midwestern united states. *J. Natl. Cancer Inst.* **84**: 246–252.
- 90 Spyratos F. (1993): DNA content and cell cycle analysis by flow cytometry in clinical samples: application in breast cancer. *Biol. Cell.* **78**: 69–72.
- 91 Stål O., Brisfors A., Carstensen J., Ferraud L., Hatschek T., Nordenskjöld B. (1992): Interrelations between cellular DNA content, S-phase fraction, hormone receptor status and age in primary breast cancer. *Acta Cytologica* **31**: 283–292.
- 92 Stål O., Wingren S., Carstensen J., Rutquist L. E., Skoog L., Klintenberg C., Nordenskjöld B. (1989): Prognostic value of DNA ploidy and S-phase fraction in relation to estrogen receptor content and clinico-pathological variables in primary breast cancer. *Eur. J. Cancer Clin. Oncol.* **25**: 301–309.
- 93 Stanbridge E. J. (1990): Human tumor suppressor genes. *Annu. Rev. Genet.* **24**: 615–657.
- 94 Steinarsdóttir M., Pétursdóttir I., Snorradóttir S., Eyfjörd J. E., Ögmundsdóttir H. M. (1995): Cytogenetic studies of breast carcinomas: different karyotypic profiles detected by direct harvesting and short-term culture. *Genes Chrom. Cancer* **13**: 239–248.
- 95 Tavtigian S. V., Simard J., Rommens J., Couch F., Shattuck-Eidens D., Neuhausen S., Merajver S., Thorlacius S., Offit K., Stoppa-Lyonnet D., Belanger C., Bell R., Berry S., Bogden R., Chen Q., Davis T., Dumont M., Frye C., Hattier T., Jammulapati S., Janecki T., Jiang P., Kehrer R., Leblanc J. F., Mitchell J. T., McAthur-Morrison J., Nguyen K., Peng Y., Samson C., Schroeder M., Snyder S. C., Steele L., Stringfellow M., Stroup C., Swedlund B., Swensen J., Teng D., Thomas A., Tran T., Tran T., Tranchant M., Weaver-Feldhaus J., Wong A. K. C., Shizuya H., Eyfjord J. E., Cannon-Albright L., Labrie F., Skolnick M. H., Weber B., Kamb A., Goldgar D. E. (1996): The complete BRCA2 gene and mutations in chromosome 13q-linked kindreds. *Nature Genet.* **12**: 333–337.
- 96 Thompson A. M., Anderson T. J., Condie A., Prosser J., Chetty U., Carter D. C., Evans H. J., Steel C. M. (1992): p53 allele losses, mutations and expression in breast cancer and their relationship to clinico-pathological parameters. *Int. J. Cancer* **50**: 528–532.
- 97 Thompson F., Emerson J., Dalton W., Yang J.-M., McGee D., Villar H., Knox S., Massey K., Weinstein R., Bhattacharyya A., Trent J. (1993): Clonal chromosome abnormalities in human breast carcinomas I. Twenty-eight cases with primary disease. *Genes Chrom. Cancer* **7**: 185–193.
- 98 Thor A. D., Moore D. H., Edgerton S. M., Kawasaki E. S., Reihsaus E., Lynch H. T., Marcus J. N., Schwartz L., Chen L.-C., Mayall B. H., Smith H. S. (1992): Accumulation of p53 tumor suppressor gene protein: an independent marker of prognosis in breast cancers. *J. Natl. Cancer Inst.* **84**: 845–855.
- 99 Thoralcius S., Børresen A.-L., Eyfjord J. E. (1993): Somatic p53 mutataions in human breast carcinomas in an Icelandic population: a prognostic factor. *Cancer Res.* **53**: 1637–1641.
- 100 Thorlacius S., Jonasdottir O., Eyfjord J. E. (1991): Loss of heterozygosity at selctive sites on chromosomes 13 and 17 in human breast carcinoma. *Anticancer Res.* **11**: 1501–1508.
- 101 Tsuda H. and Hirohashi S. (1995): Identification of multiple breast cancers of multicentric origin by histological observations and distribution of allele loss on chromosome 16q. *Cancer Res.* **55**: 3395–3398.
- 102 Tsuda H., Uei Y., Fukutomi T., Hirohashi S. (1994). Different incidence of loss of heterozygosity on chromosome 16q between intraductal papilloma and intracystic papillary carcinoma of the breast. *Jpn. J. Cancer Res.* **85**: 992–996.

- 103 Umekita Y., Kobayashi K., Saheki T., Yoshida H. (1994a): Nuclear accumulation of p53 correlates with mutations in the p53 gene on archival paraffin-embedded tissues of human breast cancer. *Jpn. J. Cancer Res.* **85**: 825–830.
- 104 Umekita Y., Takasaki T., Yoshida H. (1994b): Expression of p53 protein in benign epithelial hyperplasia, atypical ductal hyperplasia, non-invasive and invasive mammary carcinoma: an immunohistochemical study. *Virchows Archiv* **424**: 491–494.
- 105 Wada T., Shimabukuro T., Matsuyama H., Naito K., Skog S., Tribukait B. (1994): Optimal conditions of fixation for immunohistochemical staining of proliferation cell nuclear antigen in tumour cells and its cell cycle related immunohistochemical expression. *Cell Prol.* **27**: 541–551.
- 106 Waseem N. H. and Lane D. P. (1990): Monoclonal-antibody analysis of the proliferating nuclear antigen (PCNA). Structural conservation and the detection of a nuclar form. *J. Cell. Sci.* **96**: 121–129.
- 107 Weidner N., Moore D. H., Ljung B.-M., Waldman F. M., Goodson, W. H., Mayall B., Chew K., Smith H. S. (1993): Correlation of bromodeoxyuridine (BRDU) labeling of breast carcinoma cells with mitotic figure content and tumor grade. *Am. J. Surg. Pathol.* **17**: 987–994.
- 108 Witzig T. E., Ingle J. N., Cha S. S., Schaid D. J., Tabery R. L., Wold L. E., Grant C., Gonchoroff N. J., Katzman J. A. (1994): DNA ploidy and the percentage of cells in S-phase as prognostic factors for women with lymph node negative breast cancer. *Cancer* **74**: 1752–1761.
- 109 Wolman S. R., Pauley R. J., Mohamed A. N., Dawson P. J., Visscher D. W., Sarkar, F. H. (1991): Genetic markers as prognostic indicators in breast cancer. *Cancer Suppl.* **70**: 1765–1774.
- 110 Wong W. W., Vijayaakumaar S., Eichselbaum R. R. (1992): Prognostic indicators in node-negative early stage brast cancer. *Am. J. Med.* **92**: 539–548.
- 111 Wooster R., Bignell G., Lancaster J., Swift S., Seal S., Mangion J., Collins N., Gregory S., Gumbs C., Micklem G., Barfoot R., Hamoudi R., Patel S., Rice C., Biggs P., Hashim Y., Smith A., Connor F., Arason A., Gudmundsson J., Ficenec D., Keisell D., Ford D., Tonin P., Bishop D. T., Spurr N. K., Ponder B. A., Eeles R., Peto J., Devilee P., Cornelisse C., Lynch H., Narod S., Linoir G., Egilsson V., Barkadottir R. B., Easton D. F., Bentley D. R., Futreal P. A., Ashworth A., Stratton M. R. (1995): Identification of the breast cancer susceptibility gene BRCA2. *Nature* **378**: 789–792.
- 112 Wooster R., Neuhausen S. L., Mangion J., Quirk Y., Ford D., Collins N., Nguyen K., Seal S., Tran T., Averill D., Field P., Marshall G., Narod S., Gilbert M., Lynch H., Feunteun J., Devilee P., Cornelisse C. J., Menko F. H., Daly P. A., Ormiston W., McManus R., Pye C., Lewis C. M., Cannon-Albright L. A., Peto J., Ponder B. A. J., Skolnick M. H., Easton D. F., Goldgar D. E., Stratton M. R. (1994): Localization of a breast cancer susceptibility gene, BRCA2, to chromosome 13q13–13. *Science* **265**: 2088–2090.
- 113 Zafrani B., Gerbault-Seureau M., Mosseri V., Dutrillaux B. (1992): Cytogenetic study of breast cancer: clinicopathologic significance of homogeneously staining regions in 84 patients. *Hum. Pathol.* **23**: 542–547.
- 114 Zhang R., Wiley J., Howard S. P., Meisner L. F., Gould M. (1989): Rare clonal karyotypic variants in primary cultures of human breast carcinoma cells. *Cancer Res.* **49**: 444–449.

References 2.3.2

- 1 William L., Donegan M. D. (1992): Prognostic Factors, Stage and Receptor Status in Breast Cancer. *Cancer Suppl.* **70/6**.
- 2 Bässler R., Schnürch H.-G. (1994): Standards der pathohistological Aufarbeitung des Mammakarzinoms (Standards of Pathohistological Reappraisal in Breast Cancer). *Gynäkologe* **27**: 23–36.
- 3 Nealon T. F., Nkongho A., Grossi C., Gillooley J. (1979): Pathological Identification of Poor Prognosis Stage I ($T_1N_0M_0$) Cancer of the Breast. *Ann. Surg.* **190**: 129–132.

- 4 Dutrillaux B., Gerbault-Seureau M., Remvikos Y., Zafrani B., Prieur M. (1991): Breast Cancer genetic evolution: I. Data from cytogenetics and DNA-Content. *Breast Cancer Res. Treat* 19: 245–255.
- 5 Harada Y., Katagiri T., Ito I., Akiyama F., Sakamoto G., Kasumi F., Nakamura Y., Emi M. (1994): Genetic Studies of 457 Breast Cancers. Clinicopathologic Parameters Compared with Genetic Alterations. *Cancer* 74: 2281–2286.
- 6 Wolman, S. R., Pauley, R. J., Mohamed, A. N., Dawson, P. J., Visscher, D. W., Sarkar, F. H., Genetic Markers as Prognostic Factors in Breast Cancer. *Cancer* 70: 1765–1774.
- 7 Hedley D. W., Clark G. M., Cornelisse C. J., Killander D., Kute T., Merkel D. (1993): Consensus Review of the Clinical Utility of DNA Cytometry in Carcinoma of the Breast. *Cytometry* 14: 482–485.
- 8 Kunze W.-P., Willeboordse S., Ambrosius C.-A., Peka B., Zender-Reinhardt C., Velehorschi V., Bollmann R., Brightman I. (1994): Immunocytophotometric controlled flow-cytophotometry for DNA in Breast Cancer. *Int. J. Surg. Pathol.* 2: 72.
- 9 Witzig T. E., Ingle J. N., Cha S. S., Schaid D. J., Tabery R. L., Wold L. E., Grant C., Gonchoroff N. J., Katzmann J. A. (1994): DNA Ploidy and the Percentage of Cells in S-Phase as Prognostic Factors for Women with Lymph Node Negative Breast Cancer. *Cancer* 74: 1752–1761.
- 10 Böcking A., Chatelain R., Biesterfeld S., Noll E., Biesterfeld D., Wohltmann D., Goecke C. (1989): DNA Grading of Malignancy in Breast Cancer. Prognostic Validity, Reproducibility and Comparison with other Classifications. *Analyt. Quant. Cytol. Histol.* 11: 73–80.
- 11 Fallenius A. G., Auer G. U., Carstensen J. M. (1988): Prognostic Significance of DNA Measurements in 409 Consecutive Breast Cancer Patients. *Cancer* 62: 331–341.
- 12 Marchevsky A. M., Bartels P. H. (1994): *Image Analysis. A Primer for Pathologists.* Raven Press New York.
- 13 Böcking A., Giroud F., Reith A. (1995): Consensus Report of the ESACP task force on Standardization of Diagnostic DNA Image Cytometry. *Analyt. Cell. Pathol.* 8: 67–74.
- 14 Böcking A., Füzesi L., Striepecke E. (1993): Indikationen und tumorzytogenetische Grundlagen der diagnostischen DNA-Zytometrie (Indications and Tumour-Cytogenetic foundations of diagnostic DNA cytometry) *Verh. Dtsch. Ges. Zyt.* 18: 70–82.
- 15 Biesterfeld S., Gerres K., Fischer-Wein G., Böcking A. (1994): Polyploidy in neoplastic tissues. *J. Clin. Pathol.* 47: 38–42.
- 16 Honnef D. (1997): Computergestützte bildanalytische DNA-Zytometrie von invasiven Mammakarzinomen. Klinische Bedeutung einer objektiven Histogrammtypisierung. (Static DNA-cytometry of mammacarcinonmas. Clinical meaning of an objective classification of the histogrammtype) Inaugural Dissertation, Münster.
- 17 Verderio P., Valentina C., Boracchi P., Gambacorta M., Giardini R. (1996): Evaluation of the reproducibility of Auer's classification of DNA histogram in breast carcinoma. *Analyt. Cell. Pathol.* 11: 97–106.
- 18 Kindermann D., Mallmann P., Stark G. B., Hültenschmidt D., Bischoff M., Sasse C., Schmitz C., Knapp M., Pfeifer U. (1992): Histopathologische und bildzytometrische (statische DNS-Zytometrie) Kriterien in Hinblick auf die prognostischen Aussagewerte bei 115 Patientinnen mit Mammakarzinom unter besonderer Berücksichtigung des "Frührezidiv-Risikos" (Histopathological and image-cytometric (static DNA-cytometry) Criteria with Reference to Prognostic Value in 115 Patients with Breast Cancer, with particular reference to the "Early Relapse Risk"). *Pathologe* 13: 25–38.
- 19 Silverstein J., Lewinsky B. S., Waismann J. R., Gierson E. D., Colburn W. J., Senofsky G. M., Gamagami P. (1994): Infiltrating Lobular Carcinoma. Is it different from infiltrating Ductal Carcinoma? *Cancer* 73: 1673–1677.
- 20 Weidner N., Semple J. P. (1992): Pleomorphic Variant of Invasive Lobular Carcinoma in Breast. *Hum. Pathol.* 23: 1167–1171.

- 21 Weidner N., Bennington J. (1994): Correlation of DNA Ploidy, DNA S-Phase, and Nuclear Diameter with Classical and Pleomorphic Variants of Invasive Carcinoma, 1994 Annual Meeting, United States and Canadian Academy of Pathology.
- 22 Schenck U., Burger G. †, Jütting U., Gais P., Rodenacker K., Schenck U. B., Eiermann P. (1994): Cell Image Morphology and Hormone Receptor Analysis in Breast Carcinoma. In: Wied G. L., Bartels P. H., Rosenthal D. L., Schenck U.: Compendium on the Computerized Cytology and Histology Laboratory. *Tutorials of Cytology*, Chicago, Illinois, USA, 211–233.
- 23 McGuire W. L., Tandon A. K., Allred D. C., Chamness G. C., Ravdin P. M., Clark G. M. (1992): Prognosis and Treatment Decisions in Patients with Breast Cancer without Axillary Node Involvement. *Cancer* **70**: 1775–1781.
- 24 Silverstein M. J., Gierson E. D., Waismann J. R., Senofsky G. M., Colburn W. J., Gamagani P. (1994): Axillary Lymph Node Dissection for T1a Breast Carcinoma. Is it indicated? *Cancer* **73**: 664–667.
- 25 Wazer D. E., Erban J. K., Robert N. J., Smith T. J., Marchant D. J., Schmid C., DiPetrillo G. T., Schmidt-Ullrich R. (1994): Breast Conservation in Elderly Women for Clinically Negative Axillary Lymph Nodes without Axillary Dissection. *Cancer* **74**: 878–883.

References 2.3.3

- 1 Sneige N., Staerkel G. A., Caraway N. P., Fanning T. V., Katz R. L. (1994): A plea for uniform terminology and reporting of breast fine needle aspirates. *Acta Cytol.*: 971–972.
- 2 Giard R. W. M.; Hermans J. (1992): The value of aspiration cytological examination of the breast. *Cancer* **69**: 2104–2110.
- 3 Ballo M. S., Sneige N. (1996): Can core needle biopsy replace fine-needle aspiration cytology in the diagnosis of palpable breast carcinoma? *Cancer* **78**: 773–777.
- 4 Hees K., Bollmann R. (1997): Validity of DNA-image-cytometry in cytologically doubtful aspirates of the breast. *Pathol. Res. Pract.* **193**: 123.
- 5 Locker A. P., Dilks B., Gilmour A., Ellis I. O., Elston C. Q., Blamey R. W. (1990): Aspiration cytological diagnosis of breast lesions by nuclear DNA content and morphometry. *Br. J. Surg.* **77**: 707.
- 6 Martelli G., Daidone M. G., Mastore M., Gabrielli G. M., Galante E., Pilotti S., Silvestrini R., (1993): Combined analysis of ploidy and cell kinetics on fine-needle aspirates from breast tumors. *Cancer* **71**: 2522–2527.
- 7 Seigneurin D., Louis J., Villoud M.-C. (1994): The value of DNA image cytometry for the cytological diagnosis of well-differentiated breast carcinomas and benign lesions. *Analyt. Cell. Pathol.* **7**: 115–125.
- 8 Carpenter R., Gibbs N., Matthews J., Cooke T. (1987): Importance of cellular DNA content in pre-malignant breast disease and pre-invasive carcinoma of the female breast. *Br. J. Surg.*: 905–906.
- 9 Spyratos F., Briffod M., Tubiana-Hulin M., Andrieu C., Mayras C., Pallud C., Lasry S., Rouesse J. (1992):Sequential cytopunctures during preoperative chemotherapy for primary breast carcinoma. *Cancer* **69**: 470–475.

References 2.3.4

- 1 Miller B. A., Feuer E. J., Hankey B. F. (1993): Recent incidence trends for breast cancer in women and the relevance of early detection: an update. *Ca. Cancer. J. Clin.* **43**: 27–41.
- 2 Early Breast Cancer Trialists' Collaborative Group (1992): Systemic treatment of early breast cancer by hormonal, cytotoxic, or immune therapy. *The Lancet* **339**: 1–15, 71–85.
- 3 Harris J. R., Morrow M., Bonadonna G. (1993): Cancer of the Breast. In: DeVita V. T., Hellman S., Rosenberg S. A. (editor): *Cancer: Principles and Practice of Oncology*. J. B. Lippincot Company, Philadelphia, 1264–1332.
- 4 Goldhirsch A., Castiglione M., Gelber R. D. (1992): A single perioperative adjuvant chemotherapy course for node negative

breast cancer: five-year results of trial V. International Breast Cancer Study Group (formerly Ludwig Group). *Monogr. Natl. Cancer Inst.* **11**: 89–96.
- 5 Rosen P. P., Oberman H. A. (1993): Tumors of the mammary gland. Rosai J.: *Atlas of tumor pathology.* Armed Forces Institute of Pathology, Washington D. C.
- 6 World Health Organization (1981): *Histologic typing of breast tumours.* International histological classification of tumours. World Health Organization, Geneva.
- 7 National Institutes of Health (1991): NIH consensus conference. Treatment of early-stage breast cancer. *J. Am. Med. Ass.* **265**: 391–395.
- 8 Fisher E. R., Redmond C., Fisher B. (1992): Prognostic factors in NSABP studies of women with node negative breast cancer. National Surgical Adjuvant Breast and Bowel Project [Prior annotation incorrect]. *Monogr. Natl. Cancer. Inst.* **11**: 151–158.
- 9 Stierer M., Rosen H., Weber R. (1992): Nuclear pleomorphism, a strong prognostic factor in axillary node negative small invasive breast cancer. *Breast Cancer Res. Treat.* **20**: 109–116.
- 10 Bloom H. J. G., Richardson W. W. (1957): Histological grading and prognosis in breast cancer: a study of 1409 cases of which 359 have been followed for 15 years. *Br. J. Cancer* **11**: 359–377.
- 11 Elston C. W., Ellis I. O. (1991): Pathological prognostic factors in breast cancer. I. The value of histological grade in breast cancer: experience from a large study with long-term follow-up. *Histopathol.* **19**: 403–410.
- 12 Frierson H. J., Wolber R. A., Berean K. W., Franquemont D. W., Gaffey M. J., Boyd J. C., Wilbur D. C. (1995): Interobserver reproducibility of the Nottingham modification of the Bloom and Richardson histologic grading scheme for infiltrating ductal carcinoma. *Am. J. Clin. Pathol.* **103**: 195–198.
- 13 Harvey J. M., de Klerk N. H., Sterrett G. F. (1992): Histological grading in breast cancer: interobserver agreement, and relation to other prognostic factors including ploidy. *Pathology* **24**: 63–68.
- 14 Delides G. S., Garas G., Georgouli G., Jiortziotis D., Lecca J., Liva T., Elemenoglou J. (1982): Intralaboratory variations in the grading of breast carcinoma. *Arch. Pathol. Lab. Med.* **106**: 126–128.
- 15 Robbins P., Pinder S., de Klerk N., Dawkins H., Harvey J., Sterrett G., Ellis I., Elston C. (1995): Histological grading of breast carcinoma: A study of interobserver agreement. *Hum. Pathol.* **26**: 873–879.
- 16 Dalton L. W., Page D. L., Dupont W. D. (1994): Histologic grading of breast carcinoma: A reproducibility study. *Cancer* **73**: 2765–2770.
- 17 Aubele M., Auer G., Voss A., Falkmer U., Rutquist L. E., Hofler H. (1995): Different risk groups in node-negative breast cancer: prognostic value of cytophotometrically assessed DNA, morphometry and texture. *Int. J. Cancer* **63**: 7–12.
- 18 Dawson A. E., Cibas E. S., Bacus J. W., Weinberg D. S. (1993): Chromatin texture measurement by Markovian analysis. Use of nuclear models to define and select texture features. *Anal. Quant. Cytol. Histol.* **15**: 227–235.
- 19 Komitowski D. D., Hart M. M., Janson C. P. (1993): Chromatin organization and breast cancer prognosis. Two-dimensional and three-dimensional image analysis. *Cancer* **72**: 1239–1246.
- 20 Breiman L., Friedman J. H., Olshen R. A., Stone C. J. (1984): *Classification and Regression Trees.* Wadsworth International, Belmont, California. 1–358.
- 21 Albert R., Müller J. G., Kristen P., Kneitz S., Harms H. (1996): A new nuclear grading method on tissue sections by means of digital image analysis with prognostic significance for node negative breast cancer patients. *Cytometry* **24**: 140–150.
- 22 Harms H., Aus H. M. (1987): Tissue image segmentation with multicolor, multifocal algorithms. In: Devijver P. A., Kittler J.: *Pattern Recognition: Theory and Applications.* Springer-Verlag, Berlin, 519–528.
- 23 Castleman K. R. (1979): *Digital image processing.* Oppenheim AV: Prentice-Hall Signal Processing Series. Prentice-Hall, Inc., Englewood Cliffs, New Jersey. 357–360.

- 24 Harms H., Gunzer U., Aus H. M. (1986): Combined local colour and texture analysis of stained cells. *Computer Vision, Graphics, and Image Processing* **33**: 364–376.
- 25 CART (1985): *User Documentation*, Version 1.1. California Statistical Software, Inc., Lafayette, California.
- 26 Lachenbruch P. A. (1975): *Discriminant analysis*. Hafner Press, New York.
- 27 Leitner S. P., Swern A. S., Weinberger D., Duncan L. J., Hutter R. V. (1995): Predictors of recurrence for patients with small (one centimeter or less) localized breast cancer (T1a,b N0 M0). *Cancer* **76**: 2266–2274.
- 28 Nordén T., Lindgren A., Bergström R., Holmberg L. (1994): Defining a high mortality risk group among women with primary breast cancer. *Br. J. Cancer* **69**: 520–524.
- 29 Rosen P. P., Groshen S., Kinne D. W., Norton L. (1993): Factors influencing prognosis in node-negative breast carcinoma: analysis of 767 T1N0M0/T2N0M0 patients with long-term follow-up. *J. Clin. Oncol.* **11**: 2090–2100.

References 2.3.5

- 1 Hansemann D. (1890): Über asymmetrische Zellteilung in Epithelkrebsen und deren biologische Bedeutung. *Virchows Arch (A)* **119**: 299–326.
- 2 Greenhough R. B. (1925): Varying degrees of malignancy in cancer of the breast. *J. Cancer Res.* **9**: 452–463.
- 3 Bloom H. J. G., Richardson W. W. (1957): Histologic grading and prognosis in breast cancer. A study of 1409 cases of which 359 have been followed for 15 years. *Brit. J. Cancer* **11**: 359.
- 4 Frierson H. F., Wolber R. A., Berean K. W., Franquemont D. W., Gaffey M. J., Boyd J. C., Wilbur D. C. (1995): Interobserver reproducibility of the Nottingham modification of the Bloom and Richardson histologic grading scheme for infiltrating ductal carcinoma. *Am. J. Clin. Pathol.* **103**: 195–198.
- 5 Black M. M., Opler S. R., Speer S. D. (1955): Survival in breast cancer cases in relation to structure of the primary tumor and regional lymph nodes. *Surg. Gynecol. Obstet.* **100**: 543–551.
- 6 Scarff R. W., Torloni H. (1968): *Histological typing of breast tumours* (international histological classification of tumours, no 2). World Health Organization, Geneva.
- 7 Delides G. S., Garas G., Georgouli G. (1982): Intralaboratory variations in the grading of breast carcinoma. *Arch Path. Lab. Med.* **106**: 126–128.
- 8 Haybittle J. L., Blamey R. W., Elston C. W. (1982): A prognostic index in primary breast cancer. *Br. J. Cancer* **45**: 361–366.
- 9 Böcking A. (1993): *Zytogenetische Grundlagen der diagnostischen DNA-Zytometrie.* 29. Symposium der International Academy of Pathology, Bonn.
- 10 Mellin W. (1990): Cytophotometry in tumor pathology. A critical review of methods and applications, and some results of DNA analysis. *Path. Res. Pract.* **186**: 37–62.
- 11 Auer G., Caspersson T. O., Wallgren A. S. (1980): DNA content and survival in mammary carcinoma. *Anal. Quant. Cytol. Histol.* **2/3**: 161–165.
- 12 Haroske G., Kunze K. D., Theissig F. (1991): Prognostic significance of image cytometry DNA parameters in tissue sections from breast and gastric cancer. *Anal. Cell. Path.* **3**: 11–24.
- 13 Schapers R. F. M., Ploem-Zaaijer J. J., Pauwels R. P. E., Smeets A. W. G. B., Brandt P. A. van den, Tanke H. J., Mosman F. T. (1993): Image cytometric DNA analysis in transitional cell carcinoma of the bladder. *Cancer* **72**: 182–189
- 14 Coulsen P. B., Thornthwaite J. T., Woolley TW, Sugarbaker EV, Seckinger D (1984): Prognostic indicators including histogram type, receptor content, and staging related to human breast cancer patient survival. *Cancer Res.* **44**: 4187–4196.
- 15 Fallenius G., Auer G., Carstensen J. M. (1988): Prognostic significance of DNA measurements in 409 consecutive breast cancer patients. *Cancer* **62**: 331–341.
- 16 Kallioniemi O. P., Blanco G., Alavaikko M., Hietanen T., Mattila J., Lauslahti K., Lehtinen M., Koivula T. (1988): Improving the prognostic value of DNA flow cytometry

in breast cancer by combining DNA index and S-phase fraction. *Cancer* **62**: 183–2190.
- 17 Noguchi M., Koyasaki N., Ohta N., Kitagawa H., Earashi M., Thomas M., Miyazaki I., Mizukami Y. (1993): Internal mammary nodal status is a more reliable prognostic factor than DNA ploidy and c-erb B-2 expression in patients with breast cancer. *Arch Surg.* **128**: 242–246.
- 18 Toikkanen S., Joensuu H., Klemi P. (1990): Nuclear DNA content as a prognostic factor in T1–2 N0 breast cancer. *Am. J. Clin. Path.* **93**: 471–479.
- 19 Owainati A. A. R., Robins R. A., Hinton C., Ellis I. O., Dowle C. S., Ferry B., Elston C. W., Blamey R. W., Baldwin R. W. (1987): Tumour aneuploidy, prognostic parameters and survival in primary breast cancer. *Br. J. Cancer* **55**: 449–454.
- 20 Hitchcock A., Ellis I. O., Robertson J. F. R., Gilmour A., Bell J., Elston C. W., Blamey R. W. (1989): An observation of DNA ploidy, histological grade, and immunoreactivity for tumour-related antigens in primary and metastatic breast carcinoma. *J. Path.* **159**: 129–134.
- 21 Böcking A., Adler C. P., Common H. H., Hilgarth M., Auffermann W. (1984): Algorithm for a DNA-cytophotometric diagnosis and grading of malignancy. *Anal. Quant. Cytol. Histol.* **6**: 1–8.
- 22 Böcking A. (1990): DNA-Zytometrie und Automation in der klinischen Diagnostik. *Beitr. Onkol.* **38**: 298–347.
- 23 Ghali V. S., Liau S., Teplitz K., Prudente R. (1992): A comparative study of DNA ploidy in 115 fresh-frozen breast carcinomas by image analysis versus cytometry. *Cancer* **70**: 2668–2672.
- 24 Longin A., Fontaniere B., Pinzani V., Catimel G., Souchier C., Clavel M., Chauvin F. (1992): An image cytometric DNA analysis in breast neoplasms. Parameters of DNA-aneuploidy an their relationship with conventional prognostic factors. *Path. Res. Pract.* **188**: 466–472.
- 25 Böcking A., Chatelain R. (1988): Diagnostic and prognostic value of DNA cytometry in gynecological cytology. *Anal. Quant. Cytol. Histol.* **11**: 177–186.
- 26 Kindermann D., Mallmann P., Stark G. B., Hülenschmidt D., Bischoff M., Sasse C. M., Schmidt C., Knapp M., Pfeifer U. (1992): Histopathologische und bildzytometrische (statistische DNS-Zytometrie) Kriterien in Hinblick auf die prognostischen Aussagewerte bei 115 Patientinnen mit Mammacarcinom unter besonderer Berücksichtigung des Frührezidivrisikos. *Pathologie* **13**: 25–38.
- 27 Susnik B., Poulin N., Phillips D., LeRiche J., Palcic B. (1995): Comparison of DNA measurement performed by flow and image cytometry of embedded breast tissue sections. *Anal. Quant. Cytol. Histol.* **17**: 163–171.
- 28 Lee A. K. C., Dugan J., Hamilton W. M., Cook L., Heatley G. Kamat B., Silverman M. L. (1991): Quantitative DNA analysis in breast carcinomas: A comparison between image analysis and flow cytometry. *Mod. Pathol.* **4/2**: 178–182.
- 29 Crissman J. D., Visscher D. W., Kubus J. (1990): Image cytophotometric DNA analysis of atypical hyperplasias and intraductal carcinomas of the breast. *Arch Path. Lab. Med.* **114**: 1249–1253.
- 30 Christov K., Milev A., Todorov V. (1989): DNA aneuploidy and cell proliferation in breast tumors. *Cancer* **64**: 673–679.
- 31 Winter K. (1994): *Geburtsh. u. Frauenheilk.* **54**: 291–294.
- 32 Schlotter C.M, Bosse U., Vogt U., Bosse A. (1996): DNA Image Cytometrie (ICM), Onkogene und Prognosefaktoren bei primären Mammakarzinomen. *Arch Gynecol. Obstet.* **258/1**: 94.
- 33 Schlotter C. M., Bosse U., Bosse A., Vogt U., Brandt B. (1996): DNA Image Cytometrie und Onkogenbestimmungen bei Mammakarzinom. *Verh. Dtsch. Ges. Path.* **80**: 603.
- 34 Schlotter C. M., Bosse U., Bosse A., Vogt U., Brandt B., Brüning Th. (1996): DNA Image Cytometrie (ICM), Oncogenes and prognostic factors in breast cancer. *European Journal of Cancer A (Suppl. 2)* **32**: 56.
- 35 Beerman H., Kluin P. M., Hermans J., Velde C. J. H. van de, Cornelisse C. J. (1990): Prognostic significance of DNA ploidy in a series of 690 primary breast patients. *Int. J. Cancer* **45**: 34–39.

- 36 Brüning T., Vogt U., Schlotter C. M., Bosse U. (1996): A comparative study of DNA content and proliferation (S-SG2M-phase, Ki 67) measured by flow cytometry and image analysis in breast cancer. Annual breast cancer meeting, San Antonio TX, USA.
- 37 Rosen A. von, Rutqvist L. E., Carstensen J., Fallenius A., Skoog L., Auer G. (1989): Prognostic value of nuclear DNA content in breast cancer in relation to tumor size, nodal status, and estrogen-receptor content. *Breast Cancer Res. Treat.* **13**: 23–32.
- 38 Killeen J. L., Namiki H. (1991): DNA Analysis of ductal carcinoma in situ of the breast. *Cancer* **68**: 2602–2607.
- 39 Mittra I., MacRae K. D. (1991): A meta-analysis of reported correlations between prognostic factors in breast cancer: Does axillary lymph node metastasis represent biology or chronology? *Eur. J. Cancer* **27/12**: 1574–1583.
- 40 Berryman I. L., Harvey J. M., Sterrett G. F., Papadimitriou J. M. (1987): The nuclear DNA content of human breast carcinoma. *Anal. Quant. Cytol. Histol.* **9/5**: 429–434.
- 41 Hedley D. W., Rugg C. A., Gelber R. D. (1987): Association of DNA index and S-phase fraction with prognosis of nodes positive early breast cancer. *Cancer Res.* **47**: 4729–4735.
- 42 Coumbos A., Kühn W., Fleige B., Weitzel H. K. (1993): DNA-Analyse und Karyometrie als Prognosefaktor beim Mammacarcinom. Vortrag auf der 13. Wissenschaftlichen Tagung der Deutschen Gesellschaft für Senologie. Berlin, 1993.
- 43 Sharma S., Mishra M. C., Kapur B. M.L, Verma K., Nath I. (1991): The prognostic significance of ploidy analysis in operable breast cancer. *Cancer* **68**: 2612–2616.
- 44 Olszweski W., Darzynkiewicz Z., Rosen P. P., Schwartz M. K., Melamed M. R. (1981): Flow cytometry of breast carcinoma: 1. Relation of DNA ploidy level to histology and estrogen-receptor. *Cancer* **48**: 980–984.
- 45 Raju U., Zarbo R. J., Kubus J., Schultz D. S. (1993): The histologic spectrum of apocrine breast proliferations: A comparative study of morphology and DNA content by image analysis. *Hum. Pathol.* **24**: 173–181.
- 46 Moran R. E., Black M. M., Alpert L., Straus M. J. (1984): Correlation of cell-cycle kinetics, hormon receptors, histopathology and nodal status in human breast cancer. *Cancer* **54**: 1586–1590.
- 47 Elston C. W. (1987): Grading of invasive carcinoma of the breast. In Page D. L. and Anderson T. J.: *Diagnostic histopathology of the breast*, 300–311, Churchill Livingstone, Edingburgh, London, Melbourne and New York.
- 48 Davey D. D., Banks E. R., Jennings D., Powell D. (1993): Comparison of nuclear grade and DNA cytometry in breast carcinoma aspirates to histologic grade in excised cancer. *Am. J. Clin. Path.* **99**: 708–713.
- 49 Arnerlöv C., Emdin S. O., Roos G., Angström T., Bjersing L., Änquist K. A., Jonsson H (1990): Static and flow cytometric DNA analysis compared to histologic prognostic factors in a cohort of stage T2 breast cancer. *Eur. J. of Surg. Oncol.* **16**: 200–208.
- 50 Dhingra K., Hittelman W. N., Hortobagyi G. N. (1995): Genetic changes in breast cancer – consequences for therapy? *Gene* **159**: 59–63.
- 51 Azavedo E., Fallenius A., Svane G., Auer G. (1990): Nuclear DNA content, histological grade, and clinical course in patients with nonpalpable mammographically detected breast adenocarcinoma. *Am. J. Clin. Oncol.* (CCT) **13/1**: 23–27.
- 52 Keyhani-Rofagha S., O'Toole R. V., Farrar W. B., Sickle-Santanello B., DeCenzo J., Young D. (1990): Is DNA ploidy an independent prognostic indicator in infiltrative node-negative breast adenocarcinoma? *Cancer* **65**: 1577–1582.
- 53 McGuire W. L., Tandon A. K., Allred C., Chamness G. C., Clark G. M. (1990): How to use prognostic factors in axillary node-negative breast cancer patients. *J. Natl. Cancer Inst.* **82**: 1006–1015.
- 54 Gasparini G., Pozza F., Harris A. L. (1993): Evaluating the potential usefulness of new prognostic and predictive indicators

in node-negative breast cancer patients. *J. Natl. Cancer. Inst.* **85**: 1206–1219.
- 55 Harris J. R., Morrow M., Bonadonna G. (1993): Cancer of the breast. In: DeVita VT, Hellman S, Rosenberg SA (eds.), *Cancer: Principles and practice of oncology*, 4th ed., 1264–1332, Lippincott, Philadelphia, PA.
- 56 Atkin N. B. (1964): Nuclear size in carcinoma of the cervix: its relation to DNA content and to prognosis. *Cancer* **17**: 1391–1399.
- 57 Fossa S. D., Marton P. F., Knudsen O. S., Kaalhus O., Bormer O., Vaage S. (1982): Nuclear Feulgen DNA content and nuclear size in human breast cancer. *Hum. Pathol.* **13**: 626–630.
- 58 Horsfall D. J., Tilley W. D., Orell S. R., Marshal V. R., Cant E. L. M. (1986): Relationship between ploidy and steroid hormon receptors in primary invasive breast cancer. *Br. J. Cancer* **53**: 23–28.
- 59 Rondez R., Yoshizaki C., Pirozynski W. (1990): Determination of nuclear DNA content and hormone receptors in breast cancer by the CAS 100 Cell Analysis System as related to morphologic grade and biochemical results. *Anal. Quant. Cytol. Histol.* **13/4**: 233–245.

References 2.3.6

- 1 Schwab et al. (1983): *Nature* **305**: 245–248.
- 2 Escot et al. (1983): *PNAS* **83**: 4834–4838.
- 3 Berns et al. (1995): *Gene* **159**: 11–18.
- 4 Klijn et al. (1993): *Cancer Treat. Rev.* **19**: 45–63.
- 5 Slamon et al. (1987): *Science* **235**: 177–182.
- 6 Slamon et al. (1989): *Science* **244**: 707–712.
- 7 Ro et al. (1989): *Cancer Res.* **49**: 6941–6944.
- 8 Paterson et al. (1991): *Cancer Res.* **51**: 556–567.
- 9 Clark et al. (1991): *Cancer Res.* **51**: 944–948.
- 10 Gusterson et al. (1992): *J. Clin. Oncol.* **10**: 1049–1056.
- 11 Paik et al. (1990): *J. Clin. Oncol.* **8**: 103–112.
- 12 Allred et al. (1990): *J. Natl. Cancer Inst.* **82**: 1006–1015.
- 13 Muss et al. (1994): *N. Engl. J. Med.* **330**: 1260–1266.
- 14 Wright et al. (1992): *Br. J. Cancer* **65/1**: 118–121.
- 15 Brandt et al. (1995): *Gene* **159**: 35–42.
- 16 Vogt (1994): *TW Gynäkologie* **7**: 355–358.
- 17 Brandt et al. (1995): *Gene* **159**: 29–34.
- 18 Vogt (1994): Methods in DNA Amplifications, Plenum Press, 55–63.
- 19 Dawson et al. (1990): *Am. J. Pathol.* **136**: 1115–1124.
- 20 Sinn et al. (1997): *Der Pathologe* **18**: 19–26.
- 21 Schenk et al. (1994): *Computerized Cytology a. Histology Lab.*, ToC, 211–233.

References Appendices 2.1.2

Appendix 1

- 1 Press M. F., Greene G. L. (1987): Recent developments in the use of anti-receptor antibodies to study steroid hormone receptors. In: Clark C. R. (editor): *Steroid Hormone Receptors: Their Intracellular Localisation.* Ellis Horwood.
- 2 Gaskell D. J. et al. (1989): Relation between immunocytochemical estimation of oestrogen receptor in elderly patients with primary breast cancer and response to tamoxifen. *Lancet* **I**: 1044–1046.
- 3 Andersen J., Poulsen H. S. (1989): Immunohistochemical oestrogen receptor determination in paraffin-embedded tissue: prediction of response to hormonal treatment in advanced breast cancer. *Cancer* **64**: 1901–1908.

Appendix 2

- 1 Frazier T. C., Wong R. W., Rose D. (1989): Implications of accurate pathologic margins in the treatment of primary breast cancer. *Arch. Surg.* **124**: 37–38.
- 2 Anderson T. J. (1989): Breast cancer screening: princioles and pacticalities for histopathologists. In: McSween A. P. R. (editor): Churchill Livingstone, *Recent Advances in Histopathology* **14**: 43–61.
- 3 Carter D. (1986): Margins of "lumpec-

tomy" for breast cancer. *Human Pathol.* **17**: 303.
- 4 Connolly J. L., Schnitt S. J. (1988): Evaluation of breast biopsy specimens, patients considered for treatment, conservative surgery and radiation therapy for early breast cancer. In: Rosen P. P., Fechner R. E. (editors): *Pathology Annual*. Appleton and Lange, Norwalk, Connecticut, 1–24.
- 5 Davies J. D., Armstrong J. S., Paterson D. A. (1989): Marking planes of surgical excision on specimens with a mixture of India ink and acetone. *J. Clin. Pathol.* **42**: 893.
- 6 Chan K. W., Lui I, Chung W. B. (1989): Marking planes of surgical excision on specimens with a mixture of India ink and acetone. *J. Clin. Pathol.* **42**: 893.
- 7 Armstrong J. S., Weizwieg I. P., Davies J. D. (1990): Differential marking of excision planes in screened breast lesions by organically coloured gelatins. *J. Clin. Pathol.* **43**: 604–607.
- 8 Harris M. D. (1990): Tipp-ex: a novel marker for resection margins. *J. Pathol.* **160**: 168A.
- 9 Birch P. J., Jeffrey M. J., Andrews M. I. J. (1990): *J. Clin. Pathol.* **43**: 608–609.
- 10 Paterson D. A., Davis J. D. (1988): Marking the planes of surgical excision on breast biopsy specimens: use of artists' pigments suspended in acetone. *J. Clin. Pathol.* **41**: 1013–1016.

Appendix 3

- 1 Bartelink H., Borger J. H., van Dongen J. A. et al. (1988): The impact of tumour size and histology on local conrol after breast-conserving therapy. *Radiotherapy & Oncology* **11**: 297–303.
- 2 Calle R., Vilcoq J., Zafrani B. et al. (1986): Local control and survival of breast cancer treated by limited surgery followed by irradiation. *Int. J. Radiation Oncol. Biol. Phys.* **12**: 873–878.
- 3 Fentiman I. S., Fagg N., Millis N., Hayward J. L. (1986): In situ carcinoma of the breast: implications of disease pattern and treatment. *Eur. J. Surg. Oncol.* **12**: 261–266.
- 4 Fourquet A., Campana F., Zafrani B. et al. (1988): Prognostic factors of breast recurrence in the conservative management of early breast cancer. A 25 year follow-up. *Int. J. Radiation Oncol. Biol. Phys.* **17**: 719–725.
- 5 Holland R., Connolly J. L., Gelman R. et al. (1990): The presence of an extensive intraduct component following a limited excision correlates with prominent residual disease in the remainder of the breast. *J. Clin. Oncol.* **8**: 113–118.
- 6 Jacquemier J., Kurtz J. M., Amalric R. et al. (1990): An assessment of extensive intraductal component as a risk factor for local recurrence after breast-conserving therapy. *Br. J. Cancer* **6**: 873–876.
- 7 Lindley R., Bulman A., Parsons P. et al. (1989): Histologic features predictive of an increased risk of early local recurrence after treatment of breast cancer by local tumour excision and radical radiotherapy. *Surgery* **105**: 13–20.
- 8 Lagios M. D., Westdahl P. R., Margolin F. R. et al. (1982): Duct carcinoma in situ. Relationship of extent of non-invasive disease to the frequency of occult invasion, multicentricity, lymph node metastases, and short-term treatment failures. *Cancer* **63**: 618–624.
- 9 Lagios M. D., Margolin F. R., Westdahl P. R. (1989): Mammographically detected duct carcinoma in situ. Frequency of local recurrence following tylectomy and prognostic effect of nuclear grade on local recurrence. *Cancer* **63**: 618–624.
- 10 Schnitt S. J., Connolly J. L., Harris J. R. et al. (1984): Pathologic predictions of early local recurrence in stage I and II breast cancer treated by primary radiation therapy. *Cancer* **53**: 1049–1057.
- 11 Schnitt S. J., Connolly J. L., Khettry U. et al. (1984): Pathologic findings on re-excision of the primary site in breast cancer patients considered for treatment by primary radiation therapy. *Cancer* **59**: 675–681.
- 12 Schnitt S. J., Silen W., Sadowsky N. L., Connolly J. L. et al. (1988): Current concepts. Ductal carcinoma in situ (intraductal carcinoma) of the breast. *N. Engl. J. Med.* **318**: 898–903.
- 13 Van Dongen J. A., Fentiman I. S., Harris

J. R. et al. (1989): In-situ breast cancer: the EORTC consensus meeting. *Lancet* **II**: 25–27.
- 14 Price P., Sinnett H. D., Gusterson B. et al. (1990): Duct carcinoma in situ: predictors of local recurrence and progression in patients treated by surgery alone. *Br. J. Cancer* **61**: 869–872.
- 15 Holland R., Hendriks J. H. C. L., Verbeek A. L. M. et al. (1990): Extent, distribution, and mammographic/histological correlations of breast ductal carcinoma in situ. *Lancet* **335**: 519–522.

Appendix 4

- 1 O'Reilly S. M., Richards M. A. (1990): Node negative breast cancer. *Br. Med. J.* **300**: 346–347.
- 2 Huvos A. G., Hutter R. V. P., Berg J. W. (1970): Significance of axillary macrometastases and micrometastases in mammary cancer. *Ann. Surg.* **173**: 44–46.
- 3 Fisher E. R., Palekar A., Rockette H., Redmand C., Fisher B. (1978): Pathological findings from the National Surgical Adjuvant Breast Project (Protocol No. 4) V. Significance of axillary nodal micro and macro metastases. *Cancer* **42**: 2032–2028.
- 4 Gusterson B. A., Ott R. (1990): Occult axillary lymph-node micrometastases in breast cancer. *Lancet* **336**: 434–435.
- 5 International Breast Cancer Study Group (1990): Prognostic importance of occult axillary lymph node micrometastases from breast cancers. *Lancet* **335**: 1565–1568.
- 6 Apostostolikas N., Petrai C., Agnantis N. J. (1989): The reliability of histologically negative axillary lymp nodes in breast cancer. *Path. Res. Pract.* **184**: 35–38.
- 7 Fisher E. R., Swamidoss S., Lee C. H., Rockette H., Redmond C., Fisher B. (1978): Detection and significance of occult axillary node metastases in patients with invasive breast cancer. *Cancer* **42**: 2025–2031.
- 8 Trojani M., Mascarel I. D., Bonichon F., Coindre J. M., Delsol G. (1987): Micrometastases to axillary lymph nodes from carcinoma of breast: detection by immunohistochemistry and prognostic significance. *Br. J. Cancer* **55**: 303–306.
- 9 Wells C. A., Heryet A., Brochier J., Gatter K. C., Mason D. Y. (1984): The immunocytochemical detection of axillary micrometastases in breast cancer. *Br. J. Cancer* **50**: 193–197.
- 10 Springall R. J., Ryina E. R. C., Millis R. R. (1990): Incidence and significance of micrometastases in axillary lymph nodes detected by immunohistochemical techniquie. *J. Pathol.* **160**: 174A.
- 11 Galea M., Athanassiou E., Bell J. et al. (1991): Occult regional lymph node metastases from breast carcinoma immunohistological detection with antibodies CAM 5.2 and NCR 11. *J. Pathol.* **165**: 221–227.
- 12 Trojani M., Mascarel I. D., Coindre J. M., Bonichon F. (1987): Micrometastases to axillary lymph nodes from invasive carcinoma of the breast: detection by immunohistochemistry and prognostic significance. *Br. J. Cancer* **55**

Appendix 5

- 1 Bettelheim R. et al. (1984): Prognostic significance of peritumoral vascular invasion in breast cancer. *Br. J. Cancer* **50**: 771–777.
- 2 Davis B. W. et al. (1985): Prognostic significance of peritumoral vascular invasion in clinical trials of adjuvant therapy for breast cancer with axillary lymph node metastasis. *Human Pathol.* **16**: 1212–1218.
- 3 Pinder S. E., Ellis I. O., Galea M., O'Rouke S., Blamey R. W., Elston C. W. (1994): Pathological prognostic factors in breast cancer. III. Vascular invasion: relationship with recurrence and survival in a large study with long-term follow-up. *Histopathology* **24**: 41–47.
- 4 Roses D. R. et al. (1982): Pathological predictors of recurrence in stage I (TINOMO) breast cancer. *Am. J. Clin. Pathol.* **78**: 817–820.
- 5 Lee A. K. C. et al. (1981): Prognostic significance of peritumoral lymphatic and blood vessel invasion in node-negative carcinoma of the breast. *J. Clin. Oncol.* **8**: 15–25.
- 6 Rosen P. P. et al. (1981): Predictors of recurrence in stage I (TINOMO) breast carcinoma. *Ann. Surg.* **193**: 15–25.

- 7 Weigand R. A. et al. (1982): Blood vessel invasion and axillary lymph node involvement as prognostic indicators for human breast cancer. *Cancer* **50**: 962–969.
- 8 Sears H. F. et al. (1982): Breast cancer without axillary metastases. *Cancer* **50**: 1820–1827.
- 9 Dawson P. J., Ferguson D. J., Karrison T. (1982): The pathologic findings of breast cancer in patients surviving 25 years after radical mastectomy. *Cancer* **50**: 2131–2138.
- 10 Cote R. J. et al. (1988): Monoclonal antibodies detect occult breast carcinoma metastases in the bone marrow of patients with early stage disease. *Am. J. Surg. Pathol.* **12**: 333–340.
- 11 Lee A. K. C. et al. (1988): Lymphatic and blood vessel invasion in breast carcinoma: a useful prognostic indicator? *Human. Pathol.* **17**: 984–987.
- 12 Berger U. et al. (1988): The relationship between micrometastases in bone marrow, histologic features of the primary tumor in breast cancer and prognosis. *Am. J. Clin. Pathol.* **90**: 1–6.
- 13 Gilchrist K. W. et al. (1982): Intraobserver variation in the identification of breast carcinoma in intramammary lymphatics. *Human Pathol.* **13**: 170–172.
- 14 Rosen P. P. (1983): Tumor emboli in intramammary lymphatics in breast carcinoma. Pathologic criteria for diagnosis and clinical significance. *Pathol. Annual.* (Part 2) **18**: 215–232.
- 15 Lee A. K. C., DeLellis F. A, Wolfe H. J. (1986): Intramammary lymphatic invasion in breast carcinomas. Evaluation using ABH isoantigens as endothelial markers. *Am. J. Surg. Pathol.* **10**: 589–594.
- 16 Ordonez N. G. et al. (1987): Use of ules europaeus agglutinin I in the identification of lymphatic and blood vessel invasion in previously stained microscopic slides. *Am. J. Surg. Pathol.* **11**: 543–550.
- 17 Bettelheim R., Mitchell D., Gusterson B. A. (1984): Immunocytochemistry in the identification of vascular invasion in breast cancer. *J. Clin. Pathol.* **37**: 364–366.
- 18 Saigo P. E., Rosen P. P. (1987): The application of immunohistochemical stains to identify endothelial-lined channels in mammary carcinom. *Cancer* **59**: 51–54.
- 19 Martin S. A., Perez-Reyes N., Mendelsohn G. (1987): Angioinvasion in breast carcinoma. An immunhistochemical study of factor VIII-related antigen. *Cancer* **59**: 1918–1922.
- 20 Orbo A., Stalsberg H., Kunde D. (1990): Topographic criteria in the diagnosis of tumor emboli in intramammary lymphatics. *Cancer* **66**: 972–977.

Index

A
Abscess 65
Adenoma
– ductual 30
– of the nipple 30, 84
Adenosis
– apocrine 30
– metaplasia 30
– microglandular 31
– sclerosis 30
ADH 9–11
Antigenes, proliferation-associated 110, 112

B
Benign lesions 65
Benignancy, criteria of 64
Biological markers 57, 148
Biopsy 24 ff.
– fixation 25
– frozen sections 25
– localization 24 ff.
– naked eye examination 25
– open 28
– specimens 15, 24
BRCA1, BRCA2 115 ff.
BrdU 110
BrdUrd 113
Breast 9–11
– anatomy and physiology 1–7
– cancer, see carcinoma
Breast Sceening Program, NHSBSP 19

C
C-myc amplification 147
Calcification 18
Carcinoma in situ
– ductal, DCIS 8–9, 14, 34–36, 50–57, 67, 85
– lobular, LCIS 36, 50
Carcinoma, invasive mammary
– 10-year-survival 9, tab. 1.1
– adenoid cystic 63
– apocrine 64, 84
– ductal 37, 145
– excision 39
– grading 39, 118
– histopathology and biology 7 ff.

– infiltrating lobular 37
– invasive lobular 64
– lobular 8, 84, 145
– medullary 37, 63
– metaplastic 64
– microinvasive 36
– mitosis 40, fig. 2.3
– mixed tumours 38
– mucinous 37
– papillary 63
– prognosis 9, tab. 1.2, 132
– tubular 37, 63
– types 8
– typing 8, fig. 2.44
– vascular invasion 8, 41
Core biopsies 69
Cyst
– aspiration of 31
– duct ectasia 65
– solitare 18
Cystfluid 18, 84
– aspiration of 18
– examination 18
– residual mass 18

D
Diploid mammary carcinoma 142
DNA
– comparison between all DNA-parameters 133
– content 112
– cytometry 117, table 2.22
– degree of malignancy 141
– grading of mammary carcinoma 117, 118
– imaging 132, fig. 2.42
– index (DI) 118, 119, 132, 141
– investigative material and methods 132
– malignancy grade 118, 119, table 2.20
– parameters 132, 145, table 2.25
– ,–correlation of DNA-parameters with classic prognosis factors 135, tables 2.26–2.28
– ploidy 111
– proliferative fraction 118, 119
– SPF (S-phase-fraction) 111
– typing of mammary carcinoma 117
Duct ectasia 31

E
EGF-R 148
Epithel proliferation 32
Erb B-1 149
– deletion 151, fig. 2.49
Erb B-2 148
– amplification 151, fig. 2.49
Estrogen 3
– receptors 86, 134, 145

F
Fat necrosis 66
Fibroadenoma 28–29, 66, 82
Fibrocystic change 31
Fine Needle Aspiration, FNA 18, 57, 101–102, 109, 122
– aspiration 57
– contraindications 102
– criteria for the recognition of benign and malignant conditions 81
– cytopathology reporting form 78
– diagnostic criteria for malignancy and benignancy 59, tab. 2.7–2.8
– diagnostic pitfalls 82–84
– equipment 73, 97
– impalpable lesions 72, 95
– indications 95, 102
– needle tract implantation 102
– needles and syringes 73, 98
– palpable lesions 71, 95
– patterns of malignant breast lesions 65
– potential false negative diagnosis 84–86
– pre-FNA-requirements 96, 103
– recommended procedure 75
– sampling 72, 103
– smear 58
– technical considerations 104
– training and education of personnal 87–88, 103
– triple diagnosis 62, 68
– triple-test 97
  – ,–post-triple-test 101, 106
– use of 70
Fine Needle Aspiration Cytology, FNAC 71
– complications 76
– equipment 76
– ultrasound guided procedures 76
– X-ray guided procedures 74
FISH (fluorescence in situ hybridization) 109
Fistula
– mammary duct 32
– sub-areolar abscess 32
Flow cytometry 110, 111, 117

G
Genetic parameters 109
– chromosomal aberrations 109
– genetic markers 109
– prognostic markers 109

H
Hormon receptor status 152
Hormone Receptors 148, fig. 2.45
HSR (homogeneously staining regions) 110
Hypermasty 3
Hyperplasia
– apocrine 31
– atypical 9 ff., fig. 1.6
– ductal 33, tab. 2.3
– fibroadenomatoide 28
– juvenile 28
– sclerosing lobular 28

I
Image analysis 110
Inflammation 65

K
Ki 67 110, 112
Ki S1 112

L
Li-Fraumeni syndrome 114
LOH (Analysis of loss of heterocygosity) 113

M
Mammography
– equipment 26
– quality assurance guidelines 24
Manpower 23
Mastitis 31
Metaplasia
– apocrine 31, 65
Mib-1–3 112
Mitotic figures, counting of 110

N
National Health Service
Non-Hodgkin-Lymphomas 64

O
Oncogenes 147
Oxytocin 6

P
p53 113
Paget's disease 36, 67
Papilloma 30
PCNA (Proliferating-cell nuclear antigene) 112

PCR 149, fig. 2.50
– differential 150, fig. 2.47
Phylloides tumours 29, 66, 85
Progesterone receptor 86, 133
– average value 139, fig. 2.41
– status 146
Prognostic information 86
Prognostic parameters 158
Prolactin 3, 5
Proliferation
– activity of tumour cells 110
– rate in breast carcinoma 110

Q
Quality Assurance 19, 90
– biopsy quality assurance 22
– cytology (CQA) 22 ff.
– education and cytology training 20, 90
– external (EQA) 19 ff.
    – ,–national scheme 21
    – ,–participation in 20
    – ,–software systems 21
– managing 19
– quality improvement programs (Q1) 108
– regional coordinators 21
– standards 16, tab. 2.1
– suspicious category 107
– suspicious diagnosis 107
– technical quality 19

R
Radial scar 30 ff.
Radiotherapy 66
Reporting of breast carcinoma 47 ff.
– diagnostic information 47
– gross description 47
– histologic grade 48
– invasive carcinoma 47
– lymph node status 48
– margins of resection 48
– microcalcifications 49
– Scarff-Bloom-Richardson grading 48
– tumour description 47, 49

RFLP (Restriction fragment length polymorphism) 113

S
Sampling 27, 103
Sclerosing lesions 30–31
Screening program 13 ff.
– guidelines 13, 24
– histological examination 17
– mammography 13, 24
– pathological reporting 15
– prognostic index 13
Short-term cultures 109
Specimens
– axillary dissection 27
– excision margins 27, 50
– fixation 25
– frozen sections 25
– large blocs 26
– mastectomy 27
– sampling 27
– segmental excision 28
– weight 28
Staining 105 ff.
– cell bloc preparation 105
– inadequate specimen 106
– Papanicolaou staining 105
– reports 106
– turnaround time (TAT) 108
– unsatisfactory smear 106
– Wright-Giemsa stain 105
Stereotaxis 92
Suppressor genes 113
– in normal cells 114
– p 53 113
– prognostic significance 114

T
T stage 143
Tetraploid carcinoma 146
Thymidine labeling 110, 113
TNM-Staging 7
Tumour labeling index 113

Colour Plates

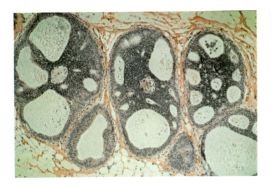

Figure 1.4, explanation see page 10 and 11

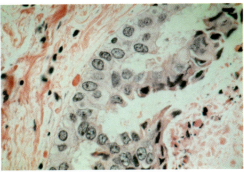

Figure 1.7, explanation see page 10 and 11

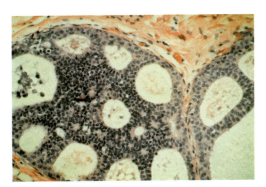

Figure 1.5, explanation see page 10 and 11

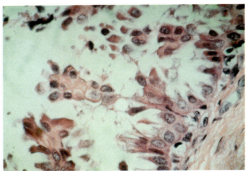

Figure 1.8, explanation see page 10 and 11

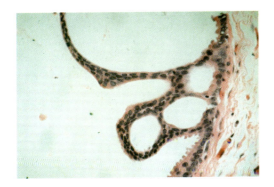

Figure 1.6, explanation see page 10 and 11

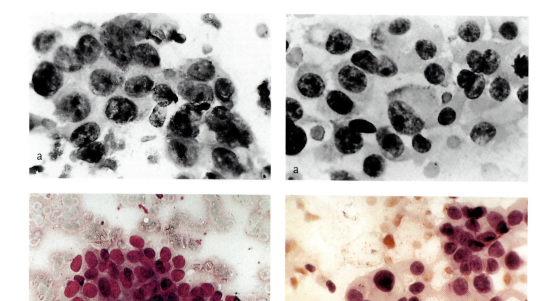

Figure 2.4: Duct cell carcinoma monomorphic type:
a) The dissociated monomorphic malignant epithelial cells are large, rounded, with fine granular sharp borders nuclei and nucleoli. Cytoplasm is scant or absent. (Pap., oil immers.) b) These malignant cells are more cohesive but the diameter of the nuclei is more than one and a half larger as an erythrocyte (MCG, x320)

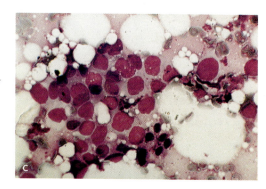

Figure 2.5: Duct cell carcinoma polymorphic type: Pleomorphic large and dissociated with irregular nucleoli and nuclei and obviously malignant.
a) Pap. x500); b) Pap. x340; c) MCG, x340

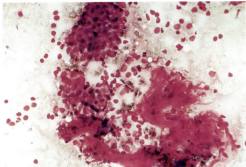

Figure 2.6: Duct cell carcinoma with mucinous component: Mucin production is better visible in MCG smears (MCG, x320)

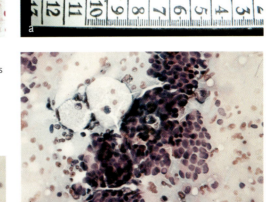

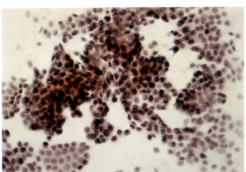

Figure 2.7: Ductal carcinoma in situ (DCIS), cribriform type (Pap., x400)

Figure 2.9: Papillary carcinoma: a) Gross specism shows an encapsulated intracystical tumour with fine granular surface. b) Pap., x400

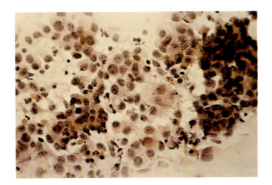

Figure 2.8: Ductal carcinoma in situ (DCIS), comedo type (Pap., x400)

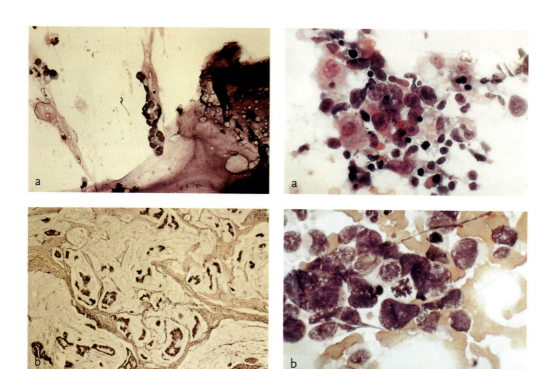

Figure 2.10: Mucinous carcinoma: a) cytological (MCG, x400); b) histological (HE, x100)

Figure 2.11: Medullary carcinoma with lymphocytric infiltration: a) & b) Pap., x400

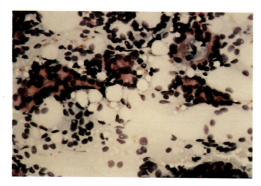

Figure 2.12: Adenoid cystic carcinoma (Pap., x400)

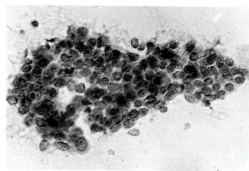

Figure 2.13: Invasive cribriform carcinoma: Our cytological diagnosis suspected precarcinomatous changes. Histological examinations revealed invasive cribriform carcinoma (Pap., x320)

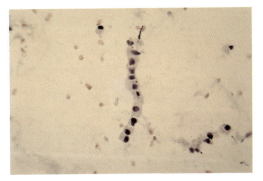

Figure 2.14: Invasive lobular carcinoma (Pap., x100)

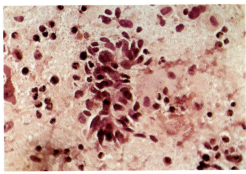

Figure 2.16: Leiomyosarcoma: Spindel-shaped, loosely cohesive, atypical cells in dirty background (Pap., x320)

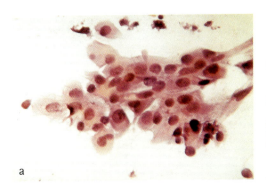

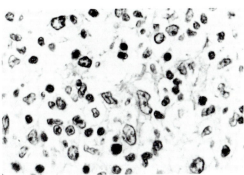

Figure 2.17: Lymphoma (Giemsa, x400)

Figure 2.15: a) Apocrine carcinoma (Pap., x320); b) Apocrine cell metaplasia (Pap., x280)

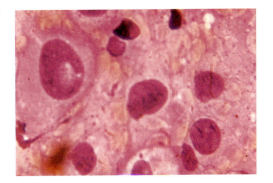

Figure 2.18: Malignant Melanoma: Large tumour cells with abundant cytoplasm. At bottom left you can see pigmentation (Pap., oil immers.)

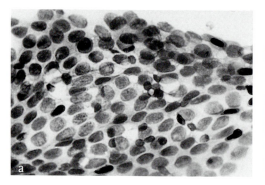

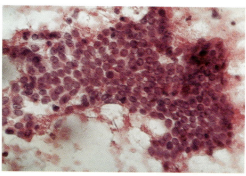

Figure 2.20: Fibroadenoma: Cohesive sheet of cells with slightly enlarged nuclei and some prominent nucleoli (Pap., x320)

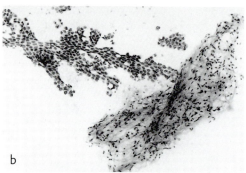

Figure 2.19: Benign epithelial and stroma cells: a) Pap., x450; b) Pap., x180

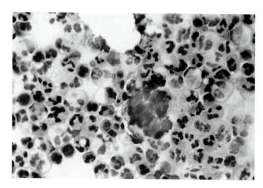

Figure 2.21: Slightly enlarged benign epithelial cells in an inflammatory background with leucocytes (Pap., x320)

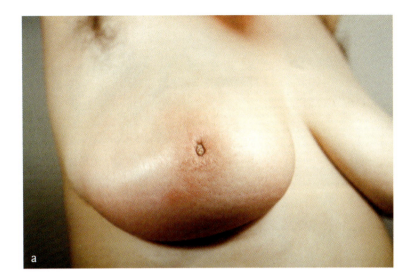

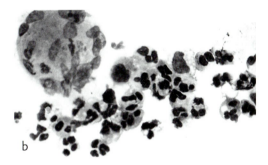

Figure 2.22: Abscess: a) Woman aged 34. The right breast is swollen, the skin is bright red and shiny, the nipple is uneven and retracted: orange-peel phenomenon appears under the nipple. The axillary lymph nodes are enlarged and painful. b) A multinucleated giant cell surrounded by granulocytes and some histiocytes (Pap., x400)

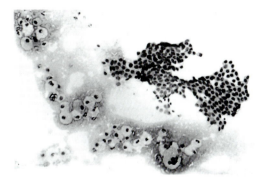

Figure 2.23: Cyst-Duct Ectasia: A cluster of regular ductal cells outlined by linearly arranged foamy cells (Pap., x180)

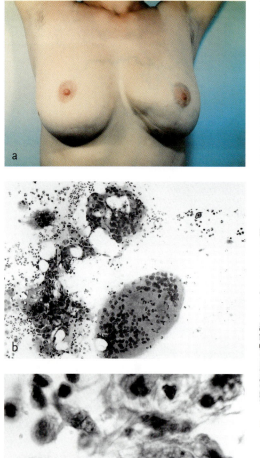

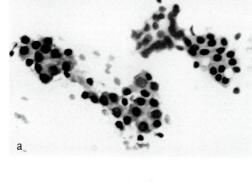

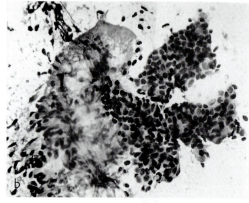

Figure 2.25: Fibroadenoma: a) Pap., x300; b) Pap., x280

Figure 2.24: Fatty necrosis. a) Woman aged 44. Some months ago the left breast was contused in a car accident. After the disappearance of the acute symptoms about 2.5 cm diameter lump localised in the lower-internal quadrant of the left breast. It was hard and tender and the skin adhered to it. In this respect it resembles carcinoma. b) Fibrocytes and clusters of round and avoid cells, histiocytes and granulocytes. On the right: a large sized multinucleated giant cell (Pap., x80).
c) Dispersed round and elongated cells with oval shaped hyperchromatic nuclei and vacuolated cytoplasm. In the background a homogeneously staining amorphous substance (Pap. oil immers.)

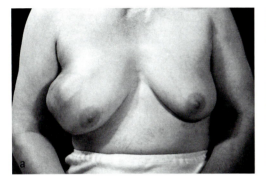

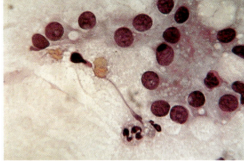

Figure 2.27: Adenoma, lactation (pregnancy) cells with vacuated fragile cytoplasms and prominent nucleoli (Pap., x340)

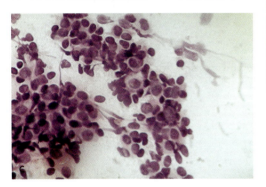

Figure 2.26: Phyllodes tumour. a) A very large lobulated tumour, involving the larger part of the right breast. It is of hard consistency and adherent to the skin. The overlying skin of the periareolar tissue displayed a prominent network of dilated subcutaneous veins (woman aged 40). b) On the right a fragment of regular mesenchymal cells; on the left grouping of ductal cells mixed with large epithelial cells consisting of large hyperchromic nuclei with distinct borders (Pap., x180); c) Pap., x320

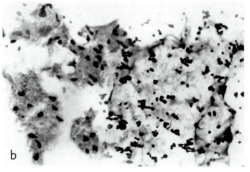

Figure 2.28: Granular cell tumour. a) 25-year-old woman: medial from the nipple a pea-sized, granulomatous swelling is seen with poor purulent discharge. The exfoliative smears contained granulocytes. Aspiration biopsy cytology from the retromamillary tumour 2 cm in diameter was palpable. b) Clustered or dissociated large-sized cells with finely granular cytoplasm, indistinct borders and round hyperchromatic nuclei. In many areas these cells are separated by connective tissue septa (Pap., x180).

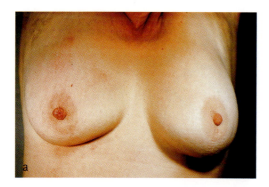
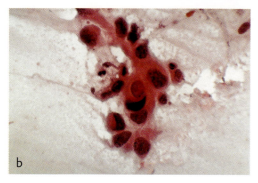

Figure 2.29: Paget's disease. a) Female patient aged 65 years. Right nipple is slightly protacted, eczematous and ulcerated. b) Large round tumour cells with pale cytoplasm and round to oval nuclei with halos (Pap., x400).